Medicine and Socie ̄ ̄ate Eighteenth-Century Berkshire: The Commonplace Book of William Savory of Brightwalton and Newbury

Edited by Stuart Eagles

Berkshire Record Society
Volume 30
2024

Published by the Berkshire Record Society
c/o Royal Berkshire Archives
9 Coley Avenue, Reading
Berkshire
RG1 6AF

Printed and bound by
Short Run Press Limited
25 Bittern Road
Sowton Industrial Estate
Exeter, EX2 7LW

ISBN 978-1-7394930-1-1

Contents

Foreword

It is more than 30 years since I first encountered the manuscript transcribed in this volume. I had embarked on researching my family history and had recently traced my ancestors to the beautiful village of Brightwalton on the Berkshire Downs. My sleuthing had taken me to the Local Studies department of Reading Central Library. It was there that I came across several shelves filled with dark green file boxes. They contained newspaper cuttings pasted onto light blue foolscap cards which were arranged alphabetically by subject, person, or place.

One of the folders included clippings relating to Brightwalton. The first item I picked up was a faded and yellowing photograph of a very overgrown churchyard, with the caption, 'SAVORYS, Eagles [*sic*], Norris's [*sic*]—all related and buried in the corner of the old churchyard, the very essence of a past Brightwalton'. I still remember the wave of goosebumps that came over me as I excitedly read these words. The accompanying report, written by Leslie North and published in the *Reading Mercury* on 15 September 1967, was full of insights into village life in the eighteenth and nineteenth century. Four paragraphs in, I read with incredulity that

> in the old churchyard, amidst its trees, Dr William [Savory] and his wife were buried together [...]. The doctor has left a manuscript book in which he dealt with not only his own family history but that of his lonely parish, with many an interesting anecdote and titbit [...].

Oh really, I thought? So where was it now?

I hurried to the enquiry desk, newspaper article in hand, and asked the assistant the question. I remember being shown some thick books loaded with paper slips containing the catalogue of the Local Studies collection. And, Eureka! Not only had Savory's 'book' survived, it was there in the library's own on-site strongroom. Unfortunately, it was too late to look at it right then. The library was about to close. I returned the next day, following a restless night, equipped with pencil and notebook. And so I began to study the rich and varied volume compiled by William Savory (1768-1824), an uncle five generations up my family tree.

I was in my mid-teens when I first read Savory's manuscript. But I was fascinated as much by it then as I am now. I jotted down what I could read, though with no scholarly sense of how to transcribe such a document accurately. Nevertheless, I explored some of the more colourful and engaging episodes in the *Berkshire Family Historian* in the 1990s. Over the years many people have expressed interest in the manuscript and have wanted to read more. And well they might.

Savory's commonplace book is full of wonderful things. Anecdotes and lyrics nestle with family history and witchcraft. Tales of daily life are interspersed with horoscopes. The activities of a modest rural parish contrast with those of a market-town and – more starkly still – with London. Savory's sense of fun is as much in evidence as his insatiable appetite for learning. We follow him from school to medical practice, via apprenticeship and hospital study. The bulk of his diary covers what we would now think of as his teenage years. Although, when I first read it, I was separated from him temporally by a little over two centuries, most of the experiences he describes occurred at the same stage of life which I had then reached myself.

Yet there is something for everyone in Savory's book. Over the years I have kept coming back to it and have re-discovered and better understood its contents. Inevitably, re-reading it at a later point in my life, carrying more years of experience and having attained a doctorate in history from the University of Oxford, opened up new perspectives and revealed new dimensions. It only re-affirmed my belief in the manuscript's value and worth. When Peter Durrant showed an interest in my proposal to bring it to print, and the council of the Berkshire Record Society gave the project the go-ahead, I could not have been more delighted and grateful. Dr Durrant's successor as General Editor, Prof. Anne Curry, has been unfailing in her encouragement and support.

The trigger for that proposal – the thing that finally compelled me to propose the idea of a full, annotated transcript – was another chance discovery, this time on a visit to the Museum of English Rural Life on the University of Reading's London Road campus. Soon after entering the main exhibition space a dower chest was pointed out to me and the display information was read out. The chest had belonged to Dr William Savory of Brightwalton, it announced, and on further enquiry it turned out that 'W.S.' and 'W. SAVORY' are carved on one of the thin vertical end panels. It transpired that the museum is also the custodian of a glass inkwell which purportedly belonged to him, as well as two severely damaged portraits allegedly depicting him or more probably a later William Savory – one of the portraits apparently being a crude copy of the other.

Such serendipity spoke to me, and it said that it was time to visit the manuscript again and with a renewed sense of purpose. So I headed to the Royal Berkshire Archives (formerly the Berkshire Record Office) where the document is now housed. Two centuries after the death of its author, the manuscript volume has finally been transcribed and published in full, and shared with the wider readership it deserves.

Acknowledgements

For permission to publish this complete transcript of William Savory's Commonplace Book (RBA D/EX2275/1), and to reproduce images from the same source, we are indebted and grateful to the Royal Berkshire Archives (formerly the Berkshire Record Office); also for permission to quote from other material relating to the parish of Brightwalton (RBA D/EW/O8). Special thanks to King's College London Archives for permission to quote from and reproduce an image of Savory's student lecture notes, and for generously waiving the associated fee, King's College London Archives, St Thomas's Hospital Medical School, TH/PP/54/1 and /2) (see Appendix D).

Particular thanks to Dr Peter Durrant and the council of the Berkshire Record Society for their role in publishing this volume. For her expert guidance and unstinting support, I express grateful thanks to the General Editor, Prof. Anne Curry. I am also grateful to the Berkshire Family History Society for allowing me to explore some of this material in print in the 1990s. I am grateful to staff, past and present, at Reading Local Studies Library, the Royal Berkshire Archives, King's College London Archives, Wiltshire and Swindon Archives, and Hampshire Archives, for their unfailing assistance. Special thanks to Anastasiia Rozhkova for her splendid work in digitally retouching the cover image. I have benefitted from conversations with many enthusiasts and specialists too numerous to name, but Sue Sayers, a resident and historian of Brightwalton, stands out.

I was blessed to start this journey with my parents as a schoolboy. Three teachers deserve special credit and thanks: John Beasley, Prof. Robert Hewison, and Prof. Lawrence Goldman. I am personally indebted to a great many amazing people, most especially Pavel Chepyzhov, Will Fradley, James Buckley, Stuart Heslegrave, Annie Creswick Dawson, Paul Dawson, Sara Atwood, Kay Walter, Mark Frost, Marcus Waithe and Clive Wilmer.

Abbreviations

BC	*Berkshire Chronicle*
MS	manuscript
PCC	Prerogative Court of Canterbury
OJ	*Jackson's Oxford Journal*
RAI	Register of Duties Paid for Apprentices' Indentures
RBA	Royal Berkshire Archives
RM	*Reading Mercury*
TNA	The National Archives
UD	*Universal Directory of Great Britain, 1791*
WSA	Wiltshire and Swindon Archives

[*NB. References to 'Savory' are to the author of the document transcribed in this volume. Numbers in square brackets refer to the relevant page in the original MS.*]

List of illustrations

Cover image: 'Willm Savory' headpiece, the most elaborate example of Savory's version of decorated blackletter calligraphy and illustrative of his best penmanship [(1)]. Digitally retouched by Anastasiia Rozhkova.

Savory Family Tree

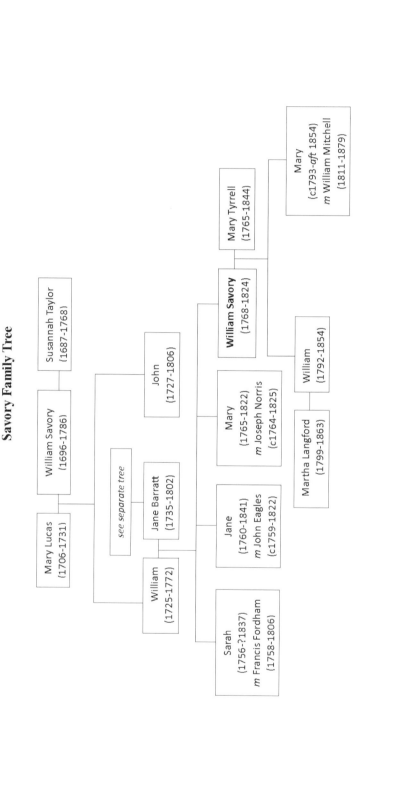

Mary Lucas (1706-1731)

William Savory (1696-1786)

Susannah Taylor (1687-1768)

see separate tree

William (1725-1772)

Jane Barratt (1735-1802)

John (1727-1806)

Sarah (1756-?1837)
m Francis Fordham (1758-1806)

Jane (1760-1841)
m John Eagles (c1759-1822)

Mary (1765-1822)
m Joseph Norris (c1764-1825)

William Savory (1768-1824)

Mary Tyrrell (1765-1844)

Martha Langford (1799-1863)

William (1792-1854)

Mary (c1793-aft 1854)
m William Mitchell (1811-1879)

Barratt Family Tree

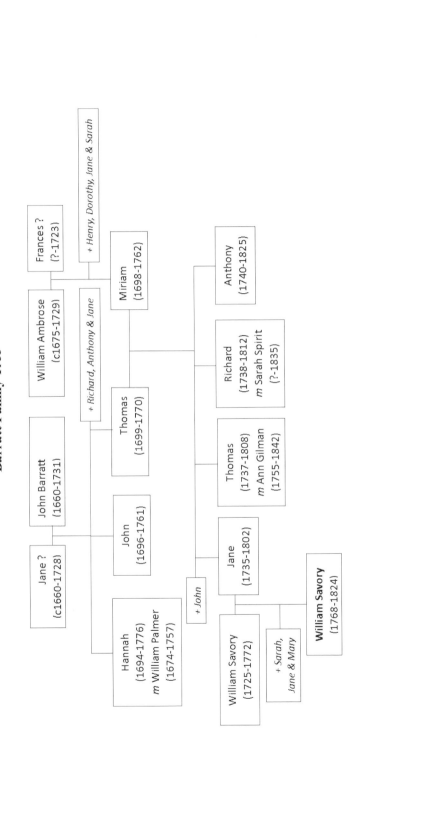

Frances ? (?-1723)

William Ambrose (c1675-1729)

+ Henry, Dorothy, Jane & Sarah

Miriam (1698-1762)

+ Richard, Anthony & Jane

Thomas (1699-1770)

John Barratt (1660-1731)

Jane ? (c1660-1728)

John (1696-1761)

Hannah (1694-1776) m William Palmer (1674-1757)

Anthony (1740-1825)

Richard (1738-1812) m Sarah Spirit (?-1835)

Thomas (1737-1808) m Ann Gilman (1755-1842)

Jane (1735-1802)

+ John

William Savory (1725-1772)

+ Sarah, Jane & Mary

William Savory (1768-1824)

Introduction

William Savory (1768-1824) was the son and grandson of village wheelwrights. He was born and brought up in the Berkshire Downland village of Brightwalton. He strove, by way of apprenticeship in Newbury and his studies in the Borough teaching hospitals in London, to become a professionally accredited surgeon-apothecary and man-midwife. At the age of 23 he set up in practice on bustling Bartholomew Street in the market town of Newbury and settled into married life. This volume presents his story in his own words. It is the fully annotated transcript of a rich and varied document of 262 pages of MS bound in full calf and preserved in the Royal Berkshire Archives.

The document is difficult to categorise. It resembles a commonplace book in most respects. It is a miscellany of prose and verse material collected and copied by one person into a single volume.[1] Yet although Savory's MS sits in that tradition, very little of it originates in identifiable printed sources. As Savory announces on his title-page, it contains 'Memorandums[,] Memoirs, Remarks &c on the Nativity of William Savory' with 'an Account of his Predecessors, place of Nativity, Birth[,] Education &c' and 'Notes on Anatomy, Surgery, Medicine, Midwifery, Chymistry, Astrology, Geomancy, Hystory, poetry, palmestry, Farriery'. If he intended it to touch seriously on the last two subjects, he did not get around to writing anything down. Insofar as his 'notes' reflect on any of these topics, they are not philosophical but autobiographical in nature. His own title and sub-title, then, if not particularly illuminating, sufficiently summarise the volume's scope, indicate its variety, and underline its rootedness in his personal experience. In many ways Savory's life, though undoubtedly interesting, was not especially remarkable, but that is what makes his account so valuable to historians. He was unusual, if not unique, in recording the everyday life of an ordinary but intelligent boy growing into early adulthood in the second half of the eighteenth century.

A more precise, roughly sequential, summary of the contents of the volume will serve as an initial introduction to its writer. Savory starts, logically enough, with his own birth. He proceeds to an account of his native parish, Brightwalton, and nearby villages, and here he indulges in some idiosyncratic toponymical speculations for Brightwalton, Blewbury and Newbury [(1)-4]. This is followed by pen-portraits of his closest relatives: his grandfather William Savory (1696-1786) [4-10]; his father William Savory (1725-1772) [16-21, 29]; his mother Jane, née Barratt (1735-1802) [32, 34], which includes an account of her ancestors and relatives [34-36]; Savory's uncle John Savory (1727-1806) [30-32, 34]; and his sisters Sarah (1756-?1837) [36], Jane (1760-1841) [42], and Mary (1765-1822) [42-43]. Interspersed with these pen-portraits are some notable verses: he includes inscriptions from family gravestones [8-9], comic rhymes [15, 23-25, 41-42], and a song composed by

---

1. For an exploration and analysis of the commonplace-book genre, see J. M. Hess, *How Romantics and Victorians Organized Information: Commonplace Books, Scrapbooks, and Albums* (Oxford, 2022).

his father about the art of the wheelwright [21-22], another about 'The Millar' [32-33], and a rhyme written by his uncle John and sister Jane (or Jenny) [34]. They possess little in the way of literary merit, but they are generally amusing and entertaining. Savory also reproduces an appeal written by his father in 1755 to raise a subscription towards the purchase of a musical instrument to be played in the local parish church [25-29].

Savory then turns to his own autobiography, specifically to the year 1779, in which he turned 11 [43-48]. This leads into the central feature of his book, namely his selections of highlights extracted from his diaries for 1780 [49-52], 1781 [53-55], 1782 [56-58], 1783 [58, 68-70], 1784 [70-75], 1785 [99-103], 1786 [117-129], 1787 [139-145], 1788 [152-159, 172-193], 1789 [193-215], 1790 [227-235] and 1791 (up to and including 8 September when he married) [246-258]. He thereby gives us an account of his life between the ages of 11 and 23. These diary extracts are punctuated by a variety of material copied from other sources, most of it from manuscripts belonging to himself or his father. There are verses that had been sent to his father, though by whom we are not told [59-67]; comical and curious material copied from his father's notebooks, which he describes as 'a few Questions, Rebuses, Enigmas &c' [145-151]; genitures (a type of horoscope), mostly for relatives and friends and drawn up by himself [76-98, 130-138, 259-262]; examples of witchcraft, occult writings and folk remedies [115-116, 159-171, 216-226]; songs and poetry [104-105, 236-238]; a parable mocking Prime Minister William Pitt the Younger [106-110]; a burlesque on quackery [239-245]; an incomplete account of the Archbishops of Canterbury [263-266]; and an index in roughly alphabetical order presented as a list of contents [267a-(271)].

As this crowded summary indicates, the volume is broad and varied in scope. By contrast, it is often lacking in depth and detail. Whilst the material sometimes touches on Savory's opinions and emotions, it is not generally personal in either of these senses. The book contains little in the way of introspection though psychological insights may be inferred. Its focus is on people and events – moreover, on local news and gossip. More than anything else, though, it is one young man's account of his upbringing and education, and his development into adulthood. The physical journeys it describes, particularly those between Brightwalton, Newbury and London, reflect the broadening of his cultural and professional horizons and echo his intellectual growth.

Savory begins with his birth and ends with his marriage. In fact, he compiled the document on becoming the head of his own household, newly established as a married medical professional in Newbury. On one level he was committing to paper the story of his life to date, and literally sandwiching it between two boards. On another, he was creating a reference book, an *aide-memoire* with its own handy index. And he was having a clear-out, taking the best material from old letters, diaries and notebooks, and presumably throwing the originals away. His changed professional and marital status served both as the motivation and occasion to write the book. His marriage supplied the beginning and the end of the volume: it was the event which sparked its writing, and the final thing to be noted in its pages. In what he tells us, and particularly in the way he tells it, he provides an abundance of material that reveals his personality.

The weight of internal evidence supporting the hypothesis that the document was written over a relatively short period following his marriage on 8 September 1791 is considerable. In the first fifth of the volume Savory writes of Joseph Norris (c.1764-1825) – his paternal uncle's apprentice who married Savory's sister Mary in 1784 – that 'his Mother now lives at North Moreton & is sister to Mrs Tyrell my Mother in law' [43], demonstrating that Savory was married when he wrote these words. Likewise, not quite one-fifth of the way through the volume, he writes, with reference to an excursion to Oxford in June 1780, that he was accompanied on that occasion by 'my present Wife' [50]. Not quite four-fifths of the way through the book he writes, 'I sent a Letter to Miss Tyrrell my Wife as is now' [200]. Earlier he writes of his father, who died on 24 July 1772, that 'his name still becomes a subject of Conversation which is 20 Years ago since his death' [19]. Whilst we should not take '20 Years' to be an exact or precise measurement of time, the implication for the dating of the document is clear.

Externally verifiable facts further support the dating. Savory writes that 'I got myself a little in disgrace at this time when Wm Dance was Married (who is since dead)' [156]. Dance married on 10 July 1788, and was buried on 12 July 1791. In writing a geniture for Mary Jones, the daughter of David Jones, the master under whom Savory served his apothecary's apprenticeship, he writes, 'The Native lived to be near 6 Years of Age' [97]: born on 29 April 1785, she was buried on 14 May 1791. Apparently contradictory evidence which seems to contest the notion that it was all written in a relatively short period of time following his marriage can be dismissed. When he writes between entries for May and June 1790 that 'a few Weeks ago was Married Miss Charlotte Bew of North Heath' (she married 11 May) it is fair to suppose that he used the word 'ago' as a synonym for 'before' rather than 'since' [231].

Although there is no precise evidence of how long it took Savory to complete the writing of the volume, there are no references to events from 1792 or after, so it is probable that he finished it within a matter of months, possibly even weeks. When he writes that on 8 September 1791, 'I entered the altar of Hymen, but as I entered into a new life I shall for such a memorandum enter into a new book' he clearly signals his own sense of how the shift in his status has brought an end to the first chapter of his life just as another has begun [258]. By his compilation of this volume he symbolically drew a line under his boyhood, schooling, training, studies, bachelorhood and life in the countryside. It is as if, on the point of achieving one type of independence, and at an exciting time of mixed opportunity and risk, he was minded to reflect on the path which had led him there. A certain amount of understandable anxiety seems to have stimulated in him a desire for affirmation, possibly even a need for validation. In his own past and roots he seeks to find the firm foundations on which he could build. But he also indicates his intention to continue his project to record his life. If a second volume was ever begun, it does not appear to have survived.

In the absence of direct personal testimony, it is only possible to speculate as to the intended purpose of his project. Psychologically, it was perhaps instrumental. It seems to have provided the means to assess and understand more clearly who he had become. In thus writing about his past he was certainly indulging a sense of nostalgia. This is also evident in his chronicling of changes in Brightwalton: the cutting down of trees and alterations to the church are implicitly regretted [51-52]. In a man of 23 this might suggest more than a hint of sentimentality. Yet it should be borne in mind that he was a medical practitioner with relatively little protection against the many dangers to which he was exposed. Few other professions could instil in a young man a sharper sense of the fragility of life. His consciousness of mortality was doubtless intensified by the fact that at the age of four he had lost his father to smallpox. That this had a profound effect on him is indicated by the fact that no fewer than 11 times he uses the phrase 'my father died'/'dyed'. In some respects, Savory was following his father's example. His father sold medicines and offered basic medical services, and made written notes on a range of subjects, including Brightwalton's history [145-151 and see Appendix A]. Had Savory died prematurely like his father, his own volume would at least have offered a type of immortality and would have bequeathed the most personal of legacies that might have provided comfort to the bereaved. Perhaps the thought even occurred to him that he was giving to posterity a record of his own achievements, though there is no obvious hint of egotism in his writing.

By the time Savory compiled his MS he was a medical professional and the master of his own household, with support from a wife, an apprentice and a servant for whom he was, in turn, financially responsible. Margaret Railton, in her groundbreaking history of early medical service in Berkshire, points out that the county had three orbits of medical care at this time, Windsor to the east, Reading in the centre, and Newbury to the west. The nearest hospital to Brightwalton was the Radcliffe Infirmary in Oxford, established in 1770.[1] Savory had served his five-year apprenticeship as an apothecary in Newbury. He had studied surgery and midwifery at England's leading teaching hospitals. He had earned professional accreditation, having been admitted as a member of the Corporation of Surgeons of London following an admittedly woeful and cursory *viva voce* exam and the apparently more important payment of fees. His business premises and family home were on Bartholomew Street which, with Northbrook Street, provided the town with its strength in commerce and professional services.

The transcript on the pages following this introduction is presented, as one would expect, in strict sequential order and provides straightforward access to Savory's MS. By contrast, the central purpose of this introduction is to demonstrate the document's significance and value. It therefore takes a thematic approach in order to piece together scattered references and explore additional contextual information. It shines a light on parts of the MS that might otherwise escape notice or remain obscure. Sometimes we will return, more than once, to the same incident or phrase, but will do so in order to take a look from a different angle. After examining the document's history, and following a brief consideration of William Savory (the boy and man) and his family background, this introduction will scrutinise Savory's MS in terms of

---

1. See M. Railton, *Early Medical Services: Berkshire and South Oxfordshire from 1740* (Cranbrook, 1994), 1-5.

education, health, medical apprenticeship, astrology and witchcraft, women and sexual politics, leisure, music and dance, religion, royalty and politics, transport, crime, disability, medical training, and medical practice, and will end – as the life of the MS itself began – with Savory's marriage. Whilst these themes are all strongly represented in the volume, it must be admitted that our focus on them is in part influenced by modern preoccupations and prejudices. Although it has sometimes been appropriate to acknowledge modern sensitivities, historical accounts should be read, understood and appreciated in the full context of the period in which they originate, not measured against the standards of a later period, though a description and assessment of such differences is often worthwhile. Four appendices provide additional relevant local and personal context, and the afterword explores Savory's life and legacy to extend the narrative beyond the period covered in the MS volume itself.

First, though, it is important to say something about Brightwalton and the home the Savorys occupied there. The village is known today as Brightwalton – and has been so known through most of its modern history – but Savory preferred Brightwaltham, and may have been partly responsible for a popularisation of that variant in the first half of the nineteenth century. A local population census conducted in October 1790, around a year before Savory wrote his MS, gives a population of 401, of which 191 were males, and 210 females, living in 79 households, an average of around five people per household, though in practice household sizes varied from a lone resident to a household of 13 and even 18 [see Appendix C]. This represented a growth in population since May 1768 (i.e. more or less within Savory's lifetime) of 52 [see Appendix B]. Many of the charming thatched cottages that lined the principal streets in Savory's day survive, though sometimes in radically altered form. The vast majority of residents in the eighteenth century were employed directly or indirectly in agriculture, most of it arable farming. The majority of work undertaken by local craftsmen, such as the wheelwrights, carpenters and blacksmiths in Savory's own family, sprang from the needs of agriculture. Brightwalton, high on the Downs and surrounded by trees, commands a fairly central position in the larger western portion of Old Berkshire (as defined before 1974) and is bounded on the north by Farnborough, on the east by Lilley and Catmore, on the south-east by Peasemore, on the south by Leckhampstead with Leckhampstead Thicket to its west, on the west by Chaddleworth, and by Letcombe Regis at the boundary with Woolley, a long and thinly shaped manor at the north-west edge of Brightwalton, much as Savory describes [3]. Sparrowbill is in the east of the parish towards Peasemore and Brightwalton Holt is in the south-east, the two connected by Pudding Lane. Brightwalton Green is to the south and west, and Dunmore and Brightwalton Common in the north. Inevitably, these are the villages and Brightwalton landmarks to which Savory most frequently refers. Readers wishing to contextualise Savory's MS in terms of village history should turn to *Brightwalton, A Downland Village*, by June Osment, Sue Sayers and Jean Stephens.[1]

---

1. See J. Osment, S. Sayers and J. Stephens, *Brightwalton, A Downland Village* (Oxford, 2002), especially 4, 10, 17, 29, 32-33, 50, 59, 64, 84, 98-102, and 107.

Savory informs us that his grandfather sold a house in his native South Moreton and bought his master's property, Old Grays, in Brightwalton. He implies that this may have occurred before his grandfather's apprenticeship was completed, presumably in the 1710s, but the only surviving additional source is an agreement dated 1737.[1] The house remained the family home into the nineteenth century. Savory tells us that it originally featured an orchard which had since been turned into a meadow [5]. Taking possession of the property after his marriage in 1755, Savory's father added a parlour, cellar, chamber and wellhouse [5]. Savory's uncle took possession of the property in 1772 and added a brewhouse in 1781 [5, 52]. On 15 November 1786, having acquired fruit trees from Reading, John Savory reinstated an orchard by converting a garden [128]. Though much altered, the house survives today as White Cottage.

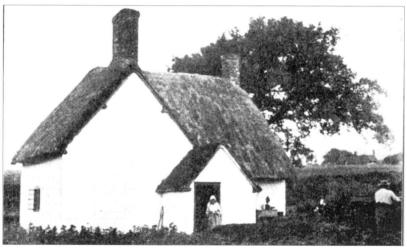

1. Old Grays, in Brightwalton, the Savory family home, as pictured in G. C. Peachey, *The Life of William Savory* (1903), 4.

(i) Document history
The likelihood that Savory intended his MS to survive him is suggested by the simple fact that he kept it safe all his life. He almost certainly passed it to his son, William Savory (c. 1792-1854). Whether by fate or fortune, or some combination of the two, it has always been in the care of trusty custodians and has survived in good condition for more than 230 years. At some point undetermined, and in a manner unknown, but probably following the death of Savory's grandson, William Savory (1828-1870), it was passed into the hands of the rector of All Saints' Church, Brightwalton. By the start of the twentieth century it was certainly in the care of Rev. Henry Fredrick Howard (1844-1938), the incumbent for an extraordinary period of more than 60 years from

---

1. RBA D/EW/T28.

1872 to 1933.[1] In 1928 Rev. Howard deposited the MS with the Reference Department of Reading Public Libraries.[2] In November 2011 it was transferred to its present home at the Royal Berkshire Archives (formerly the Berkshire Record Office).[3] In the early twentieth century, however, the MS was borrowed and carefully studied by George Charles Peachey (1862-1935), essentially Savory's successor as the village's medical practitioner, in residence by 1890. Fortunately, Peachey recognised the historical value of the MS. He selected, transcribed and published portions of the volume in 1903.[4]

Naturally enough, Peachey focused on what most interested him and what he considered of greatest historical significance. He was fascinated by Savory's medical training and professional practice, but he was also interested in his faith in folk remedies and witchcraft. He published extracts in two articles that appeared in the St Thomas's Hospital Gazette, which he later combined in a standalone pamphlet. The following year, he also transcribed the historic account left by Savory's father of the beating of the bounds of Brightwalton c. 1720, a processioning ceremony to stake out the extent of the parish [see Appendix A].[5] A physician and medical historian, Peachey was born in Calcutta (Kolkata), India. By 1871 he lived in Hove, Sussex, where he boarded with a large, apparently unrelated family. He was educated at Brighton and Taunton. He trained at St George's Hospital, which was founded in 1733 and located at Hyde Park Corner. The Times announced on 16 January 1885 that he had graduated in Anatomy. In 1887 he registered as a Licentiate of the Royal College of Physicians, Edinburgh, a Licentiate of the Royal College of Surgeons, Edinburgh, a Licentiate of the Faculty of Physicians and Surgeons, Glasgow, and a Licentiate of the Society of Apothecaries, London. Although Peachey had married Lincolnshire-born Alice Mary Allcroft in Somersham, Cambridgeshire, in 1888, his obituary in the British Medical Journal claimed that he 'ploughed a somewhat lonely furrow' at Brightwalton.[6] Nevertheless, he also served as one of the medical officers for the Wantage Union. When he published his extracts from Savory's commonplace book, he did so from the house Savory's son built, now known as The Lawns.[7]

Peachey wrote:

In the history of William Savory, his ancestors and descendants, we have an example of the vicissitudes of families: we shall be able to imagine what sort of medical treatment was obtainable in our country villages in the middle of the eighteenth century, and we shall see how the son of a village

---

1. For Howard's miscellaneous MS, historical notes on the parish of Brightwalton, c. 1830-1930, see RBA D/EX 1805 (formerly Reading Local Studies Library, BVH/D).
2. Reading Local Studies Library, ref. B/TU/Sav 1928.
3. RBA D/EX2275/1.
4. G. C. Peachey, 'The Life of William Savory, Surgeon, of Brightwalton' in St Thomas' Hospital Gazette, xiii:4 & 5 (May & June 1903) and G. C. Peachey, The Life of William Savory, Surgeon, Of Brightwalton (with Historical Notes) (1903). For a detailed account of what Peachey's publication includes, see the Editorial Note below.
5. G. C. Peachey, Beating the Bounds of Brightwalton (1904), originally published in The Berks, Bucks & Oxon. Archaeological Journal, x:3 (1904), 71-81.
6. British Medical Journal, ii:3889 (20 July 1935), 142.
7. See Peachey, Life of William Savory, 20.

wheelwright was able, by perseverance and application, to raise himself to the membership of the Surgeons' Company.

In the process we shall hear what he says of his doings as apprentice, and, in especial, we shall read in his own words interesting account of his short Hospital career.[1]

'Data on the daily lives of surgeon-apothecaries and general practitioners throughout the period from 1750 to 1850', the medical historian Irvine Loudon has written, 'are far from plentiful.'[2] Peachey had recognised this when he brought Savory's MS to public attention. 'It is seldom indeed that material is available for the exhibition of so complete a picture of the life of an obscure country practitioner in the eighteenth century', he wrote.[3]

Peachey's work on Savory's MS is significant also because it appears to represent his first published writing on medical history, a discipline in which he would excel after he moved away from Brightwalton sometime around 1910. At the end of his summary of Savory's account, he implores his 'professional brethren' to emulate the example of 'recording the medical history of a small country village'.[4] In a footnote, he laments that, 'There is no professional chair of medical history at any of our universities; it is included neither in the schedules of education nor examination – even as an optional subject – in any medical school, and there is no existing society which makes it a speciality!'[5] It is to his credit that he set out to remedy the deficit by means of numerous subsequent publications. Moreover, his *BMJ* obituary lauds his 'conscientious' research. Between 1910 and 1914, Peachey wrote the seminal three-volume history of his *alma mater*, St George's Hospital.[6] Later came memoirs of John Heaviside (c. 1748-1828), surgeon to George III, of William Bromfield (1713-1792), and of the surgical pioneers at St George's, the brothers William Hunter (1718-1783) and John Hunter (1728-1793) (the latter, coincidentally, an associate of Savory's principal medical teacher in London, Henry Cline).[7] Peachey appears to have been a regular speaker at the History of Medicine meetings of the Royal Society of Medicine, of which he was a member, addressing them, for instance, in 1924, on the 'Provision for Lying-in Women in London up to the Middle of the Eighteenth Century'.[8] He also produced the fifth edition of William MacMichael's *The Gold-Headed Cane*, a history of the symbol of great physicians, with biographies of its most distinguished bearers, to which he added notes and commissioned

1. Peachey, *Life of William Savory*, 3-4.
2. Irvine Loudon, *Medical Care and the General Practitioner* (Oxford, 1986), 6.
3. Peachey, *Life of William Savory*, 5.
4. Peachey, *Life of William Savory*, 5.
5. Peachey, *Life of William Savory*, 11n.
6. See G. C. Peachey, *The History of St. George's Hospital* (1910-1914).
7. See G. C. Peachey, *John Heavisde, Surgeon* (1931), idem., 'William Bromfield (1713-1792)' in *Proceedings of the Royal Society of Medicine*, viii (1915), 103-126, idem., *A Memoir of William and John Hunter* (Plymouth, 1924). Peachey also wrote an article on 'The Homes of the Hunters', *The Lancet*, ccxi:5451 (18 February 1928), 362-63.
8. See G. C. Peachey, 'Provision for Lying-in Women in London up to the Middle of the Eighteenth Century' in *Proceedings of the Royal Society of Medicine*, xvii (1923-1924), 72-76.

illustrations.[1] Additionally, he was a keen collector of books, and a particular connoisseur of medical bookplates.[2] The *Annals of Medical History* and *Janus* were among the journals to which he frequently contributed articles such as that on 'The Origin and Evolution of the Eighteenth Century Hospital Movement' (1913-14), 'Thomas Trapham (Cromwell's Surgeon) and Others' (1931) and 'The Two John Peacheys, Seventeenth Century Physicians; their Lives and Times' (1918) who were distantly related to him.[3]

Peachey clearly felt some pride in his early work on the Savory MS, remarking to Mr Slocock in a letter inserted in Reading Library's copy of his pamphlet, and addressed from Barnet, Hertfordshire, where Peachey was in practice in the 1920s, that 'it has been frequently referred to by writers on eighteenth century medicine'.[4] This was no idle boast, and his extracts continue to be cited by scholars today, testifying to his own perspicacity in recognising the value and significance of Savory's record. Peachey's burgeoning work as a medical historian nevertheless remained a sideline: he did not abandon general practice.

Peachey's *Life of William Savory*, with its medical emphasis, reproduced only a fraction of the commonplace book. The value of the complete transcript provided in the present volume is that the whole document remains intact and in context. Peachey's *Life* was a partial digest, an account of an apprentice, a hospital pupil, and a young practitioner, but it lost by its necessary selectiveness a sense of the growth of the boy into the man, the nature of someone who was as interested in the knavery of his neighbours as he was in mending a fracture, and who was as comfortable singing and playing musical instruments in the local church as he was at mixing medicinal compounds. But it is owing to Peachey that Savory's testimony has been available to a wide range of scholars including Thomas R. Forbes, writing on 'Verbal Charms in British Folk Medicine', Hilary Marland and Doreen Evenden writing on the history of midwifery, Susan Lawrence for her invaluable study of hospital training and medical practice, and historians of medical training such as Thomas Neville Bonner and John M. T. Ford.[5] Consequently, Savory has never completely slipped out of sight.

---

1. W. MacMichael, *The Gold-Headed Cane*, ed. G. C. Peachey (1923).
2. See G. C. Peachey, 'Book Plates of Medical Men' in *The Proceedings of the Royal Society of Medicine*, xxiii:4 (February 1930), 493–495.
3. See *British Medical Journal*, ii:3889 (20 July 1935), 142.
4. Reading Local Studies Library: letter from G. C. Peachey to Mr Slocock (undated, inserted inside Peachey, *Life of William Savory*).
5. T. R. Forbes, 'Verbal Charms in British Folk Medicine', in *Proceedings of the American Philosophical Society*, cxv:4 (20 August 1971), 293-316; H. Marland, *The Art of Midwifery: Early Modern Midwives in Europe* (1993); D. Evenden, *The Midwives of Seventeenth-Century London* (Cambridge, 2000); S. C. Lawrence, *Charitable Knowledge: Hospital Pupils and Practitioners in Eighteenth-Century London* (Cambridge, 1996); T. N. Bonner, *Becoming a Physician: Medical Education in Britain, France, Germany, and the United States, 1750-1945* (Oxford, 1995); J. M. T. Ford (ed.), *A Medical Student at St Thomas's Hospital: The Weekes Family Letters* (1987).

(ii) William Savory, boy to man

William Savory was born, he tells us on the opening page of his MS, at 12.25pm on Tuesday, 28 June 1768, and was baptised four weeks later on 25 July (his father's 43rd birthday and his parents' 13th wedding anniversary). The name William had been predominant for three generations, and would remain so for two generations to come. All references to Savory in the introduction and afterword, however, refer exclusively to the author of the MS. Savory was one of four children, the last of his generation and the only son. His father, William Savory, was a wheelwright who ran a village store which sold hardware and an impressive stock of medicines [17-18]. The father also performed (presumably minor) surgery, bled patients and drew teeth, and Savory's uncle also later drew teeth. Savory's mother, Jane, was the daughter of Thomas Barratt, a yeoman farmer in Great Shefford in the Lambourn Valley, and his wife, Miriam. Savory's paternal grandfather had settled in Brightwalton after leaving his native South Moreton about half a century before Savory was born. In May 1768 Brightwalton was home to 349 people (178 males and 171 females) living in 70 different households [see Appendix B]. This gives a mean average of almost five per residence, though in practice the variation ranged from a lone inhabitant to a household of 16, the latter consisting of the Lord of the Manor and his 15 servants.

Savory leaves off his personal narrative and picks it up again 42 pages later when he embarks on 'a little Account of myself to the time my father died' which occurred on 24 July 1772 when the boy was only four years old [43]. Savory's christening, which took place on St James's Day, the patron of the church in the neighbouring parish of Leckhampstead, was conducted at the modest Saxon All Saints' Church, Brightwalton, with its short tower topped with a pointed roof, by the Rev. Dr Richard Eyre, Rector from 1743 until his death in 1778. Two uncles served as godfathers: John Savory, a wheelwright, who would be an important influence in Savory's life, particularly after the premature death of his father; and Richard Barratt (1738-1812), a blacksmith in East Garston, later of Eastbury, Lambourn. His godmothers were young friends of the family: Elizabeth Trumplett (c.1743-1814), who would marry Arthur Whiter in 1772; and Sarah Mouldy (b. 1744), who would marry Richard Bird in 1771.

The birth of a son was greeted as an occurrence worthy of particular celebration. 'My father', Savory reports, 'kept a great merryment & invited most of his Neibours' [44]. Social, legal and cultural biases favoured the arrival of boys in the eighteenth century, and Savory's father seems to have seen in his son the promise of vicariously fulfilled ambition, a point underlined by Savory when he informs us that his father wanted to call him 'Doctor Jack': Jack referred to his paternal uncle, but Doctor was meant to signify his father's medical dabblings and expectations. 'Doctor' would represent a generational rise in status, a definite step up from the druggist father who performed minor medical procedures in surgery, dentistry and bleeding (the drawing of blood then commonly practiced as a medical intervention) [17-18]. There is no record that the father received any formal training. Few gestures could have competed with the conferment of the baptismal name 'Doctor' in instilling in a child a sense of professional destiny. In the end, though, Grandfather Savory's wish to preserve tradition prevailed, and the boy was simply named William. Nevertheless, Savory would indeed grow up to become a qualified and professionally accredited medical man. Having climbed far above his father's amateur status, to become a registered surgeon-apothecary and man-midwife, the professional antecedent of the general practitioner (GP) that would emerge in the nineteenth century.

Savory barely gives us any clue as to his own physical appearance. The few comments he makes all relate to his hair. He writes in June 1783, when he was nearly 15, that he 'first had my hair dressd at Walsh and was to pay him 3/- pr Q[uarte]r for once a Week' [68]. At 17, in February 1786, he wrote about going to a different hairdresser and explained the reason for the change: it was 'the first time of going to Nathaniel Winters to have my hair dressd. Old Walsh lately died and his Grandson John (Son of the present Walsh in Northbrook Street) not minding the business as he ought to do for his Grand Mother, she declind business' [118]. On 7 June 1786, just before his 18th birthday, Savory writes that he 'had my hair tied the first time' [142]. It was then the fashion for young men to wear their hair long. He refers to only one item of clothing: 'a pair of Blue Leather britches' (i.e. leggings that usually stopped above the knee) which he purchased when he was 17 in May 1786 from 'Jones a Britches Maker' and 'methodist preacher' with a 'Crooked Leg' and a penchant for telling falsehoods [119]. As an adult Savory presumably wore the professional black cloak and hat associated with the medical profession, though he never mentions it. He may not have worn a wig: they were beginning to go out of fashion in the 1790s.

As to Savory's personality, the quality that consistently shines through is his good humour and keen sense of fun. A twinkle never seems far from his eye. Perhaps this in part reflects the fact that Savory was a young man just starting out in life and writing about what we would now call his teenage years and youth. It is evident that he was quick to recognise a sense of humour and a cheerful disposition in others. He comments that Grandfather Savory would 'tell Stories or Jests' and praises his father's 'Merry Chearfull disposition' [10, 19]. He writes of his sister, Jane, that she was 'a chearfull Affable creature' [82], describes his schoolmaster, Richard Aldridge, as 'Merry' among other things [45], and reckons Dr Cooper Sampson 'a very merry Companion' [48]. John King was 'a very merry Joking man' who 'could play a great many funny tricks', one of which Savory proceeds to record, also adding a quip – a humorous semantic paradox – which begins with the daring assertion that it is 'no harm [...] to Swear, lie or take advantage': 'its no harm to swear to the truth, its no harm to lie with your Wife, & its no harm to take advantage of a Horse to get upon it' [103]. He even confides his astonishment at how 'chearfull' a 14-year-old patient at St Thomas's Hospital proved to be whilst having his leg amputated, an unimaginable ordeal in the days before general anaesthesia [187].

Savory certainly enjoyed a trick, prank or practical joke. Of John Nelstone or Nelson, his father's schoolmaster at Chaddleworth, he writes that as he became infirm and 'almost for the 2nd time a Child [...] the schollars used to play tricks with him: put pins in his Cushion &c, Dumbledors &c. in his Wig' [16]. Given that Savory was only four when his father died, this story, dating to the 1730s, was presumably told to him by relatives or friends. After visiting a Catholic Church in Holborn he records a story about how someone blackened the holy water so that everyone who entered and crossed their face marked themselves black [204]. At 17, in October 1785, he purchased 'a pack of Cards which is divided from Corner to Corner' and he quotes some mumbo-jumbo intended 'to deceive the Company' [102]. He describes how he sent Miss H. Lovelock of Grange Farm, Shaw, 'a Love Letter written backwards in the name of Wm Rolfe for this Rolfe wanted to be in her Company' adding, in mirror-writing, the words 'My Dearest Miss' [153] to demonstrate his meaning. Lest the reader should suppose Savory was merely being a tricksy Cupid, he adds that, having sent the letter by post, 'the next Markett day Rolfe went as usual into the butter Markett very innocent of the matter but they was att him like so many Birds at an Owl' [153]. He confides, with evident satisfaction, 'It was never found out'. On 10 September 1790, then fully qualified and aged 22, he records how, as he walked down a lane to visit a patient,

> I met John Deacon Collar maker at Brightwalon with a firkin of Tar at his back & <a> head of the Firkin was out. he thought I meant to throw something at it, went to stoop to pick up a stone to throw at me, and great part of the Tar run over him. he was obliged to go back after more Tar & his Wife went after his Coat with a prong[.] [233]

The fact that Deacon sought to anticipate the throwing of a stone suggests that the young doctor had a reputation as a prankster.

Savory could also be so blunt and frank at times that it is difficult to believe that he was not trying to amuse with dry wit, however seriously he felt the sentiment expressed. Such instances are ambiguous and invite multiple readings. This is particularly so in instances where his descriptions of others veer into sarcasm. Thus he says of his maternal uncle, Anthony Barratt, that he was 'what we may call an Oddity, no companion, neither good for himself nor nobody else' [36]. Of his paternal uncle, John, he writes that after badly cutting his finger, 'Mr Work and my Uncle disagreed' and 'on that account he made a Vow never to wear an Apron any more' [30]. When Mary Coxhead got married, and Savory sent a notice to the *Reading Mercury*, he realised that he did not know her father's name so simply made one up. His caustic post-script to this story perhaps explains his inattentiveness: 'she was a very disagreeable Woman both in her personal & mental accomplishments' [120]. Many of his most sarcastic comments involved his sister Mary, as we shall see: 'she was always of a contrary disposition to myself by which reason we could never agree' [43]. Of Thomas Iremonger (c1720-1784) he writes, 'this Old Iremonger used to Carry Victuals in his pockett to Markett and sometimes his heart would be open enough to spend a penny' [69]. He writes of James Pettit Andrews (1737-1797), Justice of the Peace for Berkshire, author, and a member of the Andrews family of Shaw House and Donnington Grove, that he was 'a very troublesome man to the Country' [58]. Of his father's schoolmaster, Nelstone, he writes, 'he used to wear a great Coat in the Winter to keep the Cold out and a great Coat in the Summer to keep the Sun off' [16]. Of the Rev. Edward Jones, whom Savory regarded as an 'excellent Minister' and particularly liked, he writes, with shades of Henry Fielding, that he was 'a person very much addicted to Drinking & Swearing' [231]. What all of these examples demonstrate is that, whatever Savory intended to convey, he consciously or otherwise had a comic turn of phrase.

Savory was also prone to gossip and sometimes gave a sarcastic twist to his account of other people's opinions. He comments that 'it was the general opinion' that Richard Bird set his own house on fire [52], and later alleges that Bird was 'a Crafty roaguish person' who overreached himself, squandered his fortune, and spent time in Reading Gaol in August 1787 [144]. When Savory managed to get his chaise stuck by poor steering, and caused his passenger, Mrs Trulock, to ruin her shoes in scrambling up a bank, he seizes the opportunity to take a barbed verbal swipe at her, at least in the pages of his MS: 'this Mrs Trulock is a very particular Old Lady of a Tall slender shape – a proud, Conceited, fancifull Queen. she lives now at Newbury and noticed by every one but respected by none' [101]. He demonstrates the point a couple of pages later by copying out a particularly caustic and bawdy song lampooning a relationship conducted in Mrs Trulock and her lover, Messetter's, twilight years [104]. The song, which Savory judged to have been written by an 'injenious person', provides the only instance of swearing in the MS ('shite') [103, 104] (see below).

Occasionally the drawing up of a geniture – the type of horoscope that was Savory's preferred astrological device – provided the opportunity for personal comments, often speculative and frequently catty. For example, he writes of his master's son, David Jones, that the signs denoted 'some dangerous fluxes & Cold Rhumes or Colds perhaps by being too great a friend to Bacchus', i.e. a drunk [93]. Young David's future wife, moreover, would be 'rather slovenly inclined' and the couple would 'disagree' [94]. Indeed, he could look forward to having 'few friends and those he seldom agrees with' [95]. One can only hope for Savory's sake that he kept such prognostications to himself. It has proved impossible to confirm or contradict these predictions.

What strikes one above all about Savory's MS is its readability. He is gossipy and conversational, traits that are amplified by his pre-Victorian inconsistencies and inaccuracies of grammar, punctuation, spelling ('beleive', 'wheelright', 'apprentiship', 'chearfull' etc), and his haphazard use of upper and lower-case letters. Contradictory spellings sometimes occur within single phrases. The most amusingly ironical example comes when he boasts, '[…] by the Year 1779 I was the first Schoolar in the Schoold and so remaind till I left School' [48]. Presumably 'Schoold' was simply a mistake, and 'Schoolar' contrasts with his more common misspelling of scholar: 'a great schollar' and 'the schollars' [16]; 'a good Schollar' [19]; and 'his Schollars' [45]. Of his brother-in-law, John Eagles (c.1759-1822), he writes, 'since he has been Married to my Sister he is got very religious' [83] where 'is got' should presumably, in the vernacular of the day, have been 'has gotten'. Peachey commented caustically, 'His surgery was happily of a higher quality than his English'.[1] Nevertheless, Savory imparts one pertinent pearl of wisdom that was given him: 'The Revd E[dwar]d Jones sais there is but one Rule without

---

1. Peachey, *Life of William Savory*, 10.

exception which is u after q in the English Language' [232]. Yet if Savory's use of English was doubtful even by eighteenth-century standards, then his grasp of Latin was decidedly eccentric, as he repeatedly demonstrates.

Savory's life spanned the so-called 'long eighteenth-century'. There is a strong case for arguing that in one sense it began with the birth of his paternal grandfather in 1696. Savory was just four years old when his father died aged 47 in 1772, but 17 when his grandfather died aged 89 in 1786. Partly in consequence, the influence on him of his grandfather, who lived in the same house, was particularly strong. Savory himself died in 1824 at the age of 56. The sense of how far back Savory's personal contact with the past reached is underlined by his account of how his grandfather, accompanied by a friend, travelled from South Moreton to London where, in a market, they found a potato:

> I remember of hearing my Grandfather talk of going to London the first time with Thos Finmore (who was a Lad about the age of my Grandfather and was father to this present Thos Finmore of Fulscot in the parish of South Moreton)[.] they seeing some potatoes in a Markett thought that they were strange Turnips & my Grandfather brought the first potatoes into Brightwalton[,] which was sent by him from London as a present from the Lord of the Manor to Mr Selwood (the late Colonel Selwoods father)[.] [5-6]

This was probably around the year 1715. Even allowing for the exaggerated romance of a tale such as this, it gives a palpable sense of how long it could take for items, which were common in the capital, to reach rural communities.

(iii) Family background

Seniority and influence justify Savory's choice to begin his family pen-portraits with his paternal grandfather, William. Savory tells us that his grandfather was born in South Moreton on 4 October 1696 and was the son of 'William and Joan Savory' [4]. The parish register, which gives the surname as 'Savoury', confirms his parentage, but states that he was born on 3 October, and baptised a week later on the 10th. Savory points out that, including himself, the name William christened the eldest son in four generations of his family. The first William *Savery* had married *Jone* Taylor at Appleton with Eaton on 26 December 1695. Grandfather Savory in fact also had a younger brother, John, born 20 February 1698, baptised the 22nd, and buried the 28th. William Savoury Snr died the following month and was buried on the 9th. What happened to Joan/Jone remains obscure, but Savory was aware that his grandfather's 'friends dying' he 'apprenticed himself to one Gray', a wheelwright in Brightwalton, though unless he was already of age himself by then he would have needed sponsorship by an adult [4]. When Gray died, or left off business, Savory's grandfather, we are informed, commenced as a master wheelwright. This was possibly before he had completed his apprenticeship, yet he quickly took on his own apprentice, Thomas Mashall [5]. Grandfather Savory married Mary Lucas (1706-1731), then resident in Peasemore, at St Leonard's Church, Wallingford, on 7 September 1724. Savory informs us that his grandmother was from Sheeplease, and, probably as a result, he believed that the wedding had taken place at Beedon [6]. The Lucas family certainly lived in Sheeplease between Beedon and Peasemore and it was at St Nicholas's Church, Beedon, that Savory's grandmother was baptised on 2 April 1706 and buried on 17 August 1731. Savory later tells us that Mary had a brother, and that Savory's paternal uncle, John, was 'to have been a Watchmaker had his Uncle Lucas been according to his Word who was a Watchmaker in Newbury' [30]. This was John Lucas (1708-1741), a clockmaker in Newbury. The Royal Berkshire Archives have a copy of a lease assigned to John Lucas, heir of John Lucas, late of Standmore [*sic*], Beedon, yeoman, entrusting to Thomas Parsons of Oare, in the parish of Chieveley, yeoman, and John Merriman, of Speenhamland, gentleman, the freehold messuage and its appurtenances, and two grounds called Sheepleazes,[1] consisting in 34 acres in the parish of Peasemore (formerly part of Peasemore Farm, the property of Thomas Coward, clerk, deceased.).[2] Mary and John Lucas were the children of John and Elinor Lucas: John Lucas Senior died when his daughter was only six and a half years old and was buried at St Nicholas's Church, Beedon, on 14 October 1712, and Elinor, his widow, joined him more than 22 years later, on 27 November 1734.[3] Savory's great uncle, John Lucas, who married Elizabeth Dowset at Wantage on 10 September 1737, made a deathbed will on 26 June 1741 'labouring at present under some indispositions of Body'.[4] He bequeathed all his goods to his wife, his estate having been already entrusted to Parsons and Merriman, Francis Leicester, Elizabeth Dowsett (possibly his mother-in-law), and his apprentice Anthony Lynch or Linch. A codicil made the following day, 27 June, stipulated that the estate should pass to any children of his marriage or, there being no survivors, to William and John Savory 'sons of my only Sister Mary Savory' as tenants in common. Probate was proved at Newbury on 16 July 1741 by his widow, Elizabeth. He was buried at Beedon on 5 July 1741.

Savory's father, William, and uncle, John Savory, were the only children of the Savory-Lucas marriage. As Savory comments, his grandfather 'soon grew tired of being a Widower' [6]. On 24 August 1732, just over a year after losing his wife, Grandfather Savory married Susannah Taylor (1687-1768). He was a 35-year-old widower, and she was a 44-year-old spinster. Savory's description of the wedding, which took place at St Mary's Church, in North Fawley, is particularly instructive and entertaining:

> they were Married very private unknown to any of the Neibours for Mr Bridegroom[,] taking the Baskett of Tools at his back pretending to mend the Church Rails & Mrs Bride no way at a loss to be likewise private & when the ceremony was finishd he went home with his baskett of Tools at his back and she to her brothers at fawly. now her brother Thomas Taylor

---

1. RBA D/EL/T116 (Peasemore).
2. RBA D/EX 464/37.
3. For John Lucas's will, see RBA D/A1/95/39.
4. WSA P1/9Reg/99.

with whom she lived was gone to Markett & did not know of it till a few days after. [6-7]

The Taylor family of Fawley was a large one. Susannah was one of ten children born to John Taylor (1651-1728) and his wife Susannah (d. 1728), of whom six were brothers: Thomas (b. 1686), Elizabeth (1689-1709), Amy (b. 1690), Anne (b. 1692), Mary (1693-1694), John (b. 1695), William (b. 1698), twins Benjamin (1701-1732) and Joseph (1701-1739) and Henry (b. 1704).[1] Of his step-grandmother, Savory, who never knew her, comments that she was 'a very good living Woman' and a 'tender' step-mother, though he also mentions the fortune of £100 and the 'great many Goods' that went with her into the marriage, and a staggering £2,199 that Grandfather Savory inherited on her behalf, a payout allegedly received after her death [7, 8-9]. When Savory's parents married in 1755, the senior Savorys relocated to a small tenement belonging to Dame Hatt. Susannah was 80 when she died, and was buried at Brightwalton on 21 February 1768. Savory quotes the verse on her original gravestone which was replaced with a horizontal stone on the instruction of Savory's uncle after Grandfather Savory died on 5 February 1786 [8] (and Savory provides a short description of his funeral [117]). That stone has survived, though the inscription is badly worn, and the stone is cracked in two from side to side.

Grandfather Savory was tall, big-boned, but in 'no way inclind to Corpulency'; he was also handsome, with a 'King Wms Nose' [10]. His chief work duties in Savory's lifetime were

> sawing[,] Cleaving & Cording Wood for sale & keeping the Tools & shop in good Condition and what was very singular he could see to whet & sett a saw without spectacles almost to the day of his death [10].

Three times a day he would read the Bible or other devotional texts. Aspects of the old man's personality evidently rubbed off on his grandson. He was 'a good living Man, Charitable &c[,] was a great smoaker', and he was a 'good Companion' who 'could sing Songs' and 'tell Stories or Jests', many of these personal characteristics being qualities Savory seems to have greatly admired [10]. Savory's father was similarly tall and handsome, but 'raw bon[e]d' and thin-faced and 'so much study cast a Care on his brow' [19]. He even made a copy of the parish register and kept the parish accounts. Bright and capable, he quickly established himself as one of his father's 'Quickest & best' workmen [17]. Following his marriage on his 30th birthday, Savory's father succeeded his own father as a master wheelwright, but also sold hardware and patent medicines. Most importantly for Savory himself, it seems, his father 'was of a Merry Chearfull disposition[,] a real friend to every one[,] beloved by all that knew him' [19].

Paradoxically, Savory's father was only present in his son's conscious life in the sorrowful absence caused by his premature death. Apart from the vaguest of memories, everything he knew of his father must have come from his

---

1. For John Taylor's will, see RBA D/A1/130/38.

mother, sisters, uncle, grandfather, and family friends. His story, and theirs, will emerge as we turn to a thematic analysis of the MS but it should be observed that Savory writes of his bachelor uncle, John Savory, that he 'bred myself & sisters up very handsome and behaved like a father to us' [31]. He would remain a fatherly presence well into their adulthoods.

When it comes to Savory's forebears and wider family, it remains for us to consider here his maternal ancestors and relatives. Neither of his grandparents, Thomas Barratt (1699-1770) nor Miriam, née Ambrose (1698-1762), would have been known to him personally. They had married in Great Shefford on 15 June 1729. Savory refers to his great grandfather, who died nearly 40 years before he himself was born, as 'Farmer Ambrose of Maidencourt farm in Eastgarston parish' [34]. Miriam was one of the five children of William Ambrose (c.1675-1729) and his wife, Frances (d. 1723), and was baptised at East Garston on 18 September 1698. Ambrose was a successful farmer whose wealth had no doubt passed down the generations helping to keep alive his memory. It is owing to Ambrose's detailed will, made in January 1728, and the accompanying inventory of his estate, that we can build a picture of Maidencourt Farm and the upbringing Savory's maternal grandmother experienced there.[1] It emerges that Maidencourt Farm had a garret bedroom and seven other bedrooms: one over the hall, one over the kitchen, one over the brewhouse, one over the pantry, two over the stables, and one other. The value of the estate was calculated at £1,234 16s. This included £80 worth of wearing apparel and ready money; two hogsheads of ale, eight of small beer and 'some other liquors' in the cellar; two tables and two chairs in the hall; £30 worth of books in the 'Bookroom'; 'in the kitching [*sic*] one dozen and an half of powles + dishes one dozen & half of plates five chairs + two Tables'; a 'furnace and breweing Vessells' in the brewhouse; a cheese-press and cheese tub in the millhouse; a good table and some chairs in the pantry; and cheese shelves in the 'cheeseroom'. There was timber and part timber, hay, and 'apparel of faggots' and other (non-itemised) objects in the granary. On the farm, Ambrose had 15 horses (worth £100); 30 cattle (worth £80), 400 sheep (worth £200), 40 hogs and pigs (worth £40), six waggons (worth £40), four dung carts, six ploughs, 11 harrows, and four bowsers. There were 60 acres of 'wheate'; 120 acres of barley; 35 acres of 'pease'; 35 acres of 'oates'; and 20 acres more. There was a harness, a saddle and other items 'in and about the sheddes'; shovels in the barns; poultry; eight dozen hurdles, and three dozen cages. This clearly betokens a comfortable standard of living, and the bulk of the estate was inherited by Ambrose's only son, Henry (1690-?1762). Ambrose provided legacies of £200 each to his daughters, Dorothy and Miriam (Savory's grandmother), and a guinea each to his daughters, Sarah and Jane, 'I haveing already given them their pportions [*sic*]', he explained. One Mary Collman, who is not identified, was to receive £30.

Savory seems to have thought that his mother was Thomas and Miriam Barratt's first child. They had at least one child before Jane was born in Fawley: John Barratt, who quickly died and was buried in East Garston on 23 August 1734. Savory tells us that his grandfather's sister, Hannah Barratt (1694-1776),

---

1. RBA D/A1/38/83.

was married to William Palmer (c1674-1757) who 'used to Occupy a Farm in little Fawly now Occupied by Pocock' [35]. Savory's grandfather moved to Fawley to go into business with Palmer, and that is how Savory's mother, Jane, came to be baptised at St Mary's Church, North Fawley, on 30 April 1735: the register gives her name as 'Jane Barrott' and her mother as 'Mariam'. In fact Barratt came more frequently to be spelled Barrett as the years passed. Savory confides that 'William Palmer was 20 Years older than his Wife Hannah Barratt for when she was carrying to be Christened, Wm was threshing in the Barn & he said if ever he had a Wife that Child should be she and so it was' [35]. That such a story, apt to make us feel uneasy today, should have been remembered by Savory in 1791 testifies to the power of anecdote and the stories passed down in families by word of mouth from one generation to the next: Palmer had married Hannah Barratt on 31 May 1714, over 50 years before Savory was born. The couple had seven children together. Scrutiny of Palmer's will, made at South Fawley on 7 January 1754, reveals the extent of the family's wealth.[1] He mentions four properties: their main dwelling in Fawley; Pound's Farm leased from Sir John Moore (the Lord of the Manor) at the cost of £120 a year (which he left to his son, William); Young's or Ball's Farm, leased for £160 a year (left to his sons and executors, Richard and Anthony); and a property in East Garston, leased from William Jones (left to his wife, Hannah). Hannah was also bequeathed the bedstead, curtains, bed and bedding, and any other furniture in the chamber above the parlour at Fawley, plus homespun flaxen sheets, pillow cases, and table cloths. All the children received financial legacies: eight guineas to his son Henry, and a further £250 at the age of 21; £150 to James; £200 apiece to Hannah and Mary Palmer; and one shilling was left to his son-in-law, Thomas Blake, the husband of Jane Palmer.

The widowed Hannah Palmer subsequently moved to Catmore Farm to live with her daughter, Mary, her son-in-law Robert Stephens, and their family (see below). She made her will there on 1 March 1772.[2] The East Garston estate she inherited from her husband was left to her son, William. To her daughter Mary Stephens she left all her furniture, 'Gold Rings, plate, and wearing apparel'. To her son-in-law, Robert Stephens, and her son James Palmer, she bequeathed £80 apiece in trust for her granddaughters, Martha, Hannah, Mary and Katherine Palmer (daughters of her late son, Thomas Palmer). James Palmer and Robert Stephens, her son and son-in-law, were to act as trustees and executors, and inherited the residue of her estate. She was buried on 14 February 1776, 19 years after her husband.

After Palmer's business partnership with Savory's grandfather broke down, which seems to have occurred by May 1737, the Barratts relocated to Henley Farm, in Great or West Shefford, in the Lambourn Valley. This is where Savory's uncles were born: Thomas (1737-1808), his godfather Richard (1738-1812) and Anthony Barratt (1740-1825). The family would ultimately benefit from the Barratt inheritance, but only when John Barratt (1696-1761), the eldest brother of Savory's grandfather Thomas, died in 1761. Under the terms of John's deathbed will, Thomas was the main beneficiary: he inherited John's

1. RBA D/A1/109/203.
2. WSA P1/13Reg/109.

'free land', house, shop, garden and orchard in East Garston, and also free land known as 'Sheep Cubb Land' in Chipping Lambourn Field, provided only that he pay John's servant, Mary Butcher, 20 shillings annually.[1] John also left Thomas his stock of cattle, corn, shop, tools and 'all manner of Goods'. John and Thomas's parents are not mentioned by Savory, and necessarily fall outside the scope of this introduction, but it is important to note that Thomas's inheritance from his brother stands in stark contrast to his treatment by his father, John Barratt (1660-1731) who, for reasons not explained in his will, left Thomas only four shillings.[2] By contrast, Thomas's sister, Hannah Palmer, was bequeathed £30, and his brothers, Richard and Anthony, £90 each. John, who was executor, inherited everything else: including the 'free land in Lambourn field' and the 'free Land lying disperst in East Garston feild now in my possesion [sic] and all my Housseall [sic] Goods debts Shop Book toolls and every thing or things whatsoever'. By the terms of his brother's will, therefore, Savory's grandfather appears essentially to have inherited what had been his father's estate, but only after it had passed through his brother's hands.[3]

Savory's great uncle, Richard Barratt (1703-1769), whose death he records, is described as 'a very Choleric passionate Man and left my three Uncle Barratts, his property' [45]. Savory tells us twice that Richard lived with his brother Thomas (Savory's grandfather), and that unlike his brothers, who were all blacksmiths, he was a carpenter, and adds that he was apprenticed in Lambourn [34-35, 45]. Richard's will, dated 16 June 1764, provided legacies of £10 apiece to his sister Hannah Palmer, his brothers Thomas and Anthony Barratt, his nephew Thomas Barratt and niece Jane Savory (Savory's mother).[4] Likewise he bequeathed £10 each to his nephews Thomas, William, Anthony and James Palmer, and to his niece Mary Stephens, all to be paid within a year of his death. A further £5 was to be shared among the poor in the parish in which he died (Great Shefford) and distributed at the discretion of the church minister and churchwardens within a week of his burial. The remainder of his property and possessions were shared between his executors, two nephews, Richard and Anthony Barratt, but not the third of them.

Savory's grandparents appear to have spent the remainder of their lives at Henley Farm. It was there that Thomas Barratt made his will on 16 September 1766.[5] He bequeathed the freehold estates in East Garston and Lambourn to his eldest son, Thomas Barratt (1737-1808), subject to the provision of a legacy of £30 for his daughter, Jane (Savory's mother). Jane would receive a further £70 legacy from the estate, the remainder of which was to be shared between Barratt's three sons, Thomas, Richard and Anthony. An interesting clause in the will stipulated that should the three brothers disagree about how to

---

1. RBA D/A1/50/102.
2. RBA D/A1/49/153.
3. John Barratt Jnr also bequeathed his nephew, William Palmer, 'a Garden of free Land', namely 'Griffins in the Common Field at East Garston', provided that he pay 20 shillings a year to John's servant, Mary Butcher, and invest £5, from the interest of which the poor of the parish of East Garston would benefit. He further bequeathed legacies of £5 apiece to his sister Hannah Palmer, and brothers, Richard and Anthony Barratt.
4. RBA D/A1/50/126.
5. WSA P1/12Reg/343B.

administer the estate, two arbitrators should be nominated, one of them by Thomas and Richard jointly, and the other by Anthony. This hints at an anxiety that suggests a clash of personalities between Anthony and his siblings. In the event there does not appear to have been any disagreement and probate was awarded at Newbury on 23 July 1770. Nevertheless, Anthony Barratt's personality is directly criticised by Savory who, as we have seen, writes that 'Anthony is what we may call an Oddity, no companion, neither good for himself nor nobody else' [36]. It is fruitless to speculate precisely what Savory means by this. In the whole of the 85 years Anthony lived – he would outlive Savory himself – he does not seem to have married or had any children. Such of his nephews and nieces who survived him shared his estate, except for £100 which was to be invested by his executors and the interest paid annually to the poor of Great Shefford.[1] By the start of the twentieth century, the Barrett Bequest, as it came to be known, was still paying out a modest annual dividend every Whitsun to about fifty poor parishioners considered sufficiently deserving.[2] Contrary to Savory's assessment, therefore, Anthony's bachelorhood probably did do others some good after all.

Of his godfather, Uncle Richard Barratt, Savory simply and correctly relates that he married Sarah Spirit of East Garston, 'by whom he had 4 Children': Hannah, John, Miriam and Richard (born between 1771 and 1779) [36]. For his uncle Thomas, who continued to live at Henley Farm, he supplies information that is probably recorded in no other source, namely that his wife, Ann Gilman (1755-1842), was 'his house keeper' [35]. He does not mention that Ann was also 18 years Thomas's junior. The couple, whose wedding at Great Shefford on 29 November 1783 Savory notes [70], had three children together, among them Miriam Barratt (1791-1869) who married Thomas Langford (1786-1857), nephew of the Thomas Langford (1758-1851) whose marriage to Mary Mitchell in 1782 Savory also registers [56]. What Savory probably did not envisage when he wrote about them is that he would have a son who himself would marry into the Langford family (see afterword). This set of circumstances probably explains how Savory's son came to be an executor of the will of Miriam's brother, John Barratt (1795-1829).[3]

Of Savory's siblings, the one he probably saw least of growing up was his eldest sister, Sarah. Born on 26 October 1756, she was nearly 12 years his senior, and she seems to have been living outside the family home, working in service, by the time Savory was little: she spent 18 months with relatives in Crowmarsh, a year with Mrs Nelson in Chaddleworth, two years with Mrs Bateman in Harwell, and then went to Lady Mary Head (1700-1792) of Langley Hall [36]. In an astrological chart Savory draws for his sister, he describes her as 'bold Witty and Stout hearted' [81]. Sarah married Francis Mead Fordham (1758-1806) at St George's, Hanover Square, on 27 December 1783 (an event curiously not recorded in Savory's diary). Fordham signed the register with a cross. He was the son of Thomas and Sarah Fordham. Francis

---

1. TNA PCC PROB 11/1708/235.
2. See RBA D/P 108/25/1 and P. H. Ditchfield and W. Page (eds.), *The Victoria History of the County of Berkshire* (4 vols, 1907), iv. 242.
3. TNA PCC PROB 11/1757/407.

was baptised in Aston, Hertfordshire, on 1 October 1758 where his father, Thomas (d. 1761), worked as a tailor. A member of a large family, Francis's siblings included Thomas Fordham (1752-aft 1795) and Edward Fordham (1760-aft 1828). When the Fordhams' first child, Jane (presumably named after her maternal grandmother), was baptised at St Mary's, Whitechapel, on 27 April 1785, the family's address was given as Catherine Wheel Alley, which survives today opposite Liverpool Street Station. There is a reasonable probability that the Fordhams ran the Catherine Wheel pub after which the alley is named; the pub burnt down in 1895. When Miriam was baptised on 7 March 1787, the family's address had changed to Lambeth Street, and it seems likely that they were by then running the Flying Horse at no. 63 (as subsequently designated), in Goodman's Fields. This is somewhere to which we shall return when we consider Savory's student days in London in 1788 to 1789 when he spent some time living with the Fordhams at the inn. In the astrological charts he draws, Savory declares that his sister Jane had a 'a hard pimpled Complexion' [82]; whilst Mary was '[o]f a Middle Stature[,] lean and spare, Long Visage, light hair' [84]. While Jane was 'a chearfull Affable creature, hurtfull to none[,] delight in decency &c' and 'an agreeable Companion' who enjoyed a harmonious relationship with her husband John Eagles [82], Mary was 'very hasty and Choleric' and could yet be overcome by others 'as a Mouse before a Catt who would get at the Cheese was she not under the paws of a ruling power' yet she had an antagonistic relationship with her husband, Joseph Norris [84], We will learn more of Jane and Mary as we turn to a thematic analysis of Savory's commonplace book.

(iv) Education
Savory's story is one rooted in the Age of Enlightenment. Among his possessions were the scientific instruments that were becoming the middle-class gizmos of the day – 'many Curiosities' he calls them – such as the telescope, air pump, theodolite, measuring-wheel, electrifying machine and 'Instruments for drawing &c' which he inherited from his father, as well as peep-shows, 'sl[e]ight of hand implements', and a magic lantern which provided entertainment [19]. Savory tells us that the theodolite was lost the last time his father went out measuring land, and the electrifying machine and air pump were subsequently sold by his grandfather and uncle [31]. In 1789 he bought an electrifying machine of his own from Simpson, a bookbinder in London's Lombard Street, and presumably used it to treat patients, at a time when the application of electricity in health-care was being explored with growing enthusiasm [197]. He also mentions that, 'The peep Shows, Magic Lanthorn, Books, Telescopes &c are now at Brightwaltham in the possession of my Uncle' [31-32]. The son literally followed in his father's footsteps in measuring distances between various places in and around Brightwalton after Savory had the measuring-wheel fixed in 1790 [229-230]. He records the distances between stops on a coach journey from Spenhamland to Hyde Park Corner [125]. His passion to observe, calculate and record is palpable.

    Father and son would both benefit from formal schooling in the neighbourhood, an advantage which was available to relatively few children in the eighteenth century. Given that Savory could scarcely have remembered his father, what he reveals about his parent's schooling must have come mainly from his uncle and grandfather. It is with more than a little pride that he recalls that 'the first remarkable instance I have heard tell of my father was he could read a Chapter in the Bible at 4 Years of Age and was so ready in Arithmetics that he could tell his Sums as fast as Old Mr Nelstone could set them so that at last his Scooldmaster would have him no longer' but not before the young scholar knew 'Algebra, Astronomy, Navigation, Dialling &c' [16, 19]. The schoolmaster in question was John Nelson (1673-1747) of Chaddleworth: Savory calls him Nelstone and judges him to have been 'a great schollar' who seems to have been suffering from dementia in his final years and had grown old and infirm before he retired. 'As my father encreased in Years', Savory adds, 'the same was his ingenuity' [17].

Savory recalls that he went to school himself from some time before his father's death in 1772 until he was apprenticed at the age of 14 in 1783, 'except about one Years intermission' [45]. His schoolmaster was Richard Aldridge (1744-1783), a native of Brightwalton. The classes were taught at 'a well built tile House situated at the edge of Brightwaltham Common' adjoining Farnborough Liberty [45]. It was the 'Middle tenement' between houses occupied by John Norris and John Harris. He describes Aldridge, who never married, as 'handsome as most Crooked people are but naturally peevish and Cross to his Schollars' [45]. Yet he was merry and a 'sensible conversant' in company [45]. Perhaps Savory saw this difference as Janus-faced hypocrisy, but he otherwise gives no clue as to what he means by 'Crooked'. Aldridge succeeded Savory's father in measuring land. The schoolmaster was on his way to Penclose Wood, near Winterbourne, to measure land for a local farmer, when he fell from his horse and died [46]. His loss by such an accident at the age of 39 (not 38 as Savory records) was reflected in the verse written on his gravestone, which Savory transcribes [47]. He also notes that Brightwalton's next schoolmaster was Aldridge's nephew, Samuel Mitchell (1769-1788) whom he judged 'a clever young man', and he was succeeded by his younger brother, Henry Mitchell (1771-1797) [152]. As to Aldridge's abilities, he was 'an excellent Writer and the same in Arithmetic' [45]. His 'favorite Song', as he puts it, 'was Plato' [45-46].

'I kept to my School very diligent and began to make use of the Geeses feathers in the Year 1775 before I was 7 years of Age', he recalls [48]. In February 1776, when he was not yet eight, he 'begun Arithmetic the Numeration Table' [48]. He also notes that 'My Sister Mary at that time was learning the Multiplication Table & Jenny in the Rule of Three' which suggests what for that period would have been an unusually liberal attitude among craftsmen to the education of girls, a subject to which we will return [48]. In a presumably unconscious stroke of irony, Savory then adds the remark, in his poorest English, that 'by the Year 1779 I was the first Schoolar in the Schoold and so remain till I left School' [48].[1] Although this represents the final word on his formal schooling, it is far from marking an end to his education.

---

1. For a detailed survey of schooling in Berkshire in Savory's time, see *Berkshire Schools in the Eighteenth Century*, ed. S. Clifford (Berkshire Record Society, xxvi, 2019). For Savory's

Indeed, Savory actively sought out private tutors in a range of subjects whilst serving his apprenticeship in Newbury in the mid-1780s. At the start of 1786 he was taught to etch and engrave by 'one Powell' – possibly Robert Powell, a Newbury bookbinder – but his teacher stole from him a flute, an incision knife and four books by Cornelius Agrippa: 'so thats a reward by putting to [*sic*] great confidence in a stranger', he remarks sarcastically [117]. He did not give up, however, noting in 1787 that he purchased engraving tools [145]. On 18 July 1786, shortly after turning 18, Savory began learning French. He purchased various books to help him, including a dictionary, grammar and prayer book [122-123]. He was tutored by an unnamed Frenchman who lodged in Bartholomew Street whom he saw twice a week. The lessons only lasted a month, however, because 'Monsier left Newbury without delivering the sentiments of his mind to any one I beleive [*sic*] by reason of his Debts' [123]. Despite this second misfortune in the choice of his tutors, his appetite for learning was undiminished: we will see later how he also paid for lessons in astrology, for example. It should be added that Savory, whose standard handwriting is generally neat and legible (though his vowels are sometimes difficult to distinguish), never refers to calligraphy, but it is evident from the penmanship on display in parts of the commonplace book, particularly in the headpiece on the first page (see cover illustration), and in the extant volumes of his student lecture notes, especially in their elaborate title-pages (see illustration to Appendix D), that he also spent time studying blacklettering and simple decoration.

(v) Health

The earliest incidents Savory records in his life are illnesses. After an initial (but short) period of 'very great health', he was 'extreamly Ill' aged six or seven months [44]. Aged two, he suffered 'another violent fit of Illness' [44]. In both cases he was attended by medical men based in Wantage. 'Dr [Cooper] Sampson' (1740-1776), who attended Savory's first illness, described himself as a surgeon and apothecary. He was a successful druggist who supplied the shop run by Savory's father in Brightwalton. In July 1773 when a vacancy arose for the office of local coroner, Sampson unsuccessfully advertised himself for the job.[1] Sampson was a respected family friend who agreed to serve as godfather to Savory's sister, Mary. Savory describes him as 'a very merry Companion' and 'a good Songster', but he was a 'very little Man' who, presumably to keep himself warm rather than to appear bigger, wore three or four pairs of stockings simultaneously [48]. He was nearly killed when a group of women 'put him in the Cradle' at the christening of Savory's sister, Mary [48]. Sampson was entrusted with inoculating Savory, his three sisters and seven others with smallpox in the autumn of 1772. Advertising his inoculation service in October 1768 Sampson boasted in *Jackson's Oxford Journal* that his patients had 'left his Inoculating House on Monday last in perfect Health'.[2]

---

reference to a school kept in East Hendred by Avery Hobbs, see [55]; and for his account of schools in Chaddleworth run by Daniel Whistler and his son, Daniel, see [56].

1. *RM* (2 August 1773) and *OJ* (7 August 1773).
2. *OJ* (3 October 1768).

The advert noted that he had more than one inoculating house situated near Wantage. In 1772 the cost, including medicines, was two guineas, though there was no charge for Sampson's goddaughter. Savory recalls that 'we had the SmallPox [*sic*] all of us very favorable at a House calld Collins or Sparrow Bill' which was evidently used as some sort of isolation or fever hospital because it was there that Savory's father had died of smallpox (acquired on a visit to London) a few months earlier [47]. 'Mr [Edward] Seymour', on the other hand, who attended Savory's second illness, though described at the time of his marriage in 1764 as 'an eminent surgeon' and listed as a surgeon and pharmacist based in Wantage in the *Medical Register* until at least 1779, proved unsatisfactory.[1] Having bled Savory in the arm, Seymour was not considered adequate to the task, and is never mentioned again.[2]

Having dismissed Seymour, Savory's family sent for an altogether more respected authority: 'Dr Collett of Newbury who by the blessings of God' cured him [44]. Dr John Collet (1709-1780) was an eminent physician and Newbury's leading medical practitioner. Educated at Greenwich and subsequently at Trinity Hall, Cambridge, he then studied in Paris and London and, under Herman Boerhaave, in Leiden. He graduated Doctor of Medicine in 1731 and became an Extra-Licentiate of the College of Physicians in 1733. He spent six years in Brentford and Uxbridge but settled permanently in Newbury. He had a large practice in the town and was 'looked up to with the reverence given to patriarchs of old'.[3] It was Collet who provided Savory's father with 'proper Medical Asistance' in what nevertheless turned out to be the illness that killed him on 24 July 1772 [20].

Savory notes that his uncle, John Savory, joined with the neighbouring parishioners at Farnborough to be inoculated with smallpox in April 1780 [50]. Some patients were treated by Gilbert Cowper (1755-1799), the son of the more eminent Wantage surgeon, also Gilbert Cowper (1713-1779). This is the only time Savory refers to him, however. Other patients, including Savory's uncle, were inoculated by Lucy Sampson, née Spicer (1741-1821), the widow of Cooper Sampson, who had inoculated Savory's sisters and himself. On the death of her husband, Mrs Sampson advertised her intention of 'carrying on the Grocery, Stationary, and Drug Trade in all its branches, as usual'.[4] She also continued making and selling 'Sampson's Pectoral Balsamic Drops' to cure 'Coughs, Colds, Asthmas and Consumptions' and among the other people to sell it, who were based variously in Newbury, Faringdon, Abingdon and Reading was 'Mr Savory' of Brightwalton, presumably Savory's uncle, though in practice the shop was then run by Savory's widowed mother.[5] When Savory made his first trip to London in September 1781, accompanied by his paternal grandfather, the two of them stayed the night with Mrs Sampson and proceeded

---

1. *OJ* (3 March 1764).
2. Savory also mentions in passing Richard Bew, a surgeon in Thatcham, a professional who was officially apprenticed and took his own apprentice in turn; Savory knew Bew's father, who was a schoolmaster at North Heath [49].
3. *Newbury Weekly News* (24 July 1884).
4. *OJ* (30 March 1776).
5. *OJ* (7 February 1778, 3 December 1785).

on their journey from Wantage [53]. Mrs Sampson's business was certainly still thriving in the 1790s.

Smallpox was the fifth biggest killer in Britain in the late eighteenth century. There can be little doubt that Savory was, in part, motivated to compile his MS volume by the fear that, like his father, he would succumb to the disease and die prematurely. Furthermore, it seems reasonable to suppose that this anxiety helped spur the boy almost christened 'Doctor' to strive to become a fully qualified medical man. The suggestion is not that Savory thought he could somehow recover the loss of his father or guarantee his own good health, but rather that he could protect others from similar suffering – patients and their potentially bereaved relatives and friends. Savory refers no fewer than 11 times to the death of his father, and 12 times to smallpox and inoculation. He even records how Jane Barratt, the sister of his maternal grandfather, 'dyed with the Small Pox when Young' [35]. She was baptised in East Garson on 18 July 1708 and seems to have been buried there on 20 January 1731, aged 22. That Savory was conscious of her existence let alone the cause of her premature death nearly 40 years before he was born, seems remarkable. The threat posed by smallpox was a constant concern. John M. T. Ford, the editor of the family letters of the medical man, Hampton Weekes (1780-1855), who was a student at St Thomas's Hospital 13 years after Savory, noted that smallpox was the most commonly mentioned disease in Weekes's correspondence of 1801-1802.[1]

By a twist of fate, Savory's principal teacher in the Borough Hospitals in the late 1780s was Henry Cline (1750-1827). After Savory's student days, Cline supported the work of the Gloucestershire-based physician Edward Jenner (1749-1823), who had made the immunological discovery that safe exposure to cowpox, by means of careful vaccination, protected patients against smallpox, whose virological profile was sufficiently similar. Vaccination, moreover, quickly proved itself less risky than variation – inoculation with a small amount of smallpox matter and so-called from the Latin name for smallpox – which aimed to stimulate immunity by subjecting patients to a mild infection experienced in isolation from the general population. Variolation had been discovered in Constantinople (Istanbul) in 1719 by Lady Mary Wortley Montagu (1689-1762). As Savory's testimony suggests, many people, especially those who had experienced or witnessed the effects of smallpox, embraced variolation as the safest form of protection from the disease then available. These early experiments in immunology were, however, risky and a significant number of patients developed a more severe form of the disease and were seriously affected as a result. Nevertheless, official treatment at an inoculating-house, such as the Savorys received, was far safer than having smallpox pus smeared into cuts in the skin by blacksmiths, itinerant clergymen, midwives and even tax collectors which not infrequently occurred earlier in the eighteenth century. Whilst 1/5 to 1/8 of all

---

1. Ford, *Student at St Thomas's*, 10. Weekes's family letters reveal a very similar experience of medical training to Savory's, albeit that he walked the wards at St Thomas's over a decade later. Savory and Weekes shared a similar study timetable, both went to London from rural homes, both made anatomical preparations, attended lectures and midwifery cases, and generally had little time for leisure.

people who contracted smallpox died, only 1/50-1/70 of patients medically inoculated by variolation died.[1] It is also worth bearing in mind that many sufferers of smallpox were blinded or left infertile and all were more or less pock-marked, some of them severely so. Nevertheless, as we shall see in the afterword, Savory would find out the hard way how dangerous variolation could be when he opened his own inoculating-house in Newtown, Hampshire, just across the county border and near to his Newbury practice.

There were plenty of out-and-out amateurs who offered a variety of unofficial and cheaper medical services in Berkshire. Thomas Iremonger, the yeoman farmer at Rowdown Farm, on the border between Brightwalton and Peasemore, for example, was a bone setter, presumably putting some of his amateur veterinary skills to work on his human acquaintances [69]. Another example was John Ventrice (1744-1790), the landlord of the George and Pelican Inn at Speenhamland, who 'used to Cure wounds &c' [116]. The intriguing *et cetera* is expanded on when Savory remarks later, on the occasion of Ventrice's death, 'he used to practice Surgery' [227]. As patrons waited to feel the effects of Ventrice's handiwork, no doubt quaffing his ales or downing something stronger as they did so, they might have looked above the fireplace and read the verse there which Savory records:

Stand aside 'tis every ones desire
As well as you to see and feel the fire. [116]

(vi) Medical apprenticeship
Without doubt the medical man who exerted the greatest professional influence on the young Savory was David Jones (d. 1793), a Welshman who lived in Newbury. Though Jones was nominally a surgeon-apothecary, the main focus of his business seems to have been the selling of medicines. Nevertheless, Savory relates how he met him when 'Dr Jones' visited a Mrs Price in Brightwalton to treat her for breast cancer [68]. On 24 March 1783, when Savory was aged 14, he went to live with Jones and his family in Newbury. On 28 April, following a month's trial, he was bound to him as his apprentice for a period of five years and at a cost of £60 which was met by Uncle John Savory. It has been difficult to discover much about Jones beyond the things Savory tells us. What else can be said is that he married Jenny Hughes (1750-1795) at St Nicholas's Church, Newbury, on 18 September 1780. Jenny was the daughter of Francis and Jane Hughes of Westbrook, Boxford, part of a family of moderately successful yeoman farmers. Savory refers to several of Jenny's siblings: Mary (1747-1791), the wife of Thomas Chittle, who, Savory reveals, died a week after giving birth to her first child which occurred after 18 years of marriage [254];[2] and Sarah (1759-1808), the wife of farmer, Richard Nalder [142]. Savory reveals that Jones's mother died in Wales around June 1784, but no name, place or any further details are provided [71]. David and Jenny Jones

---

1. See D. Baxby, *Jenner's Smallpox Vaccine: The Riddle of Vaccinia Virus and its Origin* (1981), 24.
2. The couple married in Boxford on 27 October 1773; their child, Thomas Chittle (1791-1867) survived and became a chemist.

had five children together: Sarah (1781-1781) David (b. 1782), Jane (b. 1783), Mary (1785-1791) and another Sarah (b. 1786). The family seems to have left Newbury for Boxford some time after Savory's apprenticeship ended, and it was there that both David and his wife died prematurely in 1793 and 1795 respectively, leaving their children reasonably well provided for (as Savory predicts in his horoscope for David Jones Jnr, see [91]). The estate – which included property in East Woodhay – was left in trust to Jenny's brother, John Hughes (d. 1809).[1]

The duties of an apothecary's apprentice – and that is what Savory essentially was – were similar to what we might now term a pharmacist's assistant. Savory's principal task was to mind the shop, especially when his master was away visiting patients or chasing supplies. He was also expected to keep the shop and its wares in good order and condition. He notes in January 1786 that 'this month the Shop and Bottles was new painted by one Powell', something he might well have arranged or supervised [117]. Nevertheless, he candidly admits a misdemeanour five months later when he broke a pane of glass in the shop window while attempting to put up the shutters in windy weather. The Joneses had not noticed the breakage, so he contrived to deflect blame on to an anonymous hooligan. He waited till it was dark, broke the glass a second time (this time deliberately) and ran off, feigning surprise when he returned home, having sneakily 'got rid of Censure from my Mas[te]r or Mrs' by his scheme [121]. Savory was then about 18, and being two-thirds of the way through his apprenticeship he must have been anxious not to upset relations with his master. Besides, glass was expensive and at the very least he might otherwise have expected to pay the punitive cost of replacing the window-pane.

The bulk of his technical training involved learning the properties of different plants, herbs and spices used as ingredients in a wide variety of medicines, and also learning how to derive, measure and mix these medicinal compounds using what is apt to strike us today as the crude and limited range of tools and equipment available. Four months after starting his apprenticeship, Savory helped his master distil peppermint oil. Classified as a carminative herb, peppermint is still widely used as a general aid to digestion. Over the course of three days such little oil came of the process that Savory confides his frustration to his notebook: 'Davids contrivance did not answer well for he had a Wooden head fixt in the great Copper & an Opening in the middle to receive the Still Head & I think this Wooden contrivance must receive a good deal of Oil' [68]. He notes that his master had 'since got a Copper head to fix in the large Copper in the room of the wooden one' though he does not tell us whether it resulted in any improvement [68-69]. In August 1786 the 'Wooden contrivance' was blamed for the repetition of a disappointing yield [123].

One of Jones's suppliers was the successful businessman, JP, and former Mayor of Newbury, Francis Page (1719-1785) of Coldwell House on the Old Bath Road, Speen, from whose gardener Savory bought peppermint, pennyroyal and savin in August 1785 [100]. Among the other plants he ground, decocted or compounded into powders, syrups, oils and so on, were

---

1. RBA D/A1/199/234.

'adderstongue' (the roots and leaves of which were typically used to induce vomiting or to treat skin ulcers) [142]; coltsfoot or coughwort (a yellow herb which acts as a diuretic and was often used in the eighteenth century to treat sore throats) [71]; horehound (an expectorant and laxative), sage (used for dietary purposes, sore throats etc), fumitory (often used for skin and digestive complaints) [71]; and buckthorn berries (a rich source of vitamins, useful in preventing infection, and often used as a purgative in cases of constipation, or as an expectorant in cases of congestion) [123]. A new 84-gallon 'Still Tub' was noted in May 1786, though its impact is not described [119]. Summarising this aspect of his work with Jones, Savory records: 'We used to distill a great many sorts of Herbs for simple Waters & Oil. We made Cordial such as Sp[iri]t Mint &c, Sp[iri]t Wine, Gin mostly from Molasses sometimes from fruit' [154]. The work was not always straightforward, as he reminds us when he complains, in November 1786, that he 'had the Misfortune of burning' his hand 'by mixing together Oil Vitriol and Sp[iri]t Turpentine in a Vial by moving the Vial to Cork it and made as loud report as a Gun' [129]. Dr Jones sold all the standard medicines produced by others, of course, such as 'Grays Salts', grandly described by his landlord Thomas Spanswick (1744-1817) – a lay methodist preacher from Eastbury – as 'the true brown salt of phylosophers' [128].

Savory seems to have successfully navigated the often tricky personal politics of being an apprentice. He had to combine aptitude in his intended profession with a willingness to learn and an ability to fit in with other members of the household, including servants and the children of the family. His geniture for David Jones Jnr, already cited for its comic value, might suggest that Savory felt irritated by the baby and/or toddler. The eighteenth-century home could also be a hazardous place, and especially so at night when there were naked flames from candles to contend with. Savory records that at 2 o'clock on the morning of Saturday, 7 July 1787:

> we was alarmd by fire in Mr Jones Bed Room occasioned by Mary Jones a Child of two Years of Age setting fire to the Bed Curtains with a Rush Light that was then burning in the Room, but fortunately it was prevented from doing any further damage than burning the Bedding &c. in that Room being computed about £10 damage. [143]

The fact that two years after Savory's apprenticeship expired he travelled to Abingdon to bear witness in a case Jones brought against a client, Thomas Hasell, for the non-payment of a bill, hints that Savory's cordial relations with his master endured [230]. That a dispute over a bill dating back more than two years took so long to reach court implies that the wheels of justice ground slow even in this period.

It was also the role of the apprentice to undertake the less skilled, routine work that would simultaneously relieve some of the pressure on the master and provide useful experience for the trainee. In July 1783, a month after turning 15, Savory drew his first tooth [68]. In April 1784 he bled his first patient [71]. In the eighteenth century, such common treatments were generally viewed as uncomplicated. Given how often Savory must have observed his uncle and mother carrying out such procedures at home in Brightwalton, it is unlikely that he felt daunted by assisting Jones in these ways. The first general medical case during his apprenticeship that Savory mentions dated to the start of 1785 and involved Edmund Goatley (1713-1789), a wood dealer from Marlborough, Wiltshire, some 17 miles from Newbury. Presenting with 'a Cancer near his Eye' from which he had suffered for 15 years, and being 'about the bigness of half a Crown', Jones found it to be incurable and the patient later died from the disease [99]. Goatley was exceptionally wealthy and his business included 'two skin or parchment drying houses in the Marsh Ward […] near Cowbridge and the River Kennet'.[1] At the end of the year, one John King, a tanner, presented with a leg wound, but Savory's account suggests that he was more attentive to King's personality than his medical needs: he was 'a very merry Joking man, and could play a great many funny tricks' [102]. Towards the end of his account of his apprenticeship, Savory notes that 'many Boys we cured with dislocated Ancles &c' no doubt incurred in the pursuit of sport and other physical activity [153].

Although Savory seems largely to have enjoyed his apprenticeship under David Jones in Newbury, he leaves no doubt that he saw it as a form of bondage or servitude, and at 19 he was keen to break free. The digest of his diary for 1788 begins, 'I am now got to the Year 1788 to the 20th Year of my Age and near the expiration of my Apprentiship which caused my Spirits to be elevated on the thought of Liberty' [152]. His apprenticeship over, he returned to Brightwalton, and his uncle hosted a dinner to which 'all the farmers and tradesmen' in the village were invited [154]. Afterwards, 'a half pint bumper went round' to these words:

Heres a health to he that is now set free
That once was a 'prentice bound
Now for his sake this holliday we'el [sic] make
So let his health go round. [154]

It was a sign of Savory's independence, professional respectability and rising status that soon afterwards he stood godfather to the first child of Francis Hill, a maltster in Leckhampstead. Nevertheless, he was still young and reveals a capacity to party into the early hours, noting that the christening celebrations continued 'till about 3 o'Clock in the Morning' [155].

(vii) Astrology and witchcraft
During Savory's apprenticeship he amassed a collection of folk remedies that owed more to witchcraft than science, and he also studied astrology. David Jones was not immune to the appeal of occult charms, either. As Savory's apprenticeship drew to an end he noted that he and his master had 'had a great many patients supposed to be under an Ill tongue and used the means laid down for Witchcraft' to cure it (but he does not describe such means) [153]. It is clear

---

1. Document dated 25 March 1775 (private collection): see
   <http://www.durtnall.org.uk/DEEDS/Wiltshire%20201-303.htm> (accessed 17 September 2023).

that many people thought of Jones, and probably his apprentice too, as fortune-tellers or what we might now call psychics: Savory mentions that they 'had a great many come to us to know the event of their future Life, things lost &c' [154].

Whilst fortune-telling might appear to be an extraordinary service for a medical practitioner and his apprentice to offer, it was not uncommon in the eighteenth century to mix magic with medicine, folk remedy with surgical intervention, and to make diagnoses based on astrology as well as sound scientific analysis founded on a knowledge and understanding of anatomy and pathology. Although scholars such as Keith Thomas have argued that supernatural beliefs enjoyed diminishing purchase with the increasing professionalisation of medical knowledge from the eighteenth century onwards, historians such as Jonathan Barry, Charles Phythian-Adams, and James Obelkevich long ago recognised its persistence even into the nineteenth century, especially in rural communities.[1] Precisely because the 1780s was a period of transition, a decade in which hospital pupil-teaching was increasingly preferred over simple apprenticeship as a model for medical education and training, it was also a decade of fluid disciplinary boundaries in which superstitious and vernacular beliefs also informed patient choice and medical practice with albeit diminishing but nevertheless enduring significance.

Savory began his study of astrology in the early years of his apothecary's apprenticeship. At the start of 1784, aged 15, he paid sixpence to attend the weekly astrology lectures given by 'Dr' William Waters 'who lived then in Maryhill by the Star' – probably the Star beer shop on St Mary's Hill in Newbury [70]. He also bought six books on astrology from Waters at a total cost of £1 8s. These were all seventeenth-century works then still in use – books by John Gadbury (1628-1704), William Ramesey or Ramsay (1626/7-1676), William Salmon (1644-1713), Henry Coley (1603-1707), and George Wharton (1617-1681). Gadbury's *Genethlialogia, or The Doctrine of Nativities Together with The Doctrine of Horarie Questions* (1658), the most expensive book at 8s, came 'with Waters Improvements', indicating that Savory's tutor had annotated or supplemented the text [70]. Savory's partiality for astrology was no passing adolescent fad. When Waters's wife died on 20 April 1786, Savory notes that he gave the widower 10/6 for a book by the eminent barber-surgeon in the sixteenth-century French court, Ambrose Parcy (Ambroise Paré) (c.1510-1590), whose works were translated into English in the seventeenth century and were still in use in England in the eighteenth, and a 'Book of [Waters's] own hand writing containing Receits for diseases &c' [118]. Whilst Savory judges that 'this Wm Waters was very well versd in Astrology & casting Urine' [i.e. for the purpose of urimancy], he confides that 'he left Newbury about this time and went to live at Reading where he soon paid the last debt of Nature. he was very much addicted to drinking & Women which was his utter ruin' [118]. So here we have a third private tutor engaged

---

1. See K. Thomas, *Religion and the Decline of Magic* (New York, 1981), J. Barry, 'Piety and the Patient' in R. Porter (ed.), *Patients and Practitioners* (Cambridge, 1986), 145-176, C. Phythian-Adams, 'Rural Culture' in G. E. Mingay (ed.), *The Victorian Countryside* (1981) 616-625, and J. Obelkevich, *Religion and Rural Society: South Lindsey, 1825-1875* (Oxford, 1976).

by Savory whose moral standards and personal behaviour seem to have fallen short of Savory's expectations. Among 'all the Charms' Savory had 'collected from Dr Waters and others' were examples of witchcraft and folk remedies for toothache, ague, warts, the 'Falling Evil', unwanted spirits and thieves: there are 15 pages of such material (page numbers 168 and 169 are used twice) [159-171]. Earlier in the volume Savory reproduces magic spells relayed to him by David Jones: 'To buy a Spirit' and 'To appear Invisible' [115-116], and there are also the 'mixt medlies', towards the end of the volume, among which are details of different methods of divining mortality and criminality, forecasting travel experiences, curing swellings, sores and warts and ridding horses of bot infestations [216-226]. The meticulous recording of such material indicates the value Savory placed in it. Yet he also alleges that the elderly Dame Harding of Shaw, who frequently visited David Jones's shop in Newbury, 'was computed a Witch. used to tell fortunes by Tea Leaves &c', an intriguing point to make for a man so evidently fascinated by witchcraft himself, perhaps suggesting a hint of snobbishness and misogyny [121].

Savory also purchased works on the occult sciences such as those written by [Henricus] Cornelius Agrippa of Nettesheim (1486-1535), which he bought in London in July 1785 [100]. His sister, Sarah, sent him Agrippa's '4th Book' in April 1786 [119]. When Savory picked up those first three books of Agrippa's, he adds that he also bought 'some Old Ephemeris & Surgeons instruments' [100]. The juxtaposition of such different items reaffirms the notion that for Savory, as for many of his contemporaries and not all of them youths like himself, there was little if any tension between science and the vernacular arts, the medical and the occult: they were complementary rather than contradictory. Savory would have used the ephemeris, which provided tables of dates charting the trajectory of astronomical objects, in order to draw up the horoscopes that feature in the volume. He provides 11 genitures for relatives, friends, King George III and the Prince of Wales, all but one clearly indexed for quick reference [267b]. Savory's preference for the geniture as a form of horoscope is in line with the seventeenth-century astrological texts he studied. He drew on the judicial astrology of forecasting the lives of individuals.

Genitures and nativities were horary, answering questions based on the position of the planets and stars in relation to an individual's time and place of birth. Whether Savory often in fact knew such precise details is doubtful, but he seems to have persuaded himself that he had sufficiently dependable information for his calculations to be worthwhile. Although he almost certainly relied in large part on printed tables to derive his data, the mathematics involved were

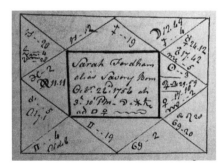

2. Savory's geniture chart for his sister, Sarah Fordham: a typical example of his preferred form of horoscope [76].

nevertheless relatively complex. If nothing else, the mental exercise must have been beneficial as his mind developed in his teenage years.

William Waters was not Savory's only teacher of astrology. In October 1784 Savory recalls that he became acquainted with Jeremiah Grant, a young clockmaker who had lived in Abingdon, but who, since his marriage in June of that year, had settled in Speen [71-72]. Savory describes him as 'very injenious. he gave me great instructions in Astrology. he was Lame & was obliged to wear an Iron to support his Leg' [72]. He then reproduces an elaborately flattering, even hyperbolic letter, addressed 'Fidelis' and signed 'Jemy Grant', which expresses a striking depth of friendly faith and feeling [72-75]. Grant evidently meant a lot to Savory. All but four of Savory's genitures follow Grant's letter [76-98]. Savory remarks of Grant beforehand, however: 'He left Newbury soon after he wrote this Letter which gave me great uneasiness for the loss of so sincere a Friend. as at this time I was very fond of studying Astrology' [75]. Grant was certainly Savory's most agreeable tutor.

Another letter to Savory is yet more noteworthy because it came from the celebrated medic and astrologer, Ebenezer Sibly (1751-1799) [134-135]. Savory had evidently written to him to ask about the relative positions of the planets and stars on the day of his birth, 28 June 1768, data which Sibly duly supplied. Presumably Savory intended to cast his own geniture horoscope, though it is perhaps telling that he does not confide it to his MS volume. He does, however, reproduce the letter among the second, smaller clutch of genitures with which he concludes his diary for 1786 [130-33, 136-8]. Sibly wrote, 'Thus Sir as you are a lover of Science I have complied with your Request. wishing you all the success as possible to be desired from being a Son of the divine Urania & remain your friend' and it is signed 'E. Sibley' [sic] [134-135]. Sibly was a physician with an MD from King's College, Aberdeen who, in the words of the scholar Patrick Curry, 'fervently believed that modern scientific knowledge, while valuable, needed to be supplemented by the vitalism of and spirituality of the natural magic tradition'.[1] Knowledge of the mystical and occult was as important to Sibly as the latest scientific and medical learning. His writings about astrology also provided a substantial income. In a post-script to his letter to Savory Sibly added, with a commercial flourish, 'If you want any Ephemeris you may have them by directing the parcell with Money to me No. 39 Castle Street Bristol [:] the price of them is 1/- each', an indication that although he had answered Savory's initial enquiry for gratis, he would expect payment in future [135].

Yet, despite Savory's apparent faith in astrology and witchcraft, he was more than content to exploit and subvert popular superstition in order to find a real-life thief, as he did in the case of the farm-servants at Brightwalton Manor in 1788 (see below). Likewise, when he planted some nightshade in June 1790 he confides that 'Pryar of Steventon', from whom he had obtained it, 'sais its good for Witchcraft given in powder or any other form', and quickly adds, 'but he could not cure his Wife with it' (though he does not say what he might have cured her of), nevertheless reporting that 'he also sais the Urine of a person that is afflicted with Witchcraft will bubble in a Glass' [231]. The fact that

---

1. P. Curry, *Prophecy and Power. Astrology in Early Modern England* (Oxford, 1989), 135.

Savory was also able to laugh at such a burlesque on quackery as the 'Pharmacopola Circumforaneus' (about a horse-doctor hawking his fake medicines across the streets of the globe), which he quotes at length, suggests that his feet were in fact planted firmly on the ground and that he viewed his own vernacular interests with a sense of good humour [239-245]. Among the funniest boasts of the fictional mountebank is his claim that he possessed a cure for 'the Venereal Disease with all its train of Gonnorrheas [sic], Buboes & Shankers, Phymosis, [and] Paraphymosis' which could be taken

> with as much pleasure as the same was contracted so that its worth any persons while to get into that modest distemper once a fortnight if it be to be had for Love or Money to enjoy the benefit of so diverting a Remedy. [243]

Savory's authentic medical knowledge contrasted starkly with such charlatanism, of course, but there is more than a hint of humility evident in quoting such material, and it is suggestive of a young man determined not to take himself too seriously.

(viii) Women and sexual politics

Savory's MS provides insights into various aspects of the role and status of women in Berkshire in the late eighteenth century. We have already seen how his mother and Mrs Sampson were able to provide some basic medical services, but they only achieved recognition as widows who had previously assisted their husbands. Savory writes, 'My Mother practices Blood letting & dressing Wounds & sells medicines &c same as when my father was living' [32]. We have also seen how Dame Harding, who told fortunes by reading tea-leaves, was considered a witch, but no such slur seems to have attached to men who did much the same thing.

We have seen, too, how Savory's sisters, Jane and Mary, were taught mathematics, apparently in the same formal setting as Savory himself: Joseph Aldridge's Brightwalton schoolroom. Savory, who blamed Mary's 'contrary disposition' for the fact that they 'could never agree' and did not get on, claims that, as a consequence of her attitude and behaviour, 'Grandfather was at the unnessesary expense of putting her to Miss Thompsons Boarding School at Wantage for a twelve month' [43]. Whether Savory would have used such terms for a brother in a similar situation is doubtful. In 1778 *Jackson's Oxford Journal* published an advert notifying readers that

> Miss Thompson begs Leave to acquaint the Public, That, for the better Accommodation of the Pupils, she has removed her School to a large commodious House in Wantage, Berks, which belonged to the late Mr Towsey, senior, Apothecary; where Young LADIES are genteelly boarded, and carefully instructed in the English Tongue, Writing, Arithmetic, Musick, Dancing, Tambour, and every Branch of Needle-Work, the Art of Painting on Silk, and many other useful and ornamental Accomplishments, on the following Terms, viz. – Board, English, and Needle-Work, Eleven Guineas per Annum, and One Guinea Entrance; Writing and Arithmetic, 5s.

6d. per Quarter; Musick 10s. 6d. per Quarter, and 10s. 6d. Entrance; Dancing, ditto; Painting on silk, (including Colours and Pencils), 7s. 6d. per Quarter. – No Entrance-Money is expected with Ladies who have been at other Boarding-Schools. N.B. The House has a handsome Garden and Outlet. – Mr Wheeler continues his Attendance, as usual.[1]

An 'unnessesary expense' clearly hints at Savory's sense of the limits of male generosity when investing in the education of girls, particularly troublesome ones. How far such schooling might be taken to indicate an enlightened or liberal attitude in the 1770s is difficult to assess because the education of girls, as of boys, was intimately bound up with social class, societal expectation and personal or familial aspiration. But it appears that Grandfather Savory, who was born in 1696, and his younger son, John, born in 1727, both of them wheelwrights, believed or were persuaded that it was worth paying people outside the household circle to educate and train the girls of the family as well as the boy, albeit that much of that education and training for girls was directed towards the acquisition of what were considered decidedly feminine accomplishments. Of Savory's sister, Jane, who lived at home until her marriage and whose 'good easy disposition' he praised and contrasted with Mary's, he tells us, 'My Uncle Apprenticed her to Mrs Bird to learn the Art of Mantua Making' [42], that is the making of the loose gown then routinely worn by women. Mrs Bird was paid three guineas for a year's training at her home at Ballard's Farm. Such work pushed no gender or class boundaries, and Jane's training might well have owed more to the need of a fatherless family to bring in some extra income than anything else. It was also no doubt motivated in part by the notion that an accomplished woman was more marriageable.

Savory writes very little about his mother, Jane, which no doubt reflects the extent to which he took her for granted. Nevertheless, early in 1789 when he was courting the woman he would marry, he told her that as she was a member of 'the softer part of the Creation' and 'out of respect to she that brought me forth into the World, and has discharged the duty of a parent by me', he 'would wish to shew' – as he puts it, 'all females' – 'all the respect and lend them all the asistance in my power when wanted' [202]. Thus he makes his case for the pureness of his heart. the rectitude of his intentions, and his sincerity [201-202]. He has nothing to say in the MS of his mother's physical appearance or character, but he does give us a few facts about her. Predictably, the dowry gets a mention, 'My father had near £300 fortune with my Mother' [20]. In a lengthy section on his mother's family background, which focuses mostly on male relatives, he tells us that she was born in Fawley [35]. In October 1781 she 'was Inoculated three or four times with the SmallPox but to no effect' [55]. He does say something of his step-grandmother's character, but he did not know her, so he was not imparting his own assessment. She is described as 'a very good living Woman' and Savory quotes the verse on her gravestone praising her (feminine) qualities of peace and composure, her virtue as a wife, faith as a friend, and tenderness as a nurse and mother [7-8].

---

1. *OJ* (12 December 1778).

When Savory describes his visit to Newgate, where he saw some men and a woman hanged opposite the prison after being convicted of treason, he comments that 'the Woman received her reward in this life opposite the 7 men & was afterwards burnt' [197]. He makes no further comment and it is a matter of speculation what he might have thought of the woman's exceptional treatment: enough to make note of it, but not enough to comment on it; moreover, the presumably ironical use of the word 'reward' is ambiguous. Was it applied because she was a woman, because she was treated differently to the men, because her treatment was particularly brutal, or any combination of these reasons, for another reason, or for no reason in particular?[1]

Modern readers of several of the verses Savory quotes – all of them songs or poems of doubtful literary merit, but apparently considered entertaining when sung or recited – are likely to be struck by their misogynistic tropes. First, the cliché of the nagging wife: the jolly blade whose wife is a dumb country maid comes to regret his efforts to set her tongue at liberty, making an ungovernable scold of her in the process [23-25]. It is a variation on the traditional, anonymous ballad, 'The Dumb Maid', dating from the late 1670s. 'Hymens Commission' is a paean to the domestic goddess: the male narrator seeks aid in choosing a 'harmless maid' to be his 'tender Wife'; 'strife' would come in the form of pride and a 'Clamorous Voice', whereas bliss consists in a good temper and a kind nature [62]. But she should also look nice, dress well, behave gracefully, and be adept at cooking, sewing and household economy. She should be healthy and happy, but: 'Let her delight at home be found/ In me and Children tatling [sic] round', though this is described as an 'uncommon comfort' [63]. She should not be envious, and she should refrain from tea and brandy which are considered foreign and are therefore implicitly condemned as objectionable, and she must enter the marriage with sufficient dowry. She should be of good lineage for the children's sake, she should be Christian, and she should be aged between 21 and 30 so that there would not be too many costly children draining the husband-father's hard-earned income (the obligation to provide being the only duty expected of him – and even that is merely implied). Then there is the saucily suggestive story about the melancholy young woman who complains to her mother, 'my husband won[']t give me time to say my prayers', presumably code for the sexual demands made on her, though her mother's reaction suggests that she should be grateful it was nothing worse [15].

Savory's personal comments about various women are also revealing. When he ruined Mrs Trulock's white shoes by getting the chaise stuck after taking the wrong road, he takes it as an opportunity to criticise her as 'a proud, Conceited, fancifull Queen [...] noticed by every one but respected by none' [101]. He then records a bawdy song about 'this Old Ewe' in which, by way of a mixed metaphor, she is pictured as an 'old Cow' [103, 104]. Whilst her caution about entering into marriage might be construed as amusing, she is nevertheless empowered, telling the 'Old Bull' pursuing her (one Messetter of Thatcham): 'you shall never familiarly feel / Until with a Lawyer you sign & do seal', an insistence on what today we would call some kind of prenuptial

---

1. For the details of the case he describes, see below.

agreement by which he was bound 'Ne'er to kiss nor to ride any other' [104, 105]. Consenting to this, he quickly 'Quenched his Amorous fire' only to be unfaithful, and although the wronged woman vows revenge, she is dissuaded from pursuing the matter when he blackmails her with the stinging accusation, 'I can prove you are not fit for my Bed / Disabled you are in your Tail not your head' [105]. It is implied that the 'old cow' deserves the stalemate that thereby ensues, and the old bull gets away with his sexual infidelity as a result. The fact that all of this is rendered comically entertaining in rhyming couplets implies generalised criticism of such behaviour, but the social and sexual norms they reflect were overwhelmingly accepted and often endorsed by the men who dominated public discourse and the institutions.

Whether Savory composed the announcement in the *Reading Mercury* of the marriage between William Steptoe, aged about 30, and Mrs Horn, aged 79, is not clear, but his delight in the ironical intimation that so unusual a union of people of such divergent ages had come about 'after a long and tedious Courtship of 14 days' is plain [57]. Savory was certainly responsible for making up the names of Mary Coxhead's parents when he sent the announcement of her marriage to the newspaper in 1786, causing offence in the process. He bluntly dismisses the bride as 'a very disagreeable Woman both in her personal & mental accomplishments' [121]. As was the case with his reaction to Mrs Trulock, where he was also guilty of personal error, he seems a little too willing to blame the innocent woman, and too reluctant to own his mistakes.

Savory details a variety of medical cases involving women: a young woman 'burnt all over as black as a Coal', a woman of 18 in great pain with a cancerous uterus, and a 'a Girl of 12 Years of Age […] under Mr Birch with the Venereal disease contracted from a Young Chimney Sweep' [188-189]. He tells us that the first midwifery case he attended was a 'Natural Labour' at Redriff, and records that he paid the mother 2/6, presumably for affording him valuable experience as a trainee midwife [192-193]. On 2 February 1789 he attended the nine-hour labour of a young, first-time mother and makes the comment: 'they were Irish people and I delivered her kneeling which is their Country way. they told me 'twas always customary with them to give the Child Rue or Black Cherry Water and not to give them the breast till 3 or 4 days after they are born' [193]. Without doubt the most upsetting entry in the entire volume involves the apparently casual use of a shocking simile to describe a foetus discovered in the womb a month after its death [194]. If this is evidence of a lack of sensitivity, it might also be a symptom of the emotional detachment widely accepted as necessary for anyone in Savory's profession.

Most of the women workers Savory mentions were servants. When he set up his own household on Bartholomew Street, Newbury, he notes that on 11 July 1791, 'I hired Leah Pointer at the Rate of 3½ Guineas pr Year but she was not fit for my service therefore staied but a few Weeks & her sister Martha came in her room' [255]. He then points out that 'they are daughters of Thos Pointer of Leckhamstead Egypt', whose home, he had told us earlier, was two miles and 20 poles from the corner of the stable at Brightwalton Manor Farm [229]. Leah Pointer, who was not yet 17 when Savory appointed her, was passed over in favour of her older sister, Martha, who was 23 and in fact older than Savory himself, and the connection between the two families was thus maintained.

During his courtship of Mary Tyrrell, the woman with whom he would spend the rest of his life, he told her in a Valentine's letter in 1789 that he had 'seen so much of the agreeable Companion shine' in her 'behaviour and Conversation' [200]. He followed this with a declaration that came close to a proposal in its echo of the marriage vows:

> dear Miss please to beleive I never felt the power of female attraction till I saw you, as the perfections of your mind are such as can never fail to please; even in sickness or in Age, when Youth and beauty is no more. [202]

Making the solemn pledge that 'the rest of my Life shall be devoted to make you happy' he signs off by calling himself her 'Affectionate Friend and Admirer till Death' [203].

(ix) Leisure

Aside from the arguable exceptions of the special studies Savory engaged in – engraving, etching, French, astrology and probably calligraphy – and the reading and writing they entailed, there is little in the MS recognisable to us today as a pastime or hobby. Nevertheless, some observations may be made. He liked to note tombstone inscriptions, for instance [7-8, 47, 119, 140-141], and he also records an amusing verse inscribed in a young lady's prayer book [145]. Measuring distances was one of his and his father's enthusiasms, as was (church) music, as we shall see. Savory's transcription of folk charms and remedies perhaps suggests a general partiality for collecting.

Savory's paternal uncle, he tells us, 'was very fond of Card playing' and presumably that involved some gambling, too [30]. Savory himself entered a raffle which won him 'a curious piece of Shell Work' in February 1786 [117]. Gambling was certainly central to the only phenomenon referred to in the MS as 'sport', namely cockfighting: Savory confides that David Jones, his 'Master at that time [*January 1785*] was very fond of Cockfighting[.] he won 2 Guineas which inclined him to follow that sport some time but at last he grew tired by reason of bad Luck' [99].[1] Even some contemporary sources referred to cockfighting as a 'cruel pastime', though Savory gives no indication that he shared in this assessment.[2] For his own part, Savory seems to have been partial to lotteries. He reports how, when he was in London, he went to 'Guild Hall to see the drawing of the Lottery ticketts' [199]. He explains that 'there are two Wheels one on each side of Guild Hall[,] one containing the Ticketts the other Blanks & prises. the Blue Coated Boys change every hour. they have one Arm tyed behind them' [199]. Prizes of £10,000 and even £20,000 in the lottery were not uncommon. Encouraged by the Government, the lottery was phenomenally popular, with 49,000 tickets sold in one state lottery alone in 1779. If not at Guildhall, tickets were drawn at one of the livery companies' halls in the City. The lottery commissioners and their president generally sat

---

1. For a reference to fox-hunting, see below.
2. *Bath Chronicle and Weekly Gazette* (7 May 1789).

on the platform to oversee the draw. Tickets were picked from two large boxes by two boys from Christ's Hospital, the first of the blue-coated schools, just as Savory describes. Rosamond Bayne-Powell has explained, 'One boy on one side thrust his bare arm into the box and drew out a number, and the boy opposite him produced a prize ticket or a blank. The body of the hall was filled with an excited mob.'[1] However, the lotteries attracted criminals and corruption and were declared illegal in 1826.

Savory had noted a little earlier in his MS that he and his sister, Sarah, 'tryd our Luck in the Lottery but proved all Blanks' [197]. Nevertheless, he confides, 'Khuns who kept the flying Horse [inn] before my Sister had half the £30-000 prise in the Lottery (viz) £15-000 amongst some poor German Sugar Bakers, about £700 each' [197]. In fact, it was reported in the press at the end of March 1789 that the £30,000 prize was paid out in shares and that half the ticket was divided among 'a club held at the Flying-horse' and that what was known of the other half was divided 1/4 to a Miss Noble, of Holborn, 1/16 to 'the dyer of the Prince's Patent Union', another 1/16 to 'two servants at Islington', and 1/8 'to a person as yet unknown'.[2]

Although Savory writes that 'during my time in London I was never at leisure', it was during his intensive months of medical study in the capital in 1788-1789 that he makes note of his most interesting excursions [204]. He recalls that on Easter Monday (13 April) 1789, for example, he 'went with three or four of my Acquaintances to Greenwich fair', though he supplies no details of what they did or what they thought of it [177]. Greenwich Fair in fact took place on *Whit* Monday, and was an extremely popular and notoriously riotous occasion. Dickens's account of it in *Sketches By Boz* (1836) is particularly evocative.

Savory describes other days out. Between 11 and 15 September 1781, then aged 13, he made his first visit to London [53]. He accompanied his paternal grandfather, who turned 85 the following month. Savory lists all the towns they passed through on the way, and tells us that on arrival they went to 'St Pauls, the Tower, Westminster Abby &c' [54]. His grandfather would go to London for a week every year and usually stayed at the Black Lion on Water Lane, off Fleet Street, towards White Friars Dock [10]. Savory's paternal uncle was in London from 4 to 17 January 1787, though the purpose of the visit is not disclosed [139]. Savory mentions visiting London on 23 July 1785, when he bought books on astrology and surgeon's instruments [101], and on 22 May and 10 July 1791, though arguably these were business trips rather than excursions or holidays [252, 254]. Savory also records a visit to Oxford at the end of June 1780, around the time of his 12th birthday, when he was accompanied by James Norris, Miss Sheppard, Miss Tyrrell and Mary Tyrrell, the last of whom he later married: 'we went to most of the Colleges' he boldly claims, and 'went to the printing Office and had our Names printed and gave them 6d each. I stood upon the Clapper of Great Tom & saw the two old Eagles' [50]. Savory means Old Tom, the bell in Tom Tower, the imposing gateway to Christ Church College, Oxford, designed by Wren and built in 1681-1682. The

1. R. Bayne-Powell, *Eighteenth-Century London Life* (1938), 189.
2. *Saunders's News-Letter* (25 March 1789).

bell is still struck 101 times every evening at five past nine to recall the traditional closure of the gates to the original 101 scholars of the college. The printing office was presumably that of Oxford University Press, then in the Clarendon Building on Broad Street. They must have had a long day if they really visited all the colleges.

Apart from the fact that Savory lodged with his sister at the Flying Horse, he seems to have had more than a passing interest in public houses. In October 1786, when the 18-year-old accompanied his paternal uncle to London to prove his grandfather's will, he notes that 'my curiosity led me to Number the public Houses that we passd by from Speenhamland to Hide Park Corner', a journey of 56 miles undertaken on the Newbury Coach; he counted 222 [124-125]. He mentions several pubs in his MS: an alehouse in Wickham, Welford [5]; the Marquis of Granby at Brightwalton, run by his step-grandmother's nephew, Thomas Taylor (c. 1731-1813) [6, 71, 129, 230]; the Black Lion on Water Lane, in London [10]; a pub in Baydon, Wiltshire [46]; the Blue Boar at North Heath [46]; the Chequers at Newbury [69]; the Three Tuns at Thatcham [101]; the Monument at Newbury [152]; the George and Pelican at Speenhamland [116, 157], and the Old Inn (later the Fox and Cubs) at Lilley [230, 251]. Whilst he only tells us definitely that he visited the last two, it is almost certain that he patronised the Granby.

Savory has very little of a specific nature to say about food and drink. He refers to breakfast four times [34. 58, 172, 204], does not mention lunch at all, and dinner is alluded to twice [154, 205]. When he was studying in London he would have his breakfast at 9am after one-and-a-half hours' work, and he 'used to get a good appetite' for his dinner around 3pm [204, 205]. Tea – the hot beverage – is mentioned three times, the first two in verse, and the last in relation to reading fortunes in tea-leaves [34, 63, 121]. Coffee is mentioned only once, in one of the verses which also mentions tea – some simple lines about breakfast written by Savory's sister Jane, and uncle John, which also states 'Uncle had Cake and Spirrit / And I had Bread & Butter' [34]. Bread is most frequently mentioned in Biblical and charitable allusions, and we have already noted the 'discovery' by Savory's grandfather of potatoes in a London market in the early eighteenth century. Savory also notes that his paternal uncle remembered cherries being sold in London for a farthing per pound in the late 1730s [30], and hints at rapid inflation in the price of wheat in the fourteenth century [61]. Beer is mentioned only a few times [4, 149, 154], and ale only once [69], whilst two references to the consumption of liquor allege intoxication [215, 252]. In writing his MS in 1791, Savory decried the passing of the good old days, lamenting the fact that every 'Labouring person had good Victuals & a Barrell of good Beer' in the past 'but now they thinks themselves well off if they can get Bread & Small Beer' [4].

(x) Music and dance

Music, though not dance, features so prominently in Savory's MS that it would merit a sub-section of its own, but the topics belong together. For Savory, music was more than a leisure interest or pastime. Rather, it was a fundamental aspect of his church-going experience.

To start with dancing, however, Savory records that his Uncle John 'was very fond of [...] Dancing &c': 'him with more of his Companions went to Morris Dancing, and ornamented themselves with Snail Shells instead of Bells' [30-31]. According to scholars such as Jameson Wooders and Michael Heaney, the use of snail shells was innovative, and Savory's MS is one of the few sources to suggest that Morris dancing took place in Berkshire in the eighteenth century.[1] Furthermore, Savory tells us, the Morris dancers' 'squire' was Robert Brown, 'who lived at a little Cottage House in the Way to farmbro' & Occupied his own land since dead' and the group's 'Musitioner' (musician) was Betty 'the Wife of Stephen Taylor now living at Brightwaltham' [31]. Wooders and Heaney point out that the inclusion in the group of a yeoman, a wheelwright and a female musician is also understood to be uncommon, and Heaney speculates that it 'suggests, perhaps, a middle- class representation that may have had a hint of self-parody about it'.[2]

Above all, it is music that resounds as one of the Savory family's key passions. Savory shared with his father a love of music: the father was 'excellent in Music' – nobody could 'excell him' in 'singing Songs & Catches' (he even composed songs, see [21-22]) – and he played the bass viol in church [19]. Dr Cooper Sampson, a particular friend of Savory's father, was described as 'a good Songster' [48]. Grandfather Savory also used to sign songs [10]. Moreover, Savory notes that though his Morris-dancing paternal uncle 'would play on no instruments' he nevertheless used 'to sing Songs & Healths very frequently in Company' [32]. Uncle John also sang in the church choir for at least 40 years ('the Bass part') [215, 31]. We are told that he bought a flute for a guinea on 12 November 1781 [55]. Its former owner, Avery Hobbs of East Hendred, had been compelled to give up the instrument after having his finger amputated following a severe cut – so he took up the violin instead. The flute was bought for Savory, who started to learn how to play it, but gave it up, at any rate temporarily, in favour of the bassoon which cost four guineas plus five shillings for the reeds and box [55]. In January 1786 he had his flute stolen from him by his tutor in etching and engraving [117], but on 2 October he bought a new one in London for £2 12s 6d [125]. On 6 January 1790 Uncle John made another purchase from Hobbs – this time a spinet costing 2½ guineas [227]. The spinet, a keyed instrument closely resembling the harpsichord, but smaller and having only one string to each note, was common in England in the eighteenth century. It was one of the instruments of the age. Given that Savory claims his uncle played on no instrument himself, we might assume that Savory was the player, as he was in the case of the flute.

Brightwalton appears to have been unusual in the variety of musical instruments played in church by the congregants, or perhaps it is simply that few parishes were as fortunate as Brightwalton in having such activity so meticulously chronicled. Churchwardens' accounts, if they allude to music at all, tend to focus on the cost of reeds and strings, the commission and repair of

---

1. See J. Wooders, '"With Snail Shells Instead of Bells": Music, Morris Dancing, and the "Middling Sort" of People in Eighteenth-Century Berkshire' in *Folk Music Journal* x:5 (2015) 550–574, and M. Heaney, *The Ancient English Morris Dance* (2023).
2. Heaney, *Morris Dance*, 374.

bells, and payments made to singers. On 31 March 1755 a petition was advanced 'For the better performance of Church Music in the parish Church of Brightwalton' and Savory copied it out from the notebook kept by his father, who led the campaign [25]. It stated that 'the Singers are very desirous of having a Bass Vial (or some instrument) for the use and ease of the Choir' [25-26]. Savory records that a subscription of £2 10s 4d was raised [26]. The bass viol cost three guineas, but as Savory's father, still single at this point, was the one who played upon the instrument in church, he contributed the rest of the funds and eventually replaced it, keeping the subscription viol which John Savory later sold [29]. In April 1791, when Savory registers the burial of John Pratt of South Moreton, he records that he also 'used to play the Bass Vial' [247].

Savory writes that in 1780, the year in which he turned 12, he 'began playing on the tenor Vial at Church and Joseph Norris the Bass Vial and one Jo. Fisher [...] playd the Hoboy' (the oboe) [49]. In her unpublished doctoral thesis, 'The Performance of English Provincial Psalmody c.1690-c.1840', the historian of church music, Sally Drage, speculated that by 'bass vial' Savory meant a violoncello and by 'tenor vial' he was referring to a viola, an uncommon if not unknown instrument in the eighteenth-century church.[1] Around 1782, Savory had mastered the bassoon sufficiently well to play it in church [55]. He evidently kept at it, noting how, during the year 1790, he 'playd the Bassoon at Brightwalton Church & never doubled one Tune & Psalm except the 55th Anthem which was when I was not there' [234]. The last observation is confusing, but presumably he meant that only one tune was doubled in the church that year, and on an occasion when the bassoon was played by someone else or not at all. He then sets out in tabular form the tunes, psalms and anthems played [235]. He also played several anthems on the bassoon at Fawley Church in July 1790, just after his 22nd birthday. On that occasion he met the 'Letcomb Singers', presumably an established group, possibly of promenading musicians, which was something more than a standard parish choir [232]. The following month he played the bassoon and met the Letcombe singers again, this time at Farnborough Church [232]. This suggests that, at least in the summer months, there was a certain amount of co-operation among neighbouring parishes to bring music to different congregations.

Most parish churches had a choir and a dedicated company of bellringers in this period. In Brightwalton, Savory was a member of both from youth. He reveals that he 'learnt to Ring at Church' four or five years before he moved to Newbury, which points to 1778 or 1779 when he was 10 or 11 years old [58]. He explains that he

> used to go with the Ringers at Christmas round the Village. we used to ring two or three peals and go to Mr Harbert [*at the Manor Farm*] to Breakfast and stay till 11 or 12 o'Clock [,] from there to Stanbrooks, Holmes, Whiters, Mrs Taylors [*presumably, the Morris dancers' musician*] & spent

---

1 S. Drage, 'The Performance of English Provincial Psalmody c.1690-c.1840', unpublished doctoral thesis, University of Leeds (2009), 164, 166.

the Eve[nin]g at my Uncles. and to Blackneys, Trumplets, South End, Birds, Mitchels &c., the following Evenings. We used to go to Comb on New Years day. the Rector gives a Crown every Christmas. on Christmas Eve we have a fire in one Corner of the Bellfree and Rang almost <all> Night. Sheepshears and Harvest homes was very much in fashion[,] particularly at Blackneys, Churchs, Horns &c. Healths [*illegible deleted word*] <were> very much used as mums [*i.e. a masked festival*]. [58-59]

These last two sentences are not easy to interpret, but the context suggests that the bellringers were in demand during the key festivals typically associated with important moments in the agricultural and church calendars. Tradition was broken at Christmas 1788, however, when John Savory gave the ringers 2/6 'instead of entertaining them at his own house' [215]. John Holmes (1729-1798), a tailor nearly 60 years old who had been a tenor in the choir with John Savory for 40 years, used to ring the peals of the psalms. He was so offended by John Savory's unwelcome innovation that 'he left the Gallery' and, 'being in the heat of Liquor', he swore 'many Oaths' and vowed never to sing in church again.

As well as ringing the bells during festivals, the group also rang them for weddings [49, 55, 57, 142, 233, 238]. Sometimes the bells seem to have been rung at Brightwalton even when a resident's wedding took place in a neighbouring parish, such as in December 1780 when Thomas Horne, a farmer in Brightwalton, married Elizabeth Nelson in Chaddleworth [49]. On another occasion, at the wedding of William Butler and Anne Cooper, in February 1790, Savory notes that 'the Bells was rung backwards' though he does not reveal why or say whether it was deliberate [238]. According to Savory the money received by the ringers ranged from 2/6 in 1790 [233] to two guineas when the marriage of Brightwalton's Rector, Richard Boucher (1752-1851), was pealed two days after his wedding in Tottenham [142]. As the amount of money received by the ringers was typically between three and five shillings, it seems likely that it constituted a voluntary donation rather than a fee, though it is probable that some contribution was expected.

(xi) Religion

Life in Brightwalton inevitably revolved around the parish church, especially for the village's majority Anglican community. The stream of christenings, weddings and funerals noted by Savory testify to that, but he reveals nothing about regular Sunday services except for the allusions to music we have already discussed. He gives the sense of the changes a new Rector could bring. Soon after his arrival Rev. Boucher cut down a 'pretty' 60-year-old yew tree near the Savory family graves towards the south wall of the churchyard, and removed other trees in the garden of what Savory calls the parsonage as well as four chestnuts trees opposite the house; the Commandments written near the gallery on the north side of the church were moved to the chancel and in their place were written verses 'taken out of the Colossians Respecting Wives & Husbands behaviour to each other' [51]. Savory seldom quotes from the Bible himself, but he does copy out the passages relating to music quoted by his father in his petition to the church in 1755 [26-28]. Savory also transcribes in full a rendering of the Lord's Prayer in verse which was among 'verses [...] sent to my father' [59] and must therefore date to 1772 or earlier, but it is of uncertain provenance [59-61]. A fragment of the Lord's Prayer in Old English is also evident at the end of a missing section of text [115], and the satire of Prime Minister Pitt the Younger is modelled on the Parable of the Rich Man and Lazarus [106-110]. Additionally, Savory includes, towards the end of the MS volume, a brief and incomplete account of the Archbishops of Canterbury [263-266]. On a personal note, he records his confirmation on 22 July 1783 by the Bishop of Salisbury, Shute Barrington (1734-1826), at a service which presumably took place at St Nicholas's Church, Newbury [69]. The sermon, Savory tells us, was preached by Brackley Kennett (1741-1795), the Rector of East or Market Ilsley.

Savory seems to have been broad-minded in his approach to nonconformism and religion generally. He hints at the more zealous attitudes of others when he writes of his brother-in-law, John Eagles, that 'since he has been Married to my Sister he is got very religious and now frequents the Methodist Meetings &[c]' [83]. In 1789, referring to a britches maker by the name of Jones, he notes that he was a lay methodist preacher with a crooked leg, adding that he was 'a very false Lying fellow &c', perhaps suggesting that he felt little sympathy for methodists, though probably indicating a specific antipathy towards Jones [119]. He also notes that David Jones's landlord, Thomas Spanswick, was a methodist preacher [129].[1] His description of the London Hospital in Whitechapel emphasises the extent of the financial contribution it received from members of the Society of Friends (the Quakers) and the impact of diminished funds when they withheld subscriptions after their preferred candidate for physician (Savory wrongly says surgeon) was not elected and, as Savory puts it, 'the Aminadabs were offended' [191]. The use of this pejorative term indicates some degree of prejudice, or at least ignorance, but Savory's implied frustration about the perceived dangers of vested interests to medical care arguably stands in mitigation, if not justification, of his attitude.

Savory recounts how, when he was training as a medic in London in 1789, he visited a 'Romish meeting in Holborn'. He writes that 'just agoing in is a pillow [sic] of Wood and a bason of Water fixd up on one side of this pillar, every Catholic as enters dips his finger in the bason of Water & Crosses their faces. I recollect hearing of a Story that some person black the Water and every person had black Crosses upon their faces.' [203-204]. Perhaps there is a hint of mockery here, but it is more likely that Savory was simply tickled by hearing of the practical joke. He does not seem to share in the violent intolerance that led to the anti-Catholic Gordon Riots in London in 1780. The fact that Savory visited a catholic church at all, and records the event, at least hints at open-minded religious curiosity.

Such an impression is reinforced by what immediately follows. 'I went also to a Jews Synagogue', he reports: 'there were 7 priests and all the people had branches of Trees in their hands & they beat them so much that at last all the

---

1. For details of the nature and extent of nonconformism in Berkshire in this period, see *Berkshire Nonconformist Meeting House Regulations 1689-1852, Part I*, ed. L. Spurrier (Berkshire Record Society, ix, 2005).

leaves were off it – it was on the Account of Joshua's taking Jericho, see Joshua Chap 6th. they went 7 times round the Meeting & the Rams Horn was blown each time in going round' [204]. This is evidently a description of the synagogue built on the edge of Whitechapel and the city at the start of the eighteenth century – the Bevis Marks Synagogue on Heneage Lane as it is known today. It served Sephardi Jews who originated in the Mediterranean (Spain, Portugal, North Africa and the Middle East). The community dates back to the readmission of the Jews in the late 1650s. They totalled about 30,000 by 1800. Specifically, Savory describes the eight-day celebration of the festival of *Sukkot*, a ritual celebration of the bounties of nature. This falls in the early autumn, involves symbols of plant fertility, and is akin to harvest festival. The 'branches of Trees' refers to the *lulav*, bound palm leaves which are shaken. Worshippers typically also hold an *esrog*, a rare type of citrus fruit.

During a visit to London with his uncle, John Savory, in October 1786, Savory went one Sunday to 'a Jews burying' and he describes how

> there was a Hearse to convey the Corpse to the burying ground [(]as is customary for the poorest person that is). and two Mourning Coaches and upwards of 20 Hackney Coaches followed. the Corpse is never caried [*sic*] on Shoulders as is customary with us but when they get to the burying Ground the Corpse is taken out of the hearse and as many as can asist [*sic*] conveys the Corpse into the Meeting House upon their Arms and then the Corpse is putt on Stools, the Lead of the Coffin is unhapsed (as they seldom use Nails or Screws) and something done to the deceased then the relations Garment is rented by Cutting the Coat with a knife[,] afterwards a few prayers &c. spoke in Hebrew, the Lead of the Coffin is hapsed on again and conveyd to the Grave. [126]

Savory expresses his astonishment at the sight of 'so many relations & friends of Deceasd […] weaping and praying over the Graves for the good of the departed Souls [*sic*]' [126-127]. He also acknowledges the numerous tombstones – 'mostly laid Horizontal [and] most of the inscriptions was in Hebrew' [127]. This is undeniably a Jewish funeral, almost certainly at the same Sephardi synagogue, in the cemetery of which the gravestones are indeed laid flat on the ground, not standing at right angles to it. The clothes of the deceased's close relatives would have been 'rent' – cut – as a sign of mourning, as Savory describes. He adds that 'its a very common custom with them to put Lime in the Graves and when the body is putt [*sic*] in [someone] throws in some water to burn the Body, sometimes there is holes at the bottom of the Coffin for the heat of the Lime to get at the body and sometimes the body is put in the ground & the Coffin broke to pieces and thrown in afterwards' [127]. In fact, this probably was not a common practice, but he is on firmer ground when he writes that 'they generally interr the Body in the Earth so soon as it has resignd its breath if it before Sun sett' [127]. Jews bury their dead very quickly, within 24 hours if possible, and the burial service itself is neither long nor elaborate, but simple and swift. The eulogies come later and elsewhere.[1]

---

1. With thanks to Prof. Lawrence Goldman for his guidance in these matters.

This account of a Jewish burial contrasts with a funeral Savory attended at the Anglican church in Whitechapel. He explains that it had become customary there for the curate to say the prayers at the graveside and only to read the service in church and admit the corpse if a payment of 17 shillings had been received [199].

(xii) Royalty and politics

The Prince of Wales, later George IV, is mentioned personally in Savory's volume, when it is noted on 10 February 1790 that 'the Prince of Wales came in these parts to Hunt with Lord Cravens Hounds' [228]. In fact, the newspapers reported that on Tuesday the 9th 'his Royal Highness the Prince of Wales paid a visit to Lord Craven at his seat at Benham, near Newbury; and on Thursday his Highness took the diversion of fox-hunting with his Lordship at Shefford.'[1] Savory mentions the 21st birthday of Lord Craven's son, William, on 1 September 1791, when 'there was a great entertainment at the Mansion house' at Benham Park, Speen, though it is unlikely Savory attended it [257]. Old Lord Craven would die less than a month later, on 26 September, upon which young William became the 7th Baron.

In the final pages of the MS Savory draws up a geniture horoscope for the Prince who was aged 29 when Savory compiled the volume [260-261]. Savory's astrological calculations reflect the low esteem in which His Royal Highness was then widely held: the universe declared him to be 'weak in substance' owing to 'Gaming, Drinking, Women, Sickness, Servants & people under his Authority &c' [260]. Moreover, 'he will not improve his partrimony' [sic] and 'he shall be little bettered thereby' [260-261]. He predicted a 'plurality of Wives providing he lives long enough' but 'small Issue' [261]. Nevertheless, the planets declared him to be of 'a good disposition' at least insofar as the Prince (and here the planets strongly echoed well-informed public gossip) 'delight[ed] in the Company of the female Sex' [261]. Yet he was 'ungratefull to his friends, a destroyer of his own substance & of a very mutable fortune &c' [261]. In common with most people of his time, Savory seems to have felt little regard for the future King.

By contrast, Savory seems largely sympathetic towards the Prince's father, King George III. He writes 'God Bless great Geo: our K[in]g / Long live our Noble K[in]g / God save the King', although he also gives George's birthday incorrectly as 24 May [133]. When he produces a horoscope based on the date of George III's coronation (22 September 1761), however, he finds the King's 'Enemies in general to be victorious' and that he is 'also in fear of his people' [259]. There was widespread public and political concern when George III fell into serious mental ill-health in November 1788. Savory tells us that 'When the King was very Ill reports spread about one Morning that he was dead and almost all the black Cloth was bo[ugh]t even old Black Cloth at Rag fair' [198-199]. In fact, the King's illness precipitated a constitutional crisis. Prime Minister, William Pitt the Younger (1759-1806), favoured by the King, refused to believe that George would not recover, and successfully resisted the appeal by Charles James Fox and the Opposition to transfer the King's powers to the

---

1. *Bath Chronicle and Weekly Gazette* (19 February 1790).

unpopular Prince of Wales. When the King recovered in the latter half of February 1789, the public largely joined with Pitt in rejoicing. Public buildings were illuminated from Hampstead and Highgate to Clapham and Tooting, and from Greenwich to Kensington. Some houses which were not reverently decorated and were deemed not to be joining in the celebrations even had their windows broken by a disapproving mob. Savory gives his own eye-witness testimony of events.

> After the Kings recovery the principal streets in London was illuminated two Nights: the Bank, Royal Exchange, Sun fire Office, India House &c. was very elegantly illuminated, on the India House were large letters of Lamps May the King live for Ever, and over it a beautifull Star set with different coloured Lamps[.] we travelled all Night to see the fire Works[.] we was 7 hours going on a Coach from Aldgate Church to the Royal Exchange on account of so many Coaches. [198]

A striking example of the celebrations inspired by the King's recovery is provided by Robert Stephens (c.1724-1801) of Catmore Farm. As mentioned earlier, Savory's mother was the cousin of Stephens's wife, Mary, née Palmer (1733-1823). The couple had married at Lambourn in 1759. Had Savory not been in London at the time he might well have attended Stephens's celebrations in Catmore. As it was, Savory might not even have been aware of them, but the *Reading Mercury* shared details. Following a service of thanks on St George's Day 1789 at the simple little late 12th-century church of St Margaret's next to the farmhouse, Stephens hosted a dinner to celebrate 'his Majesty's happy recovery' and there was reportedly 'a sufficient quantity of beer' supplied 'to all the poor of the parish'.[1] He gave all his labourers a day's paid holiday. 'The remainder of the day was spent with festivity and joy', but crucially everyone 'returned orderly to their respective habitations'. Furthermore, it was boasted that everyone was 'full of gratitude to their benefactor, and as good subjects, wishing long life to the King'. An indication of Stephens's wealth is to be found on the south wall of the chancel of Catmore Church, where an unusually large memorial consisting of a staggering 35 lines of text, gives details of the Stephens family's lives, including that of nine children and their spouses. The connection with Catmore Farm was re-established through their third daughter, Mary (1764-1800), who married George Bartholomew (?1765-1809) who later farmed there. It is also worth noting that the Stephens's only son, John (1761-1816) married Anne (1749-1805), the daughter and heiress of Richard Sellwood (1716-1776) of the Berkshire Militia whom Savory refers to earlier in the volume [3]. The Catmore memorial states that Robert and Mary Stephens resided at Catmore Farm for 38 years until 1798 when 'they retired from business to spend in quiet with their family the remainder of their days, and to prepare for eternity'. Nonetheless, such a cosy account as that found in the provincial press of universal satisfaction at Stephens's celebration of the King's restoration to health might be difficult to credit. Just two weeks later the events that came to

1. *RM* (27 April 1789).

define the ultimately regicidal French Revolution began to unfold across the Channel, causing the English authorities great anxiety. It makes no mark on Savory's account, however.

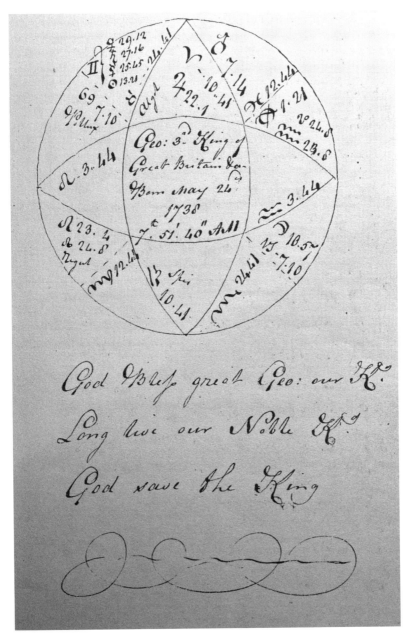

3. Savory's geniture chart for King George III, complete with patriotic chant and flourish [133].

Political controversies in Britain took a less rebellious turn. Moreover, in drawing up his horoscope based on George III's coronation, Savory finds that the King's 'parliament consisteth of very eloquent & learned Men' [259]. Yet he shows tacit approval of popular discontent when he copies out an amusing satire lampooning William Pitt the Younger, who had been Prime Minister since 1783 [106-110]. It is written in imitation of a Bible chapter with clear allusions to the Parable of the Rich Man and Lazarus (Luke 16:19-31). It expresses the exasperation felt by many members of the burgeoning middle-class at Pitt's seemingly relentless creation of taxes and hiking of rates. It is composed of 21 prose verses and casts Pitt as a self-indulgent and ungrateful spendthrift. The lifestyle and attitude of this feckless Rich Man contrasts sharply with that of the people who elected him, and more pointedly with the poor. The people are burdened by the weight of Pitt's high taxes. Among the unpopular fiscal measures alluded to are taxes on servants, windows, candles, rents on retail properties, and possibly soap and starch.[1] It is hinted that popular opposition to these taxes could threaten Pitt's continued electoral success and, if not remedied, might even result in popular riots.

(xiii) Transport

Whether Savory was travelling for business or pleasure, he required transport. On 3 September 1785, the 17-year-old drove Mrs Trulock from Thatcham to Brightwalton, as we have seen. He says nothing of the horse, and only describes the carriage as a 'chaise', a light, probably hooded vehicle, in this case for two people.

> I had the Chaise at the 3 Tuns & drove her from Thatcham to Henwick by fair Cross pond thro' Chieveley & peasemore but mistaking the right road from Peasemore to Brightwalton I drove into Yeastly Copse and could not get backwards or forwards. however we got up the Banks and got off without doing any damage to the Chaise, but spoiled the old Ladys White Shoes. [101]

He was, presumably, an inexperienced driver at this point.

His misfortunes with forms of personal transport did not end there. In the latter part of 1789, when he was 21, he reports that he 'went to farmbro' feast this Year upon the Wall Eyed Nag I bo[ugh]t at Abingdon fair' [214]. He had explained earlier that at Abingdon Fair in June he had sold a 'little poney' belonging to his uncle, John Savory, for eight guineas, and bought a 'Black Mare' for twelve [212]. However, despite taking the advice of John Holmes, his uncle's contemporary and friend, Savory found that the horse 'was what is cal[le]d Wall Eyed'. That is, the horse had exotropia, or divergent strabismus, where the eyes turn outward away from the nose, as if looking at opposing walls. He quickly took her to Crowmarsh Fair, where 'the dealer took to him [*sic*] again' [213]. On 21 June 1791, a week before his 23rd birthday, Savory laments, 'My Nag died owing to a Wound on the hollow above its Eye which was done in the stable at Lilly' [254]. This must have come as a severe blow,

---

1. I have included a more detailed commentary below [110*n*].

as the casualty was presumably the '4 Year old Gelding' which he bought from Josh Adnum of Leckhampstead for £27 only six weeks' earlier on 11 May [251]. Nevertheless, on 8 July 1791, he bought bridles from a Mr Fidler for 6 guineas [254]. The importance of keeping a healthy horse is further underlined by the fact that Savory quotes a folk remedy to cure horses infested with bots, insects which attach their eggs to the hairs of horses and other animals, causing anxiety and irritation that can so trouble the horse that it inadvertently injures itself [219].

A dependable horse that was able to transport Savory quickly was all the more vital given his status as a medical man. Early in the volume, when he describes what turned out to be his father's final illness in 1772, he points out how John Collet used his chaise as a sort of ambulance to transport the patient to the smallpox isolation house on the edge of Brightwalton [20]. Perhaps Savory was more fortunate with the third and final horse he purchased. On 25 July 1791, four days after opening his shop on Bartholomew Street, Newbury, he bought 'a Gray Horse of Mr Ward of Paughly' – probably connected with the historic Poughley Priory in Chaddleworth – for which he paid 25 guineas, and the following day he bought 'a New Saddle & Bridles' from Benjamin Ford, a Newbury saddler [255].

The volume highlights the hazards of personal forms of transport. Savory records how his schoolmaster, Joseph Aldridge, died 'from a fall of a Horse' on his way to Penclose Wood in 1780 [46]. There were also accidents caused by what today we would call drink-driving. When William Hooper (c.1759-1791), 'being intoxicated with strong Liquor' attempted to ride his horse from Farnborough to his home in Pewsey, Wiltshire, in May 1791, he 'fell from his Horse & fractured his Scul' and sternum [252]. Despite the attendance of Savory and two medical men from Pewsey, Hooper refused to be operated on until he was home, 'being of so stubborn & resolute disposition'. This resulted in premature death, caused – in Savory's judgement – by 'his own misconduct'.

Longer journeys involved commercial services. On 23 July 1785 and 1 October 1786 Savory notes that he went to London 'by Newbury Coach' [100, 124]. On the second of these journeys, he recorded the mileage as he proceeded from Speenhamland, via Thatcham, Woolhampton, Theale, Reading, Twyford, Hare Hatch, Maidenhead, Salt Hill, Slough, Colnbrook, Cranford Bridge (Harlington), Hounslow, New Brentford, and Turnham Green, to his destination at Hyde Park Corner, 56 miles from his point of departure, and, as we have seen, he counted 222 public houses along the way [125]. When he moved to London to undertake his hospital medical studies on 3 October 1788, he again went by 'Newbury Coach' [172]. Given that Savory records the death of William Clinch in November 1790, remarking that he 'drove the Newbury Coach', we can be reasonably certain what service Savory used [234]. In 1787, the *Reading Mercury* advertised W. Clinch and G. Kimber's 'Newbury Machines', travelling every day except Sunday '*to and from* LONDON, *through* READING *and* MAIDENHEAD': 'SET out from the GLOBE INN, NEWBURY, and BULL SAVAGE INN, Ludgate-Hill, London, at six o'clock in the morning', they boasted, and the passenger 'will arrive at London and

Newbury to dinner.'[1] 'A Family taking the whole coach may set out at what hour they please. Prices as usual,' they added. The coach stopped at both the Old White Horse Cellar and the White Bear, Piccadilly, both on entering and leaving London. The company also operated a post-coach, which left at eight in the morning on Monday, Wednesday and Friday from the White Hart Inn in Newbury, bringing post from London on Tuesday, Thursday and Saturday 'at the same hour'. Coach journeys could be sociable and even enlightening affairs if you met the right fellow passengers, as Savory discovered on 22 May 1791 when his companion on the coach to London, who was an artist, advised him that 'the best thing to clean an old picture was the White of an Egg beat to a froth & well rub the pictures after being well scowered with New Urine, Warm Water or Warm Water and Soap, only mind the Soap should be wiped off' [252-253]. When Savory returned to Brightwalton from London at the end of his hospital career, he notes that he took the Bristol Mail, setting off from Piccadilly at 9pm and arriving at Thatcham at 3am, a considerably faster journey than was available on the Newbury Machines [253].

Presumably Savory had some personal insight into the business of coaching via his brother-in-law Francis Fordham, who kept the coaching inn, the Flying Horse, in Whitechapel, where Savory stayed during part of the time he was in London in 1788-1789. Perhaps it helped him the better to tolerate the traffic jams which occurred during the public rejoicing in London at the news of the recovery of King George III in February 1789 [198]. Commercial services could also transport goods. When Savory left London on 3 June 1789 he points out, 'I sent my Anatomical preparations and Drugs by Clarks Waggon' [210]. John Clark & Co. operated a coach between Newbury and London for much of the eighteenth century. They pioneered the 'flying coach' in 1752 which, like the later 'Newbury Machines', travelled at four to five miles per hour, providing a journey time of about 12 hours.[2]

Most short journeys were undertaken by foot, not only in Newbury, Southwark or Whitechapel, and in Brightwalton and other villages, but also between villages. Of his father, Savory comments that he was 'such a pedestrian that no one could hardly walk with him without running' and he 'used to Measure Land for 7 or 8 Miles distant from Brightwaltham' [18]. Quite literally following in his father's footsteps, Savory set out with a measuring wheel in February 1790 and measured the distances between a variety of places around Brightwalton [229-230]. The furthest he walked was to the 'Cross Way' at Speenhamland, a distance of eight miles and 29 poles [229].

(xiv) Crime

In August 1786 Savory witnessed what happened to servants who broke the law. The Joneses' maid servant, Mary Walker, who was a few days off completing her service for the Jones family in Newbury, 'collected a few Articles together & packd it up with the cloathes' [124]. The morning before

---

1. *RM* (12 November 1787).
2. See W. Money, *A Popular History of Newbury* (1905), 17, 52.

she was due to leave she secreted 'two or three bundles' in a faggot pile in the yard. Jones noticed what she was doing because he was out of bed unusually early. The servant had tried to steal 'Hankerchiefs, Silver Spoon, Blue [china] &c'. She was 'tryed at Sessions and received 1 Months imprisonment' in Newbury [124].

Yet Savory was not above breaching the law himself, though it is a matter of opinion as to whether he was guilty of youthful over-exuberance or out-and-out hooliganism. He writes in reference to Charles Southby how he 'was a great plague to him sometime' [152]. Until the start of 1788 Southby kept a shop opposite the Monument on Newbury's Northbrook Street where he sold women's hats. Savory recounts how 'one time a Q[uar]t of Soap Lees was thrown over his Shutters and the paint came off' though he is not clear whether he was personally responsible for it [152]. On at least one occasion his behaviour resulted in what today we would surely acknowledge as criminal damage. On 10 July 1788, shortly after Savory turned 20, he and some of his friends got themselves into trouble. As a 23-year-old recalling the incident, he concedes, 'I got myself a little in disgrace' following the wedding of William Dance and Dinah Dance at Brightwalton [156]. Presumably he was intoxicated. He had been with the Brightwalton bellringers in the neighbouring hamlet of Lilley and,

> coming home with Joe Taylor & Joe Mitchel we must needs have a frolic[.] our first exploit was throwing Wood in the Well at White Lands and breaking all the gates to Sargeant Taylors. we then went to Wm Janaways who lives in the Corner of the Holt Common, and threw down his Hay Ricks & broke a new wickett gate to pieces[.] we then broke what gates we could all the Way to Trumpletts[.] we was taken up and appeared before the Justices at the pelican at Speenhamland upon susspission & likewise Jos[ep]h Mitchel Sen[io]r, but they could <do> nothing with us. [156-157]

Given that at this point in Savory's life he was establishing himself as the village's medical man, having completed his apprenticeship, such an escapade seems more than a little disgraceful. Why the Justices of the Peace could do nothing with them is not clear. Presumably the defendants denied everything and the case collapsed for want of evidence. The George and Pelican was one of the region's largest and most popular coaching inns, and dated back to at least 1658. The Irish actor, Quin, is said to have composed the quippish verse,

> The famous inn at Speenhamland,
> 　　That stands below the hill,
> May well be called the Pelican,
> 　　From its enormous bill.[1]

This was not an isolated incident of misbehaviour on Savory's part, though the others might more legitimately be categorised as 'frolics' than the gate-

---

1. See <https://www.newbury.gov.uk/history/clock-house/> (accessed 1 July 2023).

breaking. 'Another time', Savory continues, warming to his confessional theme,

> we pushed down a high pile of fellies that stood in Painters Y[art]d. Also put Old Arthur Whiters Cow Racks in the Middle of the pond in the upper street. Francis New and myself and one Norris that lived there car[rie]d Charles Whistlers plow from out of Chaddleworth field by Whitings to Chaddleworth Common and hung it up ~~the~~ A tree. and wrote on it
>
> > The Man is bad and if you can
> > Take down the plow & hang the Man. [157]

On one level, this is an extension of his predilection for pranks and practical jokes. The final verse, though comically ironical and probably written with no malice, will strike some modern readers as irresponsible, and it is difficult to believe that Savory and his chums were free of censure at the time.

During the harvest of 1788, Savory rationally manipulated the popular belief in witchcraft in an attempt to identify a criminal, specifically to collar a thief who had stolen clothes belonging to John Harbert's farm servants. His idea was to trick the criminal with a double-cross, or what Savory calls a 'pleasant devise [...] done by my orders' [158]. Precisely how many people were involved is not recorded, but the survey of Brightwalton conducted two years later, in October 1790, states that Harbert had eight male and two female servants [see Appendix C], though additional labour would almost certainly have been called in at harvest-time. John Harbert (d. 1796), whom Savory often calls Herbert, had occupied the Manor Farm at Brightwalton since 1779, Savory tells us earlier [50]. He had quickly made his mark with a programme of grubbing and ploughing, and building a new barn and granary next to the churchyard [52]. A couple of Harbert's servants are mentioned by Savory at different times: John Cook, a 'servant boy', who was killed at the chalk pit in Ash Close on 28 January 1781 [53]; and Harbert's shepherd, John Stroud, who married Ann Deacon on Christmas Day 1782 [57]. Savory's ruse to trick a thief into incriminating himself by turning his belief in witchcraft against him can only be explained in his own words.

> I ordered [the servants] to get a large Kettle or pott which was all over black and put a Cock underneath and all the Servants to go in the room which was to be made dark, and some one say, I command you to walk round three times hand in hand and then touch each of you the Kettle and as hard as you can[,] and that as is guilty the Cock will Crow when he touches. now its being dark the Guilty person will not touch, so that they was all let out of the room immediately[:] when examining the suspected persons hand he had no black on it therefore pronounced him Guilty. [158-159]

The kettle or pot was evidently not merely black, but covered in some black powder or paint. The criminal was to be caught, not red-handed, or black-handed, but clean-handed. Savory implies that the scheme was successful, though he does not name the thief. It would have required a degree of credulity on the part of the farm servants that implies a gullibility which is difficult to credit.

Savory records how, on a 'Morning in feb[rua]ry' 1789, when he was a medical student in London, he 'went to Newgate to see 7 Men and 1 Woman hangd opposite the door at Newgate' [197]. As we have noted, he adds that 'the Woman received her reward in this life opposite the 7 men & was afterwards burnt'. The only execution this can refer to in fact occurred on Wednesday, 18 *March*. Burning was not a common punishment by this time: 33 women suffered this fate between 1735 and 1789. What Savory describes would turn out to be the very last case. The punishment was formally abolished in 1790. Only women were burned for treason. Men were hanged, drawn and quartered, but as this involved nakedness it was not considered suitable as a punishment for women. The only crimes for which both men and women were burned were witchcraft and heresy. The woman Savory saw was Catherine Murphy, also known as Christian Bowman.[1] Her crime was 'coining', a form of counterfeiting which involved clipping small pieces of silver and gold off genuine coins to make fake ones. This was considered an act of treason because it involved the mutilation of the image of the King. She was led from the Debtor's Door of Newgate past the nearby gallows to the stake. Eight men hanged from the gallows, not seven as Savory states, and among them were three of her co-conspirators, including her husband. She mounted a small platform in front of the stake and an iron band was put round her body. The noose, dangling from an iron bracket projecting from the top of the stake, was tightened around her neck. When the preparations were complete, William Brunskill, the hangman, removed the platform and left her suspended for 30 minutes before the faggots were placed around her and were set alight. As principal hangman, Brunskill would hang 537 people outside Newgate.[2]

(xv) Disability

It would be unreasonable and anachronistic to look for an awareness of disability in an account dating from the late eighteenth century. Nevertheless, in a matter-of-fact way, Savory does register a number of handicaps. Of Richard Bew (d. 1780), schoolmaster since 1772 at North Heath on the border of Winterbourne and Chieveley, he remarks that he was 'a good kind of a Man and went rather lame' [49]. Of Jeremiah Grant, the 'very injenious' clockmaker who instructed him in astrology, he observes, 'he was Lame & was obliged to wear an Iron to support his Leg' [72]. After quoting a long and effusive letter from him, he regrets that Grant left Newbury shortly after writing it and confides that it 'gave me great uneasiness for the loss of so sincere a Friend' [75]. Savory notes how Jones, a britches-maker, had a 'Crooked Leg', and also alleges that he was dishonest [119]. He shows no sympathy for his father's schoolmaster, John Nelson, who had grown 'so infirm' as to be 'almost for the 2nd time a Child', recounting with apparent glee the practical jokes played on him by the schoolchildren [16]. Such a mixed response to these handicaps and

---

1. See also J. Holbert Wilson, *Temple Bar, The City Golgotha* (1853), 4.
2. For details of the case see *Proceedings of the Old Bailey*, t17880910-102, and at
   <http://www.capitalpunishmentuk.org/burning.html> (accessed 1 July 2023).

infirmities indicates that, whilst he naturally preferred some people over others, he was not obviously prejudiced about what we might now call their disabilities.

In 1782 he notes the death of Benjamin Frood or Froud (1709-1782) of Chaddleworth.

> A man both Deaf and Dumb he used to come twice or three times a Year to my mother to be let Blood[.] he knew all the news in the Country & was ready to Understand any thing by different motions. he rec[eive]d weekly pay from Chaddleworth parish & when he died had 20 or 30 Guineas conceald in his Coffer. [56]

Whilst it is possible to read this last comment as a criticism of the parish relief or benefit payment made to Frood, he might equally well have been expressing approval of Frood's thriftiness. Savory's admiration for the man in overcoming his communication difficulties is in any case palpable. Perhaps it was from Frood that Savory's father acquired knowledge of 'The silent Language' of fingerspelling that Savory copies from his father's notebooks [150-151]. Its similarity to modern British Sign Language is striking. Unfortunately, Savory does not record whether he or any other members of his family ever used it to communicate with any deaf friends or customers, Frood included.

(xvi) Medical training

Savory's account of his medical training in London is the most coherent and focused part of his MS. This is partly because his studies were concentrated in the eight months from 3 October 1788 to 3 June 1789 [172-199, 204-211]. When he began his courses of study, he was already in practice at Brightwalton, having successfully completed his apprenticeship. It was his choice to attend the Borough Hospitals of St Thomas's and Guy's in London and to apply for professional accreditation as a surgeon-apothecary and man-midwife. It was a clear sign of his ambition. His decision also reflected the significant changes then afoot in the medical profession. As the medical historian, Mary Fissell has argued:

> by the 1780s and 1790s, pupils became the large majority of trainees. Not only were traditional patterns of apprenticeship breaking down citywide [...] but the Infirmary had, without conscious intent, created a functional replacement for apprenticeship [....; it] assumed the mantle of corporate authority formerly worn by the city companies of barber-surgeons and apothecaries, and practitioners modelled themselves upon hospital men, rather than identifying themselves with a marketplace of medicine.[1]

---

1. M. E. Fissell, *Patients, Power and the Poor in Eighteenth-Century Bristol* (Cambridge, 1991), 128, 126.

Hospital study complemented but had not yet replaced the tradition of apprenticeship. Savory chose to benefit from both.

Savory spent some of the period of his studies with the Fordhams at the Flying Horse in Whitechapel, but in order to reduce travelling time and probably costs, for four months from 21 October to 25 February he paid two shillings per week to lodge with one Mrs Meakin at 32 Joiner Street, south of the Thames in Southwark [182, 195]. Joiner Street formed the eastern boundary of St Thomas's Hospital, and ran north-to-south from Tooley Street to St Thomas's Street, towards the entrance to Guy's. Joiner Street thus ran parallel to Borough High Street which was to the west. St Saviour's Churchyard, where Savory attended midwifery cases, was just the other side of Borough High Street and only a short distance away from Joiner Street. The old St Thomas's Hospital site and surrounding streets were demolished in the nineteenth century to make way for London Bridge Station which now incorporates the footprint of Joiner Street and preserves its name.

Savory complains that he was 'never at leisure' as a medical student [204]: 7.30am-9am he attended midwifery lectures at St Saviour's Churchyard; then he had breakfast; 10am-11am he attended William Saunders's medical lectures at Guy's; 11am-1pm he attended medical cases at St Thomas's (he tells us that this was when, on Monday to Wednesday, the surgeons took turns to walk the wards in order to visit patients, with all surgeons and physicians visiting the wards on Saturday, whilst Thursday was the day patients were officially admitted [179]);[1] 1pm-3pm he attended Henry Cline's lectures on anatomy and surgery at St Thomas's; then he had dinner; and thereafter he undertook dissection, attended accidents, labours and medical cases, and diligently wrote up his lecture notes [204-205; see Appendix D].[2] In addition to his formal studies, Savory also attended the Physical Society of Guy's Hospital which met at the midwifery lecture theatre at St Saviour's Churchyard, and the Medical Society of London in Bolt Court, off Fleet Street [198].

On 5 October 1788, at the start of his student experience, Savory 'breakfasted with Mr Hurlock Surgeon in St Pauls Church Yard & went with <him> to see his patients' [172]. How this came about remains obscure, and Hurlock is never mentioned again. Savory is probably referring to Joseph Hurlock (1754-1845), or possibly to his father, Philip Hurlock (1713-1801). The family was established in medical practice at St Paul's Churchyard by the mid eighteenth century. Father and son were well-regarded and respected surgeons and medical authors, and Philip was the librarian at the Medical Society in Bolt Court. That Savory's time in London should have started with a member of the Hurlock family was promising.

Savory reveals that on 6 October he visited Henry Cline at his home on St Mary Axe and paid him seven guineas to enrol as a 'perpetual pupil' of his lectures at St Thomas's Hospital and another five guineas to use the dissecting

---

1. Compare with Ford, *Student at St Thomas's*, 24-25. Susan Lawrence points out that the reasons surgeons and physicians regularly walked the wards together was because it was not always clear whether a patient should be treated by surgical intervention or medicine alone, see Lawrence, *Charitable Knowledge*, 69-70.
2. For another example of a typical student timetable c. 1800, which differs in certain respects to Savory's but not much, see Lawrence, *Charitable Knowledge*, 172.

room there [172-173]; he paid 18 guineas, plus a fee of 22 shillings, 'for seeing the practice' of St Thomas's and Guy's for six months (i.e. observing medical cases and surgical procedures) [173]; he evidently paid five guineas to attend two course of William Saunders's lectures on physic at Guy's [173]; and he paid another five guineas to attend two courses of midwifery lectures at St Saviour's Churchyard [181]. At the end of his eight months' of study in London, he calculated his total expenditure at 'upwards of 100 pounds' [211]. By some means undisclosed he also observed some operations at St Bartholomew's Hospital: an operation on the bladder for the stone and an amputation of the thigh, both on 12 October, for example [183]; scirrhous breast on 1 November [184-5]; an operation for facial fistula and one for hydrocele [189].

Joseph Warner (1717-1801), a senior surgeon at Guy's, whom Savory mentions [174], wrote an account of student life in 1792, two years after he retired from the hospital in his early 70s. It agrees with Savory's account in almost every particular, though he provides useful additional information which is worth quoting at length.

There have been lectures held in anatomy, in which observations on surgery has ever been introduced from the beginning, first by Mr Girle, then Mr Sharp, Mr Warner, Mr Else and at present by Mr Cline. The fee for these lectures and for the dissecting room is twelve guineas. There are lectures read every morning at half-past seven on Midwifery by Dr Lowder in the borough; they may continue until half-past eight. At ten o'clock in the morning Mr Babington the apothecary at Guy's gives a lecture on Chymistry which continues until eleven, when the practice begins. Those mornings that pass without the lecture in Chymistry, Dr Saunders supplies with one on the Practice of Physic. The Chymical lectures continue until there has been two courses given, which employs them from the 1st of October until the month of May. The anatomical lectures are every day from one o'clock until three. These are read at St Thomas's Theatre by Mr Cline; the former, in Chymistry and the Practice of Medicine, at the Theatre at Guy's. All the pupils that enter for the anatomical lectures pay seven guineas; if they choose to dissect and attend the dissecting room they pay five guineas extra ordinary. The terms for the Chymistry, Materia Medica and the Practice of Physic are ten guineas. I cannot take upon me to say when they were first instituted but there were lectures read before 1750. There are not any Chirurgical lectures given but those that finish each anatomical course by Mr Cline. They have amounted hitherto to twelve in number to each course. The lectures have always been delivered viva voce.[1]

St Thomas's had about 450 beds. There would be about 45 admissions a week, with a lottery being called if the waiting list exceeded the number of vacancies. The mortality rate was about 10% and if a patient was in hospital for three months she or he was generally considered incurable and was discharged.[2]

---

1. Quoted in H. C. Cameron, *Mr Guy's Hospital 1726-1948* (1954) 94.
2. See Ford, *Student at St Thomas's*, 24-25.

It is with evident enthusiasm that Savory records the names of the surgeons, physicians and wards at St Thomas's and Guy's [174-175], and gives a description of the Borough Hospitals [189-190], as well as St Bartholomew's [190], and the London Hospital [190-191]. Later he describes the operating theatre at St Thomas's [179-180], and its large lecture theatre where Cline addressed the students [181].[1] The four medical practitioners in London with whom Savory was most closely involved were Henry Cline and William Saunders, whose lectures he attended daily and wrote up with meticulous care [see Appendix D]; the surgeon, John Birch, whose operations he most often notes in his account; and William Lowder, the expert in midwifery.

As a surgeon's pupil, Savory was at the lowest end of the hospital hierarchy, beneath the status of a dresser, a house pupil and an apprentice, and there were far more surgeon's pupils than physician's or apothecary's pupils from mid-century onwards. Nevertheless, it is important to note that the numbers were still tiny. In the year Savory entered the Borough Hospitals, he became one of approximately only 100 surgeon's pupils.[2] Some 11,059 pupils walked the wards in the Borough Hospitals in the 90 years between 1725 and 1815.[3] Between 1784 and 1804, there were 1,047 surgeon's pupils at St Thomas's, and 582 at Guy's, and numbers increased roughly in line with the growth of the population, at least up to the mid-1790s.[4] As Susan Lawrence has observed, 'Ward-walking opened hospital practice to those who already had some medical knowledge, allowing more medical men to witness, discuss and (potentially) praise or criticize the bedside decisions of these elite practitioners.'[5]

Henry Cline has been described as 'probably the greatest personality the staff of St Thomas's has known'.[6] He had been educated at the Merchant Taylors' School, and in 1767 was apprenticed to Thomas Smith, surgeon at St Thomas's Hospital. Cline had been appointed lecturer in anatomy at St Thomas's in 1781 and surgeon in 1784. He stayed in both posts until 1811. He was also an examiner for the College of Surgeons in 1804, became its master in 1815, and its president in 1823. He would deliver the Hunterian Oration in 1816 and 1824. The poet John Keats, who served an apprenticeship under the surgeon Thomas Hammond of Edmonton, attended Cline's lectures as a student at the Borough Hospitals in the mid-1810s.

Savory had missed Cline's first three lectures by the time he arrived in London, but as a perpetual pupil he caught them second time round. He lists

---

1. John Flint South describes the theatre far more fully than Savory, see J. F. South, *Memorials of John Flint South: Twice President of the Royal College of Surgeons, and Surgeon to St Thomas's Hospital, 1841-61*, ed. C. L. Feltoe (1884), 29-30. Visitors to the Old Operating Theatre in the attic of the church of the old St Thomas's Hospital, which is now a museum, can still explore the successor theatre built in 1813-1814, see <https://oldoperatingtheatre.com/> (accessed 1 July 2023).
2. See Lawrence, *Charitable Knowledge*, 111.
3. Lawrence, *Charitable Knowledge*, 108.
4. Lawrence, *Charitable Knowledge*, 135.
5. Lawrence, *Charitable Knowledge*, 110.
6. F. G. Parsons, *The History of St Thomas's Hospital* (3 vols, 1934) ii. 258. But, 'it was as a teacher that Cline excelled' according to E. M. McInnes, *St Thomas's Hospital* (1963; reprinted and enlarged, 1990), 197.

all 70 of Cline's lectures on anatomy (and the 71st on the history of medicine) indicating the value he placed in them [175-177]. These were given between October and December, and repeated between January and March. The 21 surgical lectures were given only once, between April and May, and Savory also summarises their subject-matter [177-178]. These were followed by six or seven lectures on the 'gravid uterus' (i.e. pregnancy) by Lowder, Savory tells us [178]. Having observed Cline in action in the operating theatre, Savory remarks, 'this Mr Cline is an excellent Surgeon & is near sighted' [179]. This last claim is not supported by any other source and in any case seems unlikely given that Cline was widely acknowledged as a great surgeon, excelling in lithotomy: Cline recorded that between 1785 and 1797 he cut 59 patients for the stone (the operation made notorious from its painful description by the diarist Samuel Pepys) and only six of them died.[1] Yet Savory only highlights two operations of Cline's that he observed: a castration and a cataract removal [184]. Savory also discloses that Cline 'divided a Nerve in a Dogs Leg and in about 6 Weeks after the Dog was killd & the Nerve was found united again[,] so that union takes place in a tendon if Cutt & separated at some distance' [188]. This is particularly interesting because this experimental discovery of Cline's is thus shown to have predated that of his colleague, John Haighton, whom Savory also got to know and whose thesis, 'An Experimental Inquiry Concerning the Reproduction of Nerves', published in 1795, details other instances of this phenomenon. Cline only ever published one volume, *On the Form of Animals* (1805).[2] Medical and other scientific discoveries made in the course of experimentation necessarily pre-date their published documentation and the findings were often shared with pupils in lectures long before they appeared in print.

William Saunders (1743-1817) was a physician at Guy's from 1770 to 1803 and was a commanding figure. Savory seems to have attended Saunders's lectures on chemistry as well as physic [196]. He writes of Saunders, 'he is an excellent Lecturer and fine Orator' [196]. Saunders was a famously popular lecturer, and was considered both lucid and entertaining. Educated in his native Scotland, and not Oxbridge, he was elected by special grace to a Fellowship of the College of Physicians in 1790, on the intervention of his friend, Sir George Baker, its President, and Saunders subsequently served both as Goulstonian Lecturer in 1792 and Harveian Orator in 1796. His *Elements of the Practice of Physic* for students was published in 1780. Saunders argued that medicine was an art, not a science, since individual constitutions reacted in such a wide variety of ways in otherwise similar situations.[3] Hugely successful, he was appointed Physician to the Prince Regent in 1807.

Savory also gives an overview of the order and subject-matter of the midwifery lectures delivered by William Lowder (1732-1801) [192]. Lowder had a medical degree from Aberdeen, and started lecturing on midwifery at St Saviour's Churchyard in 1775, and later at the theatre at Guy's, assisted first

---

1. See Ford, *Student at St Thomas's*, 200.
2. See H. Cline, *On the Form of Animals* (1805).
3. See Lawrence, *Charitable Knowledge*, 310*n*. See also Appendix D.

by David Orme (1727-1812), and later by John Haighton (1755-1823).[1] He does not appear to have occupied any official hospital post, but was an army surgeon before becoming a lecturer, and his teaching was evidently regarded as an important complement to the courses at the Borough Hospitals. Savory mentions that Lowder used a synthetic model for demonstration purposes [193], but there were also real-life cases to give students invaluable practical experience of every aspect of pregnancy, presentation and delivery on which Lowder lectured [194]. Labours at Lowder's lying-in house (maternity hospital) were attended by the students by turn, but they also helped deliver babies in people's homes out in the community, and Savory's first was a natural labour at nearby Redriff [193]. As we have noted, he recalls the nine-hour labour of a young Irishwoman, a first-time mother, in February 1789; the baby was delivered in a kneeling position which Savory claims was 'their Country way' [193]. Other experiences must have been shocking, most notably when Savory and a fellow student, Edward Scammell, were unexpectedly confronted by a pre-natal death, and Savory describes literally handling the lifeless foetus [194]. It seems that mercifully they were accompanied on that occasion, and on some if not all others, by a female midwife called Mrs Gibson [194]. Savory gained his Certificate of Midwifery on 20 February 1789 [194]. He subsequently wrote up all of Lowder's lectures, though the volume seems to have been lost [195, see Appendix D]. Newly qualified, he proceeded to buy midwifery instruments, including forceps and catheters, from John Davenport on Whitechapel Road [196].

Savory was not too proud to admit that he initially found aspects of his medical training tough: 'The first Week I was at the Hospital my head was greatly affected by going in the fowl Wards [*i.e.* foul *wards, for women with venereal disease*] & dissecting Room' though he quickly adds, 'but afterwards it did not hurt me' [182-183]. Nevertheless, he was describing a problem that defeated some of his more sensitive fellow students. According to Benjamin Golding, 'The lectures on Anatomy and Surgery were delivered in a small and closely-confined Theatre, which (from the impurity of the air produced by its narrow capacity) was deemed so destructive to health, that many pupils were obliged to forego that most essential part of professional instruction, practical dissection, lest they should thereby endanger their health, and perhaps their existence'.[2]

Savory seems to have dived in at the deep end. A few days after enrolling as a surgeon's pupil he observed two amputations, a scalp wound and a fractured elbow [183]. He registers a variety of operations in addition to those performed at St Bart's, and those by Cline already mentioned. Operations typically took place at midday when the light was strongest. The vast majority of operations that Savory observed, at least those which he makes note of, were performed by the eminent surgeon John Birch (c.1745-1815): inguinal hernia, hydrocele, separation of the prepuce [183-184], dropsy [185], amputation of the leg [187], an ulcerated penis [188], and venereal disease [188-9] – a total of seven different procedures. Birch, appointed a surgeon at St Thomas's in

---

1. See J. Blunt, *Man-Midwifery Dissected; or, the Obstetric Family Instructor* (1793), x-xi.
2. B. Golding, *An Historical Account of St Thomas's Hospital* (1819), 128.

1784, was criticised by the celebrated surgeon and anatomist Sir Astley Cooper (1768-1841), who had studied under Cline at St Thomas's, as 'a sensual man; clever, but a bad surgeon. He had neglected anatomy, and was therefore afraid in all operations which required a knowledge of it. He devoted himself to electricity and thought he could do wonders with it'.[1] Despite Cooper's poor opinion of him, Birch became Surgeon Extraordinary to the Prince Regent.

Savory observed George Chandler (d. 1822) perform an amputation of the leg [184]. Sir Astley Cooper commended Chandler's speed and accuracy as a surgeon, and he was described by John Flint South (1797-1882), who knew the elderly Chandler in 1813-1814, as 'very active and brisk […] short in person, bald and grey-headed, careless about his dress, which however was scrupulously clean and nice […]. In his manners a perfect gentleman, kind and affable to every one, even to the poorest person'.[2] Given that Savory remarks that John Haighton was 'master of the disecting' we may assume that he also spent some considerable time observing him in the dissecting room [191].

In addition, Savory mentions, in general terms, operations for 'the Hare Lip, Stone, Fistulas, Trepanning &c.' which occurred 'two or three times a Week' [185]; the case of a nurse who choked to death on a piece of beef [185], another of a woman with severe, extensive and ultimately fatal burns [188] and yet another of 'cancerated uterus' [189]; and he notes 'three or four' cases of 'Lock Jaw' (tetanus), all of which proved fatal [185-186]. The most common operations were 'Amputations and Hernia' [187]. He also refers to some celebrated historic cases at the hospitals, such as the extraction by Samuel Sharp (1700-1778) of 214 calculi (stones) which Savory actually saw on exhibition at the theatre in St Thomas's – they were, he reckons, 'of a whitish Colour some as large as a hasel Nutt' [186].

Savory is unlikely to have practiced much medicine himself in London, besides delivering children under supervision, though he does casually mention that he 'displaced 3 large teeth for Josh. Cullum at Stratford' [199]. Apart from that he records inoculating his nephew, John Savory Fordham (1788-1826), with smallpox, and putting 'some Ear Rings in Khuns Childs Ears', Khuns being the friend of his sister Sarah who had previously kept the Flying Horse, so these cases involved a relative and a friend [203].

Among the most interesting, amusing and alarming sections in Savory's book is the account he gives of his *viva voce* examination at Surgeons' Hall in Old Bailey Street on 7 May 1789 [205-210]. Admitting that he felt 'a little timid' at the sight of three or four surgeons sat either side of the two wardens and master around a semicircular table, he nevertheless overcame his 'dread' [206]. In what reads like a verbatim transcript of his exam, he quotes the rudimentary questions he was asked and the responses he gave. The exchange is superficial in the extreme [207-209]. Called in afterwards to be told of his inevitable success, he took his Oath and was given 'a little pamphlet containing Rules & Orders', and the following day he received his diploma [210]. It is doubtful that his answers were as important as the payment of the college entrance fee of 2/6, the examination fee of £13 5s and the five shillings' cost

---

1. Quoted in McInnes, *St Thomas's Hospital*, 149.
2. South, *Memorials*, 45-46.

of the diploma, all of which he paid to become a member of the Corporation of Surgeons of London [206, 211]. Peachey asserts that the organisation was then struggling financially.[1] Savory did not pay for the certificates attesting that he had 'walked the wards' of the Borough Hospitals, presumably because he judged that they did not warrant the expense and thought them unnecessary [195]. Nevertheless, he does seem to have worked hard in the eight months he was in London, and both in the lectures he painstakingly wrote up, and his practical observations and experience of dissections, operations and labours, he was well-qualified by the (always improving) standards of his day. Savory returned to Brightwalton on 3 June, his intended departure from London having been delayed for about ten days by an attack of measles [210-211].

As John Ford has pointed out, the surgeon 'had to be able to diagnose, to drain and dress an abscess well, to draw a painful tooth with skill, and to set a fracture in a good functional position, which, badly done, could deprive a family of its breadwinner and lead to more paupers for the parish to support.'[2] He quotes Sir Astley Cooper who said that the patient could become 'a living memorial to the surgeon's ignorance or inattention'.[3] A couple of years after completing his medical studies in London, when Savory announced in the pages of the *Reading Mercury* that he had set up in practice in Newbury, he was at pains to underline his professional qualifications [256-257].

WILLIAM SAVORY,
SURGEON, APOTHECARY, and MAN-MIDWIFE,
In BARTHOLOMEW STREET, NEWBURY,

BEGS leave to inform his friends and the public, that he has attended the practice of St Thomas's and Guy's Hospitals, London, and studied the several branches of Medicine, Surgery, Anatomy and Midwifery under the most able professors, an advantage which greatly facilitated his arrival to that honour conferred on him by the Corporation of Surgeons in London, in constituting him a Member of their Body.

W. SAVORY returns his sincere thanks to his friends and the public for their past favours conferred on him at his residence at Brightwalton, and assures them no care or attention will be wanting on his part to render his endeavours satisfactory.[4]

Savory calls this notice an 'Address' in his MS, but it was of course a carefully crafted advertisement [256]. As he relates, he gave Thomas Cowslade (1757-1806) of the *Reading Mercury* 16s 6d, paid in person, to insert it three times in the newspaper [256]. That does not mean that the sentiments it expresses are less than sincere or should be mistrusted. Ward-walking was, as Susan Lawrence has pointed out, the 'mark of a better trained practitioner, one who did more than what was usually required for satisfactory expertise'.[5] Savory's pride in attending the Borough Hospitals and studying under such

---

1. Peachey, *Life of William Savory*, 18n.
2. Ford, *Student at St Thomas's*, 10.
3. Quoted in Ford, *Student at St Thomas's*, 10.
4. *RM* (1, 8, 15 August 1791).
5. Lawrence, *Charitable Knowledge*, 115.

eminent medical professionals was no doubt very real, but he also knew that such credentials were important in the eighteenth-century medical marketplace. Likewise, his membership of the Corporation and (from 1800) the Royal College of Surgeons. At the end of his 'Address', he folds his story back to his roots in Brightwalton where he had recently been in practice. This was partly out of pride, one suspects, and partly out of a sense of continuity and belonging. He was providing proof to the community that he was not an outsider who had arrived in Newbury from nowhere, or (perhaps worse) from London, but was, crucially, a local – a Berkshire man, and one of theirs. One might have expected, perhaps, that he would have mentioned his five-year apprenticeship, especially given that it was undertaken in Newbury itself, but he might have felt that this would associate him with a less exalted type of medical practitioner which he may justly have considered himself already to have surpassed.

(xvii) Medical practice

So what of Savory's initial period of practice at Brightwalton? He did, in fact, work as a medical man in the six-month period between completing his apprenticeship and starting his medical studies in London. The first thing he did was to get his brother-in-law, Joseph Norris, to paint the drawers and bottles at the shop [154], which was probably the same shop hitherto run by his mother, and previously by his father [156]. Savory calculates that between 25 March and 28 September 1788 he bled 62 people and drew 17 teeth [156]. It is with undisguised pride that he boasts that he successfully treated his first patient – a boy from Farnborough – whose 'metatarsel [*sic*] bones was very much disformed so that he could not walk for near 6 Months. I Cured him in 7 Weeks' [155].

It was after he had completed his medical studies in London and had become a Member of the Corporation of Surgeons of London, however, that his professional life really took off. On 5 June 1789, two days after arriving at Uncle John Savory's, he was treating his uncle Thomas Barratt's children for whooping cough [211]. The next day, a Saturday, he varnished his anatomical preparations and put them in a closet in the parlour [212]. Among the medical cases he refers to are a ploughboy's scalp wound [213]; a farmer's leg wound sustained while sheep-shearing [213-214]; a servant's dislocated clavicle, a flint which he cut out of an eye with his lancet, and the amputation of a finger – the three patients connected with these cases were respectively resident in Chaddleworth, Brightwalton and Farnborough – these being his 'most remarkable cases' of 1789 [214]. In his first midwifery case since his certification as a man-midwife, he safely delivered a baby boy on 21 April 1790: Richard, the son of John Brookes, a tailor, and his wife, Jane [230]. By this point, Savory was cultivating his own plants for medical use: he notes planting nightshade on 21 June, for example [231]. In the course of 1790 he bled 126 people, having bled 150 over the course of the preceding years [234]. He continues: 'during this Year I drew 29 Teeth, divided the Frenum Lingua of 3 Children. had many remarkable Cases this Year fractured Clavicle, Witchcraft, Scold Heads &c.' all of which he claims to have recorded in a medical case-book, now regrettably lost [234, and see Appendix D]. A sign of his growing status was that he assisted one of the chief constables of the county in his duties [227]. In his personal life he continued his courtship of Miss Mary Tyrrell of North Moreton.

The year 1791 started with the delivery of two stocks of bees from Mrs Jones at the Old Inn, Lilley, and on 3 May he found himself treating the same lady for extensive upper-body burns following an accident [246, 251]. Having described her as being burnt 'as black as a Coal', he immodestly claims to have made 'an excellent Cure of it' [246, 251]. Appearing to favour the notion that she had fallen into the fire as a result of 'a Giddiness in her Head', he nevertheless gives voice, albeit parenthetically, to the rumour that 'by the Essence of Sr John Barley Corn' she had 'set herself on fire with the Candle' [251]. He had some difficult cases to deal with: two ankle wounds, a burnt leg and a hand wounded by gunshot, a case of dropsy and a case of smallpox that proved fatal [246]. The associated patients lived in Fawley, Farnborough, Hampstead Norris and Chaddleworth, hinting at a gradually expanding geographical reach. The only other medical cases he mentions are two labours in Leckhampstead [253, 254]. His most significant professional breakthrough, however, came at Easter when he agreed with the Overseers of the Poor to attend the medical needs of 28 families in Farnborough (for £2 12s 6d *per annum*) and 44 in Leckhampstead (for £5 5s *per annum*), and as well as supplying names, he also copies out the Leckhampstead agreement in full [248-250]. Dated 26 April 1791, it makes it clear that, for a term of two years, Savory was to attend to the medical needs of anyone on parish relief, 'Surgery, Pharmacy & Midwifery, Fractures and Small Pox included' [250].

(xviii) A new life
Savory's marriage on 8 September 1791 was both the trigger for compiling his MS volume and the event with which its narrative would conclude. As readers, we accompany him on his journey towards independence and full maturity. He draws his account to a close by detailing his culminating preparations for his new life in Newbury as a husband, head of household, and a professionally accredited medical man with his own practice and apprentice.

Mary Tyrrell (1765-1844), the woman Savory would share the rest of his life with, makes an appearance a little under a fifth of the way through the volume, in an entry relating to the first year for which he shares highlights from his diary. This is when she accompanied him and some of his other friends on an excursion to Oxford in 'the latter end of June 1780' [50]. This demonstrates that they were already socialising when he turned 12 and she was 15. Another of their companions that day was 'Miss Sheppard', almost certainly Sarah Shepherd who would be a witness at their wedding. Savory accompanied his grandfather to London on 11 September 1781, on what was the boy's first visit to the capital. They went by the 'Wantage Stage' via Nuffield, Nettlebed, Fairmile, Henley, Hurley Bottom and Maidenhead [54]. They stayed with Savory's sister, Sarah, who was on board wages at Lady Head's London residence on Park Street, Mayfair. A couple of days earlier, on the 9th, they had visited or passed Wallingford, Crowmarsh Gifford, Ewelme, North Stoke and Hailey, and the following day they 'went to [North] Moreton to see Mr Tyrrel', presumably Savory's future father-in-law, a reference which suggests a connection between the two families [54]. After all, Savory's grandfather was born and grew up in South Moreton.

Although Savory does not refer to Mary or her family for a further seven-and-a-half years, it is evident that their attachment was romantic when, 'the day before Valentines Day' in 1789, the 20-year-old Savory, then a medical student living in London, wrote Mary a devoted love-letter [200]. After receiving the desired encouragement a week later, he quickly sent a long reply packed with ardent superlatives, despite a promise not to flatter her. He copies out both of his letters in full, but not hers [200-201, 201-203]. By June he had returned to Brightwalton as a member of the Corporation of Surgeons. He writes, 'I went to Moreton to see my Wife as is now for the first time and received such encouragement as every person ought who is sincere and behaves with Honour' [212]. His earnestness is undeniable, and the phrase 'for the first time' presumably indicates that this was their first meeting since he had declared to her the nature of his feelings. A month or two later he writes, 'I went to Moreton feast and came home to Brightwaltham the next Morn[in]g' [214]. If he went to bed, and did not party all night, there is the question of where he slept, but in the absence of evidence to the contrary we should probably assume that he continued to behave with honour (to use his word). A two-year courtship seems to have ensued, at the end of which, at a time, and in a place and manner he does not disclose, Savory presumably proposed. He bought a marriage licence on 3 September 1791 from Rev. Danvers Graves (1750-1805), the curate of St Mary's Church, Chieveley, at a cost of £1 12s 6d [257]. On the same date he records, 'Bo[ugh]t a Ring of Thomson the Jeweller for 9/' [257]. Savory refers to Thomson in 1787, when he bought some engraving tools from Thomson's apprentice, but apart from knowing that he was based in Newbury we know nothing more either of the jeweller or of what we must presume was Mary's wedding ring [145]. The expenditure seems modest – Savory spent more than three times as much on a lancet the same day – but he had many expenses at this point, as he was setting up his new medical practice and a new home in newly-purchased premises on Newbury's Bartholomew Street.

Savory made an agreement on 17 March 1791 to buy the house for £252 from William Adnam of Leckhampstead [246-247]. On 28 April he agreed to buy the washing copper, locks and bells from Adnam, too [248]. By the 23rd he had contracted local tradesmen: Charles Hamlin to do the carpentry, Thomas Whitewood the glazing, George Brown the brickwork, and Daniel Brown the painting [247]. Hamlin and George Brown were paid £31 and 19 guineas respectively on 8 July for their work [254]. In April Savory bought four 'Bath Stove grates' and contracted a Mr Davies – probably William Davis, an upholsterer and cabinet maker in Newbury – 'to paper the two Chambers', and on the 19th paid him £5 11s 8d for his work [247, 251]. On 24 August Davi(e)s 'put up' the 'new bedstead & furniture […] in the best Room' [257]. A different upholsterer and cabinet-maker, John Webb, furnished Savory's dining-room on 2 September [257]. On 2 June Savory had purchased glasses from Robert Gosling, and he comments that he had by this time moved nearly all of his belongings to his 'intended habitation' at Newbury [253]. His servant, apprentice and sister Jenny joined him at Bartholomew Street on 11 July, though probably not to stay there, since it is not until the 20th that Savory remarks, 'this Evening I slept at Newbury at my new Habitation & the 21st I opened shop being Markett Day' [255]. On 28 July all the legal matters between Adnam, Savory, and Uncle John Savory (who seems to have acted as a guarantor) were settled with the solicitor, John Blagrave, and sealed with the payment of a £200 bond [255]. Savory participated in 'Bartholomew fair' on 5 September, when the tradesmen based on Bartholomew Street, plus 'a few others keeps feast from one house to the other' [258].

When Savory married on 8 September 1791, he 'entered into a new life' and began writing the volume transcribed in its entirety and published for the first time on the following pages [258]. Full of incident and variety, it tells a revealing and entertaining coming-of-age story steeped in the life of the community. It is the record of how the son and grandson of village wheelwrights strove to become a professionally accredited, fully qualified surgeon-apothecary and man-midwife. In 1789 Savory told his future wife that it was his mission to 'study the good of [his] fellow creatures in regard to [his] business' and profession [203]. As we accompany him on his journey – on his multiple journeys – we are transported back to the late eighteenth century. We see the people, places and events of Berkshire and London through his eyes. The view he affords us is remarkable.

Editorial Note

The document

William Savory's Commonplace Book (RBA D/EX2275/1) is an octavo volume with calf boards. It is intact and in good condition. The pages of the volume were numbered sequentially by Savory from [2-268]. However, the extent of the volume is 262 pages (excluding one blank). The title-page is not numbered. Pages [11-14], [37-40], and [111-114] are missing, apparently cut out before the volume was deposited in an archive: it was noted in the catalogue entry at Reading Local Studies Library when I first consulted the document in 1993 that the pages were missing. Page numbers 168, 169 and 267 were mistakenly used twice by Savory, and are represented here as [168a], [169a] and [267a], and [168b], [169b] and [267b] respectively. The first and final two pages of the MS were not numbered by Savory but are represented here in additional standard brackets as [(1)], [(270)] and [(271)] respectively, in line with Savory's sequence.

Parts of the MS appeared in print in G. C. Peachey, *The Life of William Savory, Surgeon, of Brightwalton (with Historical Notes)* (1904). Peachey includes: Savory's list of books [70]; his letter to Ebenezer Sibly [134-135]; his breaking of David Jones's shop window [121]; his learning of French [123] and of etching and engraving [117]; the number of pubs Savoy counted on a coach journey from Speenhamland to Hyde Park Corner [125]; David Jones's witchcraft prescriptions: to buy a spirit [115], to appear invisible [116], also 'Abracadebra' [160], 'Kalendenta' [161] and 'SATOR' [159]; Savory's agreements to provide medical services to the poor of Leckhampstead and Farnborough [250] and Savory's professional advertisement in the *Reading Mercury* [256-257]. Peachey reproduces Savory's account of his medical training in London verbatim [172-211] though he excludes the full list of Cline's lectures on Anatomy and Surgery [175-178], and Savory's love-letters to his future bride, Miss Tyrrell [200-203]; additionally, Peachey omits five references for reasons of taste and decency (according to the conventions of his day) namely to a case of ulcerated penis, of venereal disease, and the discovery of a pre-natal death, plus two mentions of the penis made in lists.

Transcription rules

This transcript reproduces the MS as exactly as possible, retaining original spellings throughout. Superscript letters have been brought down and are given in standard text. The obsolete 'ye', 'yat' and 'yan' have been replaced with 'the', 'that' and 'than' except when they occur in verse. Common contractions have not been modified. However, to avoid ambiguity, and to distinguish Savory's misspellings from abbreviations he has indicated by the use of superscripts, missing letters (especially in names) have sometimes been supplied in square brackets. Where helpful, conventional spellings have been given in italics inside square brackets.

The original MS page numbers are given in italics inside square brackets at the head of every page. Words in the MS added above or below the line are indicated by enclosure in angled brackets '<thus>'. Words deleted in the MS are struck through, '~~thus~~'. Uncertain transcriptions are indicated by a question mark at the start of the doubtful word, number, or symbol and the whole enclosed in square brackets, except in the confined space available in tabular presentations.

Capitalisation
The use of uppercase and lowercase letters follows Savory's practice. Many sentences consequently begin with a lowercase letter. However, Savory sometimes uses an intermediate letter-form at the start of words which shares characteristics of both upper- and lowercase forms: occasionally a letter resembles the shape of a lowercase letter but the size of an uppercase letter; (more often) the shape of an uppercase letter but the size of a lowercase letter. I have generally interpreted these intermediate letter-forms as uppercase letters.

Punctuation
Punctuation has sometimes been modernised: dashes, underscores and implied punctuation (for example, graphologically implied by a line-break) have often been converted to commas and full-stops, and occasionally to colons and semi-colons; and sometimes they have been interpreted as paragraph breaks for ease of reading. Additional punctuation is indicated by square brackets, and is given to clarify meaning and for ease of reading.

Symbols
Astrological symbols have been rendered in words and enclosed in braces (curly brackets) thus: '{Sun}', '{Moon}', '{Mercury}', '{Mars}' etc.

Other graphological features
No attempt has been made to transcribe or interpret data set in astrological charts, but some examples have been reproduced for purposes of illustration. Savory's own narrative interpretation of his calculations is always given in full, with symbols written out in words as explained above.

Savory seems to have abhorred blank paper and often filled the bottom of pages with horizontal lines of vertically parallel loops, and other flourishes of penmanship which are generally unremarkable, but usually mark a section break or shift of focus. These have been indicated in the transcript by a series of three centred asterisks.

Footnotes
Footnotes are intended to clarify, amplify or contextualize the content of the MS. Full source information has been provided wherever possible. Details of christenings, marriages and burials have always been taken from the relevant parish register. These have been consulted extensively in order to provide corrective or additional information relating to individuals and events. Cross-references have also been provided where useful: numbers given in square brackets refer to the original page in the MS.

William Savory's Commonplace Book

[*spine and front matter*]
[*The spine, with five raised bands, bears the title* 'Common Place Book, Wm Savory'. *The rear endpaper contains several unexplained scribbled numbers, possibly astrological calculations for the geniture horoscopes featured throughout the MS. The front endpaper bears the name* 'Henry F. Howard, 1768-1791' *in a different hand from Savory's. The years 1768-1791 evidently refer to the period of William Savory's life covered by the contents of the commonplace book. The name refers to Rev. Henry Frederick Howard MA (1844-1938), a grandson of the 5th Earl of Carlisle and Rector of All Saints' Church, Brightwalton for 61 years from 1872 to 1933. George Peachey found Savory's commonplace book in Rev. Howard's care at the turn of the nineteenth century into the twentieth. Rev. Howard and George Peachey passed the volume to the Reference Department of Reading Public Libraries in 1928. It was transferred to the Berkshire Record Office (now the Royal Berkshire Archives) in Reading in November 2011.*]

[*title-page*]

Memorandums
Memoirs, Remarks &c
on the Nativity of
William Savory[1]

Containing an Account of his Predecessors, place of Nativity, Birth, Education &c[2]

also

Notes on Anatomy, Surgery, Medicine, Midwifery, Chymistry, Astrology, Geomancy, Hystory, poetry, palmestry, Farriery[3] <u>&c</u>[4]

*   *   *

[*verso: blank page*]

---

1. The title and sub-title are separated by a thick, horizontal double line.
2. The sub-title is divided by a thin horizontal double line. Although the first use of '&c' (i.e. etc) is written correctly (as above), Savory subsequently writes an almost closed 'c' with a terminating tail that resembles '&a'. For the purposes of clarity, '&c' has been used throughout the transcript.
3. Presumably farriery in the medico-veterinary sense of treating horse diseases or injuries, but the closest Savory comes to this is in his 'Botts in a Horse' remedy [219].
4. This is underlined in the original MS.

[p. (1)]

Will[ia]m Savory[1]

Was born at Brightwalton otherwise Brickleton but more properly BrightWaltham in the County of Berks on Tuesday June 28th 1768 at 25 minutes past 12 o'Clock in the Afternoon and baptized July 25th[2] following being St James's and Leckhamstead feast day,[3] but before I enter on the Hystory of myself, shall give a description of my native parish & its Vicinity[,] 2ndly of my parents & Relations &c[,] and first of the place of my Nativity which is vulgarly cal[le]d Brickleton, in old Writings Leases &c its exprest Brightwalton otherwise cal[le]d Brickleton, but its evident that neither of these names is right, but that it has undergone variations as the names itself having no signification or meaning & its not to be wondered at as for instance[:] Blewbury derived its name from Blow to the *[p. 2]* Berry or Bury; Newbury from New Berry or Bury.[4] in former days Newbury dead was carr[ie]d to Blewbury to be interrd, and by blowing a Horn or Trumpett Blewbury people used to know of the dead being near at the place so that Blewbury derivd its name from Blow to the Bury & Newbury from its being a new burial place in them days,[5] and as I said before it is not to be wondered at that any one should object to the names of Brightwalton or Brickleton as it has no meaning and to corroborate this opinion it has been inspected by Mr Boucher[6] Rector of that parish who have old writings in his possession which was written many Centurys ago that the proper name is BrightWaltham and that Bright, signifies pleasant and Waltham a Retreat among Woods (viz) a pleasant retreat among Woods, which in former days it was not wrong named (nor is it now).[7]

---

1. 'Willm Savory' is written in a form of classic blackletter Gothic calligraphy, similar in appearance to the 'Old English Text' font now widely available in digital formats: Savoy has incorporated his name into an elaborate flourish of swirling loops, tied bow motifs and wavy lines; it takes the form of a headpiece and represents some accomplished penmanship (see cover illustration).

2. Here, and occasionally elsewhere in the MS, Savory's ordinal indicator appears to spell -rd when -th, -nd or -st would be correct. For the purposes of clarity, when an ordinal indicator is supplied the correct suffix has been adopted in the transcript.

3. Leckhamsptead (nearly always spelt by Savory without the 'p') is a neighbouring and contiguous parish to the south of Brightwalton. Its church is dedicated to St James, whose feast day is celebrated on 25 July (the birthday of Savory's father and his parents' wedding anniversary).

4. Blewbury, a village five miles south-west of Wallingford, is situated on the Ridgeway.

5. This toponymy is faulty: 'bury' does not signify burial ground. Margaret Gelling traces the origin of Blewbury to *Bleoburg*, and explains that the village was 'named from the hill-fort on the parish boundary, the hill now called Blewburton Hill'. The name is a compound of Old English words meaning 'variegated' and 'fort'. The former was possibly derived from the 'creamy-white chalk soil' giving the hill a variegated appearance when it was first cultivated. She traces the origin of Newbury to *Neuberie*, straightforwardly, 'new market-town'. See M. Gelling, *The Place-Names of Berkshire, Part 1* (English Place-Name Society, xlix) (Cambridge, 1973), 151-152, 257.

6. This is Richard Boucher (1752-1841), Rector of Brightwalton from 1778 to 1841.

7. Though arguably an attractive interpretation, this is toponymically flawed. Gelling traces the origin of the name to *Beorhtwaldingtune*, i.e. 'Estate associated with Beorhtwald', see Gelling, *Place-Names of Berkshire*, 237.

The Village itself was very wooddy. Trees very numerous. Ash Close was then a Copse but now Arable Land. it is likewise situated in a very Wooddy Country which makes it very pleasant during the Hunting season.[1]

[*p. 3*] Brightwaltham is situated 9 Miles from Newbury, 6 Mile from Wantage 8 Computed Miles from Lamborn and 5 Mile from East or Markett Ilsley. its bounded on the North by Farmbro',[2] on the South by Leckhamstead[,] on the East by peasemore[,] it being computed 2 Miles to Farmbro' 2 Miles to peasemore 1½ Mile to Leckhamstead 1 Mile to Chaddleworth[.] on the west of Brightwaltham is the seat of Bartholomew Tipping Esqr cal[le]d Woolly park[.][3] at the time of my birth Sam[ue]l Eyre Esqr was Lord of the Manor of Brightwaltham and Mr Elderton his Steward.[4] Richd Selwood Esqr Captain of the Berkshire Militia[5] since Colonell, Occupied the Manor Farm[6] and Richd Eyre D.D. was Rector.[7] Brightwalton in former days <was> a very flourishing Village[.] a great many freehold and lifehold Estates were occupied by the owners but are since mostly of them fell in the Lord of the Manors hands and occupied with the Manor Farm[.] I have heard my predecessors say that Money in this place was very plenty and trade very brisk, every [*p. 4*] Labouring person had good Victuals & a Barrell of good Beer at tide time[,][8] but now they thinks themselves well off if they can get Bread & Small Beer.

I shall next treat of my parents and 1st of my Grandfather William Savory who was a Native of South Moreton[,][9] Born Oct[obe]r 4th 1696 and was

---

1. The Old Berkshire Hunt dates to 1830, but the county is said to have been hunted from 1760. See F. C. Loder-Symonds and E. Percy Crowdy, *The History of the Old Berks Hunt, 1760-1904* (1905).
2. Savory most often refers to the village of Farnborough as Farmbro', but sometimes begins with a lowercase 'f'.
3. Woolley is a tithing in the parish of Chaddleworth, on the north-west edge of Brightwalton. Woolley Park became the seat of the Tipping family in 1566. It later passed to the Wroughton family (see below).
4. Probably Joseph Elderton, an attorney.
5. Lt-Col. Richard Sellwood (1716-1776) died in Brightwalton and was buried at St Barnabas's Church, Peasemore, on 28 October 1776.
6. The Manor Farm was next to the small Saxon All Saints' Church. The house was rebuilt in the nineteenth century, and all that remains of the church, which was demolished and replaced in 1863, is the churchyard with some remarkably well-preserved eighteenth and early nineteenth-century gravestones, including Savory's.
7. The relationship between Brightwalton and the Eyre family dates back to the late seventeenth century. The first Eyre landlord was Sir Samuel Eyre (1633-1698), a judge of the King's Bench in the reign of William III, who acquired the manor through marriage to Dame Martha, one of the daughters of Francis Lucy and his wife, Elizabeth, née Molesworth. The family supplied the parish with three successive Rectors: Sir Samuel's son, Francis Eyre DD (1670-1738), served the parish from 1722 until his death. He was succeeded by Samuel Eyre, Rector from 1738 to 1743 and Rev. Dr Richard Eyre (d. 1778), mentioned by Savory, who was Rector from 1743 until his death on 1 February 1778. In 1800 Susannah Eyre (1755-1833), a great granddaughter of Sir Samuel Eyre, sold the estate to the Rev. Philip Wroughton (1758-1812), a member of an extensive landowning family who had married Mary Anne Musgrave (c1767-1841), the niece of Bartholomew Tipping of Woolley Park (Savory notes their marriage [153]).
8. i.e. at harvest time around the end of September.
9. South Moreton, a small village three miles south-west of Wallingford.

Son of William and Joan Savory[,][1] so that for four Generations the name of William has been the first in the family.[2] my Grandfather Savory's friends dying[3] he apprenticed himself to one Gray[,] a Wheelright at Brightwaltham (a predecesssor to Joseph Gray now living in the Upper street at Brightwalton[)] and at this House my Grandfather served part of his Apprentiship. his Master dying or leaving off business my Grandfather commenced Master Wheelright[,] I think before he served all his time as an apprentice and bought the House cal[le]d Old Grays (life holding) where my father & friends have lived <ever> since, and he sold a House in South Moreton at [*p. 5*] that time to pay for the new purchase.[4] at that time the Meadow was an Orchard[,] the House having no Parlour nor Cellar[,] but since my father built a Parlour, Cellar, Chamber & Wellhouse and my Uncle John Savory since my fathers decease built a brewhouse. my Grandfather soon after he commenced Master Wheelright took him an Apprentice which was one Thos Mashall and since kept an Alehouse at Wickham in the parish of Wellford[.][5]

I remember of hearing my Grandfather talk of going to London the first time with Thos Finmore[6] (who was a Lad about the age of my Grandfather and was father to this present Thos Finmore of Fulscot in the parish of South Moreton)[.][7] they seeing some potatoes in a Markett thought that they were strange Turnips & my Grandfather brought the first potatoes into [*p. 6*] Brightwalton[,][8] which was sent by him from London as a present from the Lord of the Manor to Mr Selwood (the late Colonel Selwoods father)[.] My Grandfather Wm Savory was Married to Mary Lucas of Sheeplease at Beedon Church[,][9] by whom he had two Sons (viz) William my father and my Uncle John[.] my father was the eldest and both learnt the Art of

1. According to the parish register, William Savo*u*ry, the son of 'William and *Jone* Savory' was baptised 10 October 1696: the entry notes that he was born *3* October, *not* 4 as stated here.
2. The name William would endure for a further two generations beyond Savory himself, providing six consecutive generations of William Savorys.
3. William Savoury (Savory's great-grandfather) was buried at South Moreton on 9 March 1698. Jone/Joan's burial record has not been traced.
4. RBA D/EW/T28 includes several leases and agreements relating to Old Gray's. One agreement between Gray and Robert Eyre, another between Robert Eyre and William Savory, are both dated 1737. The file also includes renewals of this latter agreement between the Savory and Eyre families dated 1770 and 1773. The house survives, though much altered, and is known today as White Cottage.
5. Wickham, near Newbury, is now divided from Welford by the M4 motorway, the two villages being joined by a viaduct. The alehouse was possibly The Five Bells.
6. Thomas Finmore was born at South Moreton on 17 April 1697, the son of William and Margaret Finmore. He appears to have died in 1771.
7. Fulscot is one of the four manors of South Moreton. Thomas Finmore Jnr, the son of Thomas and Martha Finmore, was baptised at South Moreton on 16 September 1745 and appears to have been buried there in 1799.
8. George Peachey estimates the year as 1715. See G. C. Peachey, *The Life of William Savory, Surgeon, Of Brightwalton* (1903), 4*n*.
9. In fact, William Savory, a wheelwright resident at Brightwalton, and Mary Lucas, resident at Peasemore, married by licence at St Leonard's Church, Wallingford, on 7 September 1724. Their bondsman was Paul Higgins, a basketmaker in Wallingford. Mary was, however, baptised at St Nicholas's Church, Beedon, on 2 April 1706 and buried there on 17 August 1731, aged 25. For more on the Lucas family see [30] and section iii of the introduction, and for more on 'Sheeplease', see section iii of the introduction.

Wheelright. My Grand Mother dying whilst my father and Uncle were very young which was in the Year 1731, my Grandfather soon grew tired of being a Widower[,] was Married again to Susannah Taylor of Fawly the next Year which was Aug[u]st 24 1732.[1] she was Aunt to this present Thos Taylor of Brightwaltham Holt and who keeps the Marquiss of Grandby.[2] they were Married very private unknown to any of the Neibours for Mr Bridegroom[,] taking the Baskett of Tools at his back pretending to mend [*p. 7*] the Church Rails & Mrs Bride no way at a loss to be likewise private & when the ceremony was finishd he went home with his baskett of Tools at his back and she to her brothers at fawly. now her brother Thomas Taylor with whom she lived was gone to Markett & did not know of it till a few days after. they lived together 36 Years, she dying in Feb[rua]ry 1768[.][3] she was a very good living Woman[,] was a tender Mother in law[4] to my father and Uncle & I beleive my Grandfather had £100 Fortune with her & a great many Goods. when my Father Married, Grandfather & G.Mother removd to a small tenement which belonged to one Dame Hatt her Widowhood[,] after her death to Richard Ward & at this time his Son Richard Ward who lives now at Anvills Farm. My Grand Mother in law was interrd in Brightwaltham Church Yard and a Tomb Stone was erected but since is taken [*p. 8*] down[.] on it was the following Verse –

A Vertuous Wife, A faithfull friend
A Tender Nurse and Mother
Was buried here with daily Care
Her temper was no other
Her study was for peace & love
A Quiet composed mind
Her faith was built on Jesus Christ
A place of rest to find.

When my Grandfather dyed my Uncle John had a large horizontal Stone erected & the others taken away.[5] my Grandfather lived in peace & happines till the day of his Death which was on Feb[rua]ry 5th 1786 being in the 90th

---

1. This is Susannah Taylor, daughter of John and Susannah Taylor, baptised at St Mary's Church, Fawley, on 16 October 1687. Fawley, sometimes called Great or North Fawley, is a village in the hundred of Kintbury Eagle, four miles south of Wantage. Little (or South) Fawley and Whatcombe are hamlets.
2. This is Thomas Taylor (c. 1731-1813). The Marquis of Granby at Brightwalton Holt ceased trading in the 1980s and the building was converted into two cottages. See J. Osment, S. Sayers and J. Stephens, *Brightwalton, A Downland Village* (Oxford, 2002), 56.
3. Susannah Savory, née Taylor, was buried in Brightwalton, on 21 February 1768.
4. i.e. step-mother.
5. The inscriptions on several of the Savory gravestones are recorded in a file of miscellaneous parish records for Brightwalton, RBA D/EW/O8 (Brightwalton Records), 9-10. This horizontal stone has survived, but the inscription is severely worn and only partially legible: 'Sacred / In the Memory of / WILLIAM SAVORY / who [departed this Life] 1786 / In the 90th Year of his Age / Also of SUSANNA Wife / of WILLIAM SAVORY / who departed this life 1768 / In the [*illegible words*] | Year of her Age / And also of WILLIAM son / of WILLIAM SAVORY / who departed this Life / [*illegible number*] July 1772 [*illegible words*] / also Mary [*remaining words illegible*]' (editor's transcription, 3 February 2003).

Year of his Age, having in the Year 1768 about the time of my Grandmother in laws death, the good providence to receive the sum of £2199 from a Relation deceased in London [*p. 9*] to the Taylors Family, whose name was Lennard[,] being £6653 amongst three parties (viz) My Grandfather one Share, the Taylors Family another share and Mrs Treslove the third share. had my Grandmother in law died a few days before she did my Grandfather could not have attaind none of the property. the following Letter was sent to my Grandfather respecting Lennards Estate & effects:

Sir,

I have finally got the business Valued to the claims of Mrs Savory and others out of the late Lennards Estate, settled much to my satisfaction & to the great advantage of the parties which in all have saved them many hundred pounds.

the Ballance was		£7407 4s 4d.
Due to Mr Harcourts Estate	£614 7s 0d	£754 10s 9d
Exleys Bill & expense	£140 3s 9d	(£6653 0s 0d.)
	£754 10s 9d	£6653

Mr Savorys share	£2217 13s 4d
Mrs Treslove share	£2217 13s 4d
Taylors family in 6 <parts>	£2217 13s 4d
	£6653 0s 0d

[*p. 10*] Out of Mr Savorys share his Bill for Costs in equity is £18 12s 8d.
  John Exley[1]
   Lincolns Inn, April 30. 1776.

My Grandfather Wm Savory was a person of a Tall Stature[,] big bon[e]d[,] no way inclind to Corpulency, Rather handsome countenance with a King Wms Nose[.][2] his chief employment during my remembrance was sawing[,] Cleaving & Cording Wood for sale & keeping the Tools & shop in good Condition and what was very singular he could see to whet & sett a saw without spectacles almost to the day of his death. he used to read two or three times a day[:] his chief books was the Bible, Whole-duty of Man & Beveridges Festivals & Fasts.[3] indeed he was a good living Man, Charitable &c[,] was a great smoker, good Companion, could sing Songs, tell Stories or Jests. he used to go to London every Year and stay there a Week[.] his

---

1. There appears to have been a John Exley, gent., based at Furnival's Inn in 1758: West Yorkshire Archive Services, Tong/3/632.
2. William III was renowned for his beaked nose.
3. *The Whole Duty of Man* was a popular and influential high-church devotional work, first published in 1658. William Beveridge (1637-1708), the Bishop of Asaph, Wales, was the author of several important devotional and liturgical works, including collections of his sermons.

Quarters was at the Black Lion Water lane[.][1] one time when he went to London he bought for myself & Sisters a Bible, prayer Book and Whole Duty

[pp. 11-14 are missing, cut from the MS]

[*p. 15*] There was a Young Woman who had been lately Married went home to see her relations. she seemed remarkable low in spirits so that her mother took notice of it & insisted upon knowing the reasons why she was so Melancholy. sais she, Mother I'm affraid to tell. Why do pray tell me. sais she I'm like to live a develish life. how so daughter, do pray make haste and tell me. Why if I must tell. my husband won[']t give me time to say my prayers. Ah! ha! says the Old Woman[,] make thy self contented he'll [?Come] of that.

I shall now take leave of my Grandfather Wm Savory and treat of my Father.[2]

[*p. 16*] My Father Wm Savory was born at Brightwaltham on July 25th 1725[.] the first remarkable instance I have heard tell of my father was he could read a Chapter in the Bible at 4 Years of Age and was so ready in Arithmetics that he could tell his Sums as fast as Old Mr Nelstone could set them so that at last his Scooldmaster would have him no longer (this John Nelstone was a great schollar and used to keep the free school at Chaddleworth[)].[3] a little before he resigned the school he was got so infirm and almost for the 2nd time a Child that the schollars used to play tricks with him: put pins in his Cushion &c, Dumbledors [*i.e. a cockchafer (beetle)*] &c. in his Wig. he used to wear a great Coat in the Winter to keep the Cold out and a great Coat in the Summer to keep the Sun off.[4]

[*p. 17*] As my father encreased in Years the same was his ingenuity. for soon as he left school be [*sic*] began his trade a Wheelright and in a little time he was one of the Quickest & best Workman [*sic*] my Grandfather had got. My father was Married on the 25th day of July 1755 to my Mother who was Jane Barratt[,] daughter of Thomas & Miriam Barratt of Henly farm in the parish of Shefford.[5] My father then commenced Master Wheelright and agreed to allow my Grandfather 10 pounds a Year for the use of the Stock in trade &c. when my Grand Mother in law died, Grandfather lived with my

---

1. The Black Lion was on Water Lane, which led south mid-way along Fleet Street towards White Friars Docks, west of Blackfriars Bridge. Water Lane has evolved into modern-day Whitefriars Street. John Bishop's Stage Coach used to call at the Black Lion, having departed the Crown Inn, Wantage, on Monday, Wednesday and Friday mornings at 6 o'clock. The Black Lion appears to have been a large early eighteenth-century inn: see W. Stow, *Remarks on London, being an Exact Survey of the Cities of London and Westminster, Borough of Southwark etc* (1722).

2. A horizontal dividing line separates this paragraph from what precedes and follows it.

3. Probably John Nelson (1673-1747), whose family first settled in Chaddleworth in the sixteenth century.

4. The remainder of the line, and a blank line below, are underlined.

5. A licence was granted for William Savory to marry Jane Barratt of Great Shefford on 5 August 1755. Thomas, the bride's yeoman father, was bondsman. Great or West Shefford lies in the Lambourn Valley.

father again[.] My father Sold all kinds of Nails, Locks &c & many things in the Ironmongering business, Wooden Ware. he also used to practice Surgery & Sold all kind of Apothecaries drugs & had printed on his Shop door:

[*p. 18*] Bleeding, Drawing of Teeth and Apothecaries Drugs Sold here. Also Dr James fever powders, Genuine Daffys Elixir, Manna, Batemans & Stoughtons Drops, Godfreys Cordial, Liquid Shell, Hoopers pills, Oils and Tinctures, Andersons Scott pills and Dr Hitchcocks Rochford Drops and pills. Eatons Styptic, Fryars Balsam,[1] Gums of all Sorts, best double distild Lavender and Hungary Water. Salts, Cordial Cephalic Snuff, Knives, Sissers [*i.e. Scissors*], Buckles, Buttons.[2]

My father used to Measure Land for 7 or 8 Miles distant from Brightwaltham and was such a pedestrian that no one could hardly walk with him without running & used to tell the Men what their work came to at the end of every land. [*p. 19*] he was excellent in Music. Used to play the Bass Vial [*i.e. viol*] at Church, and for singing Songs & Catches no one could excell him. he was a good Schollar[:] knew Algebra, Astronomy, Navigation, Dialling &c.[3] he had many Curiosities such as Electrifying Machines,[4] Air Pump, Magic Lanthorn [*i.e. Lantern*], Measuring Wheel, slight of hand implements, Theodolite, Peep Shows, Instruments for drawing &c.

he was a Tall raw bon[e]d person[,] thin Countenance, handsome but by so much study cast a Care on his brow. he was of a Merry Chearfull disposition[,] a real friend to every one[,] beloved by all that knew him that his name still becomes a subject of Conversation which is 20 Years ago since

---

1. Most of these items were the popular patent medicines of the day and were often marketed as cures for a wide range of ailments. Only 'Dr Hitchcocks Rochford Drops and pills' are unfamiliar. Dr James's Fever Powder was patented by Dr Robert James (1703-1776), a physician and medical author who was a friend of Samuel Johnson: see R. Porter, *Disease, Medicine and Society in England, 1550-1860* (Cambridge, 2nd edition, 1993), 43. Bottles of [Thomas] Daffy's Elixir declared that it was 'much recommended to the public by Dr [Edmund] King, physician to King Charles II, and the late learned and ingenious Dr [John] Radcliffe': see R. Bayne-Powell, *Eighteenth-Century London Life* (1938), 230. Bateman's and Stoughton's Drops were a version of Dr Bateman's Pectoral Drop (to treat the chest and lungs): the patentee was not a physician named Bateman, but a businessman, Benjamin Okell, a partner in a large medicine distribution warehouse based in Bow Churchyard which supplied many of these medicines; [Richard] Stoughton, however, was also responsible for a popular elixir (a cordial used mainly in stomach complaints). [Thomas] Godfrey's Cordial was essentially a sedative and, like Bateman's & Stoughton's Drops, contained opium. [Baron Schwanberg's] Liquid Shell claimed, among other things, to be a 'dissolvent for the stone and gravel'. Hooper's Female Pills were patented in 1743 by John Hooper, an apothecary in Reading, and were used principally to treat irregular periods. [Patrick] Anderson's Scots (or Scotch) Pills first came on to the market in 1635, and were used as a mild laxative. Dr [Robert] Eaton's Styptic was not patented until 1857, but was frequently advertised for sale from at least 1722. Though many of these medicines remained popular late into the nineteenth century and beyond, only 'Fryars Balsam', which originated in the early eighteenth century, and came to be associated with Dr Joshua Ward, is still sold today.
2. Hungary water, which was alcohol-based, was made mainly of rosemary, and like lavender water, was a perfume. The words of the shop-door advertisement are divided from what follows by a horizontal line drawn free-hand across the page. Peachey quoted the advertisement with modernised punctuation, see Peachey, *Life of William Savory*, 5.
3. i.e. concerned with the construction of sundials.
4. Electrifying machines, usually portable and made of wood, glass and metal, were then novel but were commonly used to administer mild electric shocks as a form of medical treatment.

his death. My father had three daughters & myself[.] my Sister [*p. 20*] Sarah was born Oct[obe]r 26. 1756 at 3h 10' PM, Jane was born Oct[obe]r 10. 1760 at 11h 25' Morng, and Mary was born Aug[u]st 2nd 1765, 9h 30' PM. My father had near £300 fortune with my Mother[.] he used frequently to go to London & the last time of going I beleive was owing to his death for about a Week or 10 days after he came from London he was attackd with febrile Symptoms which proved to be the Small Pox[.] he was had of in Dr Colletts[1] Chaise to a lone house in the parish of Brightwaltham cal[le]d Collins's or Sparrowbill farm[2] now belonging to John Hughes of Westbrooke and Occupied by Thos Harris.[3] notwithstanding he had proper Medical Asistance he paid the last debt of Nature on July 24th 1772 being 47 Years of Age within one day to the great grief of all who knew him. My father kept the parish Accompts [*p. 21*] And took a Copy of the Register of Marriages, Christenings & Burials in Brightwaltham parish which has been continued by my Uncle John Savory to this time[.] the following Song was composed by my father:

The Wheelright & the Blacksmith are
    Trades of great use you know
The Farmer he must have 'em both
    Before he Plow and Sow
And first a plow then he must have
    The Land then for to till
As the farmer he may sow his Corn
    His Barn then for to fill
And next a Waggon he must have
    To Carry it to the Barn
And there to make a Mow of it
    To keep it from all harm
And before the Waggon he do go,
    He must be liquord Well
[*p. 22*] By the Wheelright & the Blacksmith,

---

1. Dr John Collet (1709-1780) was, as Peachey points out, 'the most famous local physician of his time', see Peachey, *Life of William Savory*, 5. Born in London, Collet's father was a merchant and his uncle a governor in the East Indies. He was educated at Greenwich and subsequently at Trinity Hall, Cambridge. He then studied in Paris and London, and under Herman Boerhaave in Leiden. He graduated Doctor of Medicine in 1731. He became an Extra-Licentiate of the College of Physicians in 1733. He spent six years in Brentford and Uxbridge but settled in Newbury where he was a member of the Presbyterian chapel and a close friend of its pastor, David James, who published a sermon on the occasion of Collet's death entitled 'The good Christian, happy in death'. Collet was described as enjoying a large practice in the town and was 'looked up to with the reverence given to patriarchs of old', *Newbury Weekly News* (24 July 1884). See also *Correspondence of the Foundling Hospital Inspectors in Berkshire, 1757-68*, ed. G. Clark (Berkshire Record Society, i, 1994). For Savory's own successful treatment by Dr Collet, see [44].
2. Sparrowbill is in the east of the parish towards Peasemore.
3. This is Thomas Harris (1734-1813). Savory refers to the Hughes family again: Jenny Jones (1750-1795), the wife of David Jones (d. 1793), to whom Savory was apprenticed as a surgeon-apothecary in 1783, was a member of the Hughes family, see [121, 139]. For other references to the Hughes family see [142, 254].

As I to you may tell
O then this Waggon may be used
To Carry it to the Barn[1]
And there to make a Mow of it
To keep it from all harm
O then the Thresher he must come
    His frail [*sic*] must swiftly swing,
And if the Corn it does yield well
Twill make the farmer sing
Then to the Markett he must go
    His Corn there for to sell
And if it carries a good price
    Twill Chear his heart full well
Now to conclude and end my Song
    Homeward then we must go
God prosper all the farmers Works
    And likewise speed the Plows[2]

[*p. 23*]
                1
There was a Jolly Blade[3]
And he Married a Country Maid
And safely conducted her home
She was neat in every part
Which pleasd him to the heart
But Alah! and Alas! she was dumb

                2
She's as blythe as the May
And as fair as the day
And as round and as plump as a plumb
But still the silly swain
Could do nothing but complain
Because that his Wife she was dumb

                3
She could Brew and she could Bake
She could Sow and she could shape
She could sweep the house wth the Broom
She could Wash & she could Wring,
She could do any thing
But Alah and Alas she was Dumb.[1]

---

1. The inconsistent tabulation is true to the original MS.
2. The remainder of the page is filled with a simple, horizontal double-line, drawn free-hand.
3. Though no title is given, each of the eight stanzas is numbered. It is a variation on the traditional, anonymous ballad 'The Dumb Maid' dating from the late 1670s: see the *English Broadside Ballad Archive* <https://ebba.english.ucsb.edu/ ballad/31276/citation> (accessed 1 December 2022).

[*p. 24*]

4

To the Doctor then he went
To give himself Content
And to Cure his Wife of the Mums
O it is the easiest part
That belongs unto our Art
For to make a Woman speak that is Dumb.

5

To the Doctor he did her bring
And I Cut her Chattering string
And att [*sic*]t Liberty I set her Tongue
Her tongue began to Walk
And she began to talk
As tho' she had never been dumb

6

Her faculty he tries
And she fills the House wth Noise
And she Rattles in his Ears like a Drum
She bred a deal of Strife
Made him weary of his life
He'd give any thing again she was Dumb

7

To the Doctor then he goes
And thus he vents his Woes
Oh! Doctor you have me Undone
[*p. 25*] For my Wife is turnd a scold
Her tongue will never hold
I'd give any thing again she was Dumb

8

When I did Undertake
For to make thy Wife to speak
It was a thing easily done
But its past the Art of Man
Let him do what e're [*sic* he can
For to make a scolding Woman hold her tongue[2]

The following petition is a Copy written by my father & the Money gathered
by him:

---

1. The remainder of the page is filled with a single horizontal line drawn free-hand to resemble
   the shape of an elegant stretched moustache.
2. The verse is divided from what follows by a single line drawn free-hand horizontally across
   the page.

March 31st 1755

For the better performance of Church Music in the parish Church of Brightwalton the Singers are very desirous of having a Bass Vial (or some instrument) for the use and ease of the [*p. 26*] Choir, hoping it will not be disagreeable to any of the Congregation, & for the encouragement of so usefull an instrument, they had agreed to raise by subscription the money to purchase it. But the most part of them (as we call 'em) day labouring people they could not afford to give any large Sum & so not being able of themselves to purchase such an instrument. But still they are not quite in despair – hoping that the Gentlemen and farmers of the said parish will Contribute toward the purchase and in so doing the Choir will return them their most Humble thanks and be highly obliged to them for such a favour.

If Vocal Music be not full enough let the instrumental be added, they have in their hands the harps of God, and sing the Song of Moses and the Lamb,[1] saying

[*p. 27*] Great and Marvelous are thy Works Lord God Almighty Revelations Ch. xv Ver 2.3

Praise the Lord upon the Harp, sing unto him with the Psaltery and an Instrument of ten strings. Sing him a new song, play skilfully with a loud Noise.

Psalm xxxiii V.2.3

Take a Psalm bring hither the timbrel, the pleasant Harp with the Psaltery.

Psalm lxxxi V 2

It is a good thing to give thanks unto the Lord, And to sing praises unto thy name, O most high, to show forth thy loving kindness in the morning and thy faithfullness every night upon an instrument of ten strings upon the Harp with a solemn sound.

Ps. xc V I. II. III

With Trumpets and sound of Cornet make a Joyfull Noise before the Lord the King.

Ps. xcviii V. 7

[*p. 28*] Let them praise his Name in the Dance. At them sing praises unto him with the timbrel and Harp.

Ps 149. V 3

Praise him with the timbrel & Dance, Praise him with stringed Instruments and Organ, Praise him upon the loud Cymbals, Praise him upon the high sounding Cymbals[,] praise ye the Lord.

Ps cl. V iv, v, vi[2]

---

1. A song proclaiming the greatness, majesty, power and dominion of God (Revelation 15).
2. These Biblical verses are divided from what follows by a simple horizontal line drawn free-hand.

The Money subscribed from the Farmers &c.

Mr Hatt	10/6		1 3/4
Mr Blackney	5/0	L. Fulbrook	1/6
			1 4/10
Winkworth	1/6		
Wm Horn	2/0	Money subscribd from the Singers	
G. Barnett	0/6	Singers	
J. Alfridge	0/6	Wm Savory	2/6
Jn Norris	1/0	Arthur Whiter	2/6
Wm Fuller	1/0	John Savory	2/0
James White	0/3	Thos Taylor	1/6
Somebody	0/4	John Holmes	1/6
Stephen Taylor	0/6	John Venn	1/0
Ann Hind now Mrs Church	0/3	F. Purton	1/0
		Thos Coventry	1/0
	1.3.4[1]		13/0

[p. 29]

	13/0		1 1/4
Wm Wakefield	1/0	J. Aldridge	1/0
John Bird	2/6	J. Bennett	1/0
Richd Spokes	1/0	Moses Bond	1/0
Ed. Tame[2]	1/0	Thos Pettitt	1/0
Henry Horton	2/6		1 5/6
	1.0.6[3]		1 4/10

Money subscribd in all	£2 10/4

(Cost £3.3.0. & my father paid the remainder)
My father playd upon this Bass Vial some Years at Church he then bought another which is now at Brightwaltham. this subscription Bass Vial being out of repair my Uncle John sold it to John Sly of Wanbro' for 16/.[4] Uncle Jn was 6/ expense with it before he sold it besides finding Strings &c for some Years before.[5]

Soon as my father dyed my Uncle John Savory commenced Master Wheelright which brings me to consider a few remarks concerning him.

*   *   *

---

1. i.e. £1 3s 4d.
2. The RAI shows that Edward Tame was apprenticed as a wheelwright to William Savory in March 1754.
3. i.e. £1 0s 6d.
4. This is John Sly (1736-1784) of Wanborough, a village near Swindon in Wiltshire.
5. A short broken line separates this from what follows.

[*p. 30*] My uncle John Savory was born July 27th 1727 and baptized Aug[u]st 6th following. Was apprenticed to his father to learn the Art of Wheelright, tho' he was to have been a Watchmaker had his Uncle Lucas been according to his Word who was a Watchmaker in Newbury and at the time my Uncle was with him which was when he was quite young Mr Linch was at that time 'prentice to him.[1] My Uncle John went with his Uncle Lucas to London whilst he was with him at Newbury[:] he remembers hearing Cherries cryd a farthing pr lb. he is not of so ready a Genious as my father was. was a very good Workman when in his Youthfull days but Mr Work and my Uncle disagreed when he had the misfortune to Cut his finger and a profuse Haemorrhage ensued[.] on that account he made a Vow never to wear an Apron any more. he was very fond of Card playing, Dancing &c. him with more of his Companions went [*p. 31*] to Morris Dancing, and ornamented themselves with Snail Shells instead of Bells[.] their squire was one Robt Brown, who lived at a little Cottage House in the Way to farmbro' & Occupied his own land since dead[;] his land is now Occupied by a Mr Harbert with the Manor Farm.[2] their Musitioner [*i.e. Musician*] was Betty the Wife of Stephen Taylor now living at Brightwaltham. My Uncle is a single man was never married[.] he sings the Bass part at Church. My Uncle bred myself & sisters up very handsome and behaved like a father to us. G.F. and Uncle Sold my fathers Electrifying machine to Mr Knight of Newbury and likewise the Air pump. The Theodilite was lost, for the last time my father went to measuring land previous to his death which was at Jn. Wards Copse now Winkworths[,] he left it somewhere and have not been heard of since. The peep Shows, Magic Lanthorn, Books, [*p. 32*] Telescopes &c are now at Brightwaltham in the possession of my Uncle. My Uncle succeeded my father in only one branch in Surgery and that was drawing of Teeth. My Mother practices Blood letting & dressing Wounds & sells medicines &c same as when my father was living[.] my uncle would play on no instruments but used to sing Songs & Healths very frequently in Company.

The Millar

There was a Millar in Devonshire
    And he had three Sons as you shall hear
And he had a mind to make his Will
    And for to give away his mill
He sending for his eldest Son
    saying my Glass is almost run
If I to thee my Mills should make
    What Toll dost thou intend to take
Father sais he my name is Dick
    Out of a bushel I'll take a peck

---

1. The RAI shows that Anthony, son of William Linch, a clothier of Newbury, was apprenticed as a clockmaker to John Lucas (1708-1741) at Newbury in May 1735. For more on John Lucas, see section iii of the introduction.
2. This is now known as Brown's Lane. Farnborough is a small village on the Ridgeway, five miles south-west of Wantage, and nine miles north of Newbury. It lies at the highest point of the Downs, and is contiguous with Brightwalton which lies to its south.

Out of every bushel that I do grind
   That I may a good living find
Thou silly Dog the Old man Cryd,
   Now thee hast not got thee half thy trade
[p. 33] For by this Toll no man can live
My mill to thee I ne'er will give
He sending for his second Son, saying,
 Father sais he my name is Ralph
Out of a bushell I will steal half
Out of every Bushell that I do grind
That I may a good living find
Thou silly dog the Old man Cryd
Now thee has not got thee all thy trade
For:
He sending for his Youngest Son, Saying,
Father sais he I'm a Jolly Blade
By taking Toll it is my trade
Before that I will live to lack
I'll take the Corn & foreswear the Sack
Well Done Well Done the Old man Cryd
Now thou hast got thee all thy trade
The Mills be thine and all beside
So the Old man closed his Eyes & dyed.

*   *   *

[p. 34] The following Verse was composed over A cup of Tea by my Uncle
J[oh]n and Sister Jenny
One Sunday morn sometime ago
Uncle & I was at Breakfast & so
Uncle had Cake and Spirrit
And I had Bread & Butter
And besides all that we could not agree
For Uncle had Coffee & I had Tea.

    I shall now treat of my Mothers family and first of my Grandfather Thomas Barratt who was born at Eastgarison [i.e. East Garston] in this County[.][1] he had three Brothers[:] John, Richard and Anthony. they were all Blacksmiths except Richd who was apprenticed to a Carpenter at Lambourn[.] he had likewise two Sisters, Hannah and Jane. My Grandfather Barratt was Married to Miriam Ambrose[,] daughter of Farmer Ambrose of Maidencourt farm in Eastgarston parish.[2] [p. 35] Hannah Barratt was Married

---

1. For the Barratt family, see section iii of the introduction.
2. Maidencourt or Maidencott Farm on the River Lambourn and Newbury Road, East Garston, survives and lies towards Great Shefford. It was once the property of lawyer and MP, Sir

to William Palmer of Fawly who used to Occupy a Farm in little Fawly now Occupied by Pocock and Grandfather went partners with his Brother in law palmer[,] and there my Mother Jane Barratt was born[,][1] but disagreed and my Grandfather took Henly farm[2] and there my three Uncles was born. William Palmer was 20 Years older than his Wife Hannah Barratt for when she was carrying to be Christened, Wm was threshing in the Barn & he said if ever he had a Wife that Child should be she and so it was. this Wm Palmer was father to Mrs Stephens of Catmore.[3] Jane Barratt[,] sister to my Grandfather[,] dyed with the Small Pox when Young.[4] Richard Barratt always lived with my Grandfather. My Mother had three Brothers: Thos. Richd & Anthony. Thos. married Ann Gilman his house keeper.[5] [*p. 36*] Richard married Sarah Spirit of Eastgarison [*i.e. East Garston*] by whom he had 4 Children: Hannah, John, Miriam and Richard.

Anthony is what we may call an Oddity, no companion, neither good for himself nor nobody else.[6]

I shall now descend to my Sisters & first of my eldest sister Sarah who was near 16 Years Old when my father died[.] she soon after went to Cromarsh by Wallingford to live with Aunt Stiles who was my Grandfather Savorys sister in law[.][7] she lived there about a Year & a half but Wm Stiles son of Aunt Stiles was such an odd Crasy fellow she could live there no longer. she went next to Madam Nelstones of Chaddleworth [and] there lived a twelve month[.] from thence to Madame Batemans of Harwell[;] she staid there almost two Years. her next place was with Lady Head's at Langly[8] where she first

---

Francis Moore (1559-1621), who also held the manors of East Ilsley and North and South Fawley. For more on Maidencourt and Savory's ancestors (the Ambrose family), see section iii of the introduction.

1. Savory's mother was baptised 'Jane Barrott', the daughter of Thomas and 'Mariam', at St Mary's Church, North Fawley, on 30 April 1735. The following word in Savory's MS is underlined.
2. Henley or Henly Farm, Great Shefford, survives and nestles in the Lambourn Valley. For more on Savory's maternal grandparents, see section iii of the introduction.
3. This is Mary Stephens, née Palmer (1733-1823), see sections iii & xii of the introduction. She was born in East Garston to William and Hannah Palmer. The hamlet of Catmore, contiguous with Brightwalton (which lies to its west), is three miles west of East Ilsley. Under Edward I it had been a market town, and in Savory's day it was a small village, but it shrank in the nineteenth century to the size of a single farmstead. To its south is the hamlet of Lilley.
4. Jane Barratt seems to have been buried at East Garston on 20 January 1731, aged 22.
5. For more on Thomas Barratt and Ann Gilman, see [70].
6. In fact, when Anthony Barrett (1741-1826) died, he benefitted the poor of the parish of Great Shefford with an endowment of £100, and the remainder of his estate was shared by his surviving nephews and nieces. See section iii of the introduction.
7. One Elizabeth Stiles is noted in the South Moreton parish register, the daughter of Henry Stiles, a farmer and his wife, Ann, baptised on 2 May 1700 (born 25 April). One Clement Stiles, gentleman, left a will dated 1714, WSA P1/S/764. The precise connection with 'Aunt Stiles' is unclear.
8. This was Lady Mary Head (1700-1792) of Langley Hall, the widow of Sir Francis Head, 4th Baronet (1693-1768), of The Hermitage, Kent, an Anglican clergyman and landowner. Lady Mary was the daughter and heir of Sir William Boys MD (1655-1744), whom Peachey describes as 'an eminent physician of Canterbury', pointing out that she was also the 'great-granddaughter of Sir George Ent MD, the friend of Harvey'. See Peachey, *Life of William Savory*, 6n.

[pp. 37-40 are missing, cut from the MS]

[p. 41]
Old Farmer Hodge lookd desperate sour
And cryd when shall we dine
Quoth he tis almost foddering hour
Go Cicely milk the Kine
A Wag that in the Alley stood
Began to sham a Cough
Hold out as long as 'ere he could
And then movd slily off
The Clerks who tis full many a drone
Had lent a patient Ear
Was now himself impatient Grown
And could no longer bear
So when the fryar was at a stand
And could not make it out
The Clerk his PSalm Book took in hand,
And thus the PSalm gave out
All people that on Earth do dwell[1]
Then twangd it thro' his Nose
The Fryar he now perceivd full Well
Twas time the Book to Close
And tho' the day was long enough
For twas the Month of June
[p. 42]
Reservd the rest of his Choise stuff
Till time more Opportune
God prosper long Our Church & State
Our Wives and Children all
May ne'er again such tedious prate
poor Christian folks befall

*   *   *

My Sister Jane was near 12 Years of Age when my father dyed[.] she always lived at home till she was married which was on Sept[embe]r 13th 1786 to John Eagles[,] by trade a Carpenter[.][2] this Sister is of a good easy disposition. My Uncle Apprenticed her to Mrs Bird to learn the Art of Mantua Making and gave Mrs Bird 3 Guineas for ~~3~~ A Year. Bird then lived at Ballards Farm now Occupied by Fruin [i.e. *Frewin*] Wicks. My Sister Mary was 7 Years old When my father died. her Godfathers were Uncle Thos

---

1. i.e. Psalm 100.
2. In fact, the parish register gives Monday *11* September as the date of Jane Savory's marriage to John Eagles (c.1759-1822) and this is corroborated by a notice in the *Reading Mercury*: 'Last Monday was married, Mr John Eagles, of Brightwalton, to Miss Jane Savory, of the same place', *RM* (18 September 1786).

Barratt, Dr Sampson of Wantage,[1] Mrs the Wife of Thos [*p. 43*] Taylor of
Brightwalton holt & Molly Blackney. she was always of a contrary
disposition to myself by which reason we could never agree. my Grandfather
was at the unnessesary expense of putting her to Miss Thompsons Boarding
School at Wantage for a twelve month.[2] the 12th day of April 1784 she was
married to Jos[ep]h Norris my Uncles Apprentice. this Joseph Norris came
Apprentice to my Uncle in the Year 1778 from South Moreton[.][3] his father
died when he was very young[.] his Mother now lives at North Moreton & is
sister to Mrs Tyrell my Mother in law[.][4] I shall now take a little Account of
myself to the time my father died.

I was born June 28th 1768 and Baptized July 25th 1768 Leckhamstead
feast day by the Revd Dr Eyre then Rector of Brightwalton. My Godfathers
Was Uncle John Savory and Uncle Rd [*p. 44*] Barratt my Godmothers was
Elizth Trumplet now the Wife of Arthur Whiter & Sarah Mouldy the late Rd
Birds Widow.[5] My father kept a great merryment & invited most of his
Neibours. my fathers desire was to have my name William Doctor Jack but it
did not meet the Approbation of my Grandfather and the rest of the family as
Willm signified my Grandfather, Doctor my father and Jack my Uncle John. I
had very good health till I was 6 or 7 Months Old[,] then I was extreamly Ill.
Attended by Dr Sampson of Wantage and at two Years of Age had another
violent fit of Illness and was attended by Mr Seymour of Wantage.[6] my
friends thought Mr Seymour did not give proper treatmentsent sent for Dr
Collett of Newbury who by the blessings of God Cured me. Seymour during
his [*p. 45*] Attendance Bleed me in the Arm[.] about this time my Mothers
Uncle Richd Barratt died[.] he Was a very Choleric passionate Man and left
my three Uncle Barratts, his property[.] he used to live with my Grandfather

1. This is Cooper Sampson (1740-1776). He described himself as a surgeon and apothecary, and
   in July 1773 when two vacancies arose for the office of local coroner, he advertised for the
   job in the *RM* (2 August 1773) and *OJ* (7 August 1773). For more, see section v of the
   introduction.
2. On Miss Thompson's Boarding School, see section viii of the introduction.
3. The RAI shows that Joseph Norris was apprenticed as a wheelwright to John Savory in
   July 1779.
4. 'Mrs Tyrell', Savory's mother-in-law, married William Tyrrell at All Saints' Church, North
   Moreton, on 3 October 1745. She is described in the parish register as 'Elizabeth Eagleton of
   Brightwell'. The only plausible match is Elizabeth Egleton, daughter of Moses and J(e)ane
   Egleton, baptised in Brightwell on 26 September 1719. Her sister, Mary, was baptised on 13
   February 1709. She married James Batten at North Moreton on 27 October 1728 but Batten
   appears to have died the following year. Mary Batten then married Thomas Norris at
   Ardington on 20 September 1730. Though it is not clear where Joseph Norris was born, it
   would have been around the year 1765, when Mary was in her mid-50s, so the precise
   connection is unclear. Mary Norris was buried in North Moreton in 1792, but unfortunately
   her age at death was not recorded. William Tyrrell and Elizabeth E(a)gleton seem to have
   waited 20 years before having any children. Their daughter, Mary, whom Savory married in
   1791, was baptised at North Moreton in 1765. Her mother would have been in her mid-40s at
   that time. The Tyrrell gravestones at North Moreton have survived.
5. Elizabeth Trumplett married Arthur Whiter (c.1746-1829) at Brightwalton on 5 July 1772, and
   was buried, aged 70, on 5 January 1814. Sarah Mouldy appears to have been baptised at
   Chaddleworth on 29 June 1744, the daughter of Thomas and Ann Mouldy. She married
   Richard Bird in Brightwalton on 3 April 1771. For more on Richard Bird, see [144].
6. Edward Seymour, Surgeon and Pharmacist, is listed at Wantage in the *Medical Register* as late
   as 1779.

Barratt and was by trade a Carpenter[.][1] I went to School some time before my father died and continued till I was apprenticed except about one Years intermission to one Richard Aldridge[.][2] he was a Native of Brightwaltham and used to teach school at a well built tile House situated at the edge of Brightwaltham Common which Commons adjoins to farmbro' liberty. he was a single Man, an excellent Writer and the same in Arithmetic. Used to Measure Land after my father died. for his person & Qualities he was handsome as most Crooked people are but naturally peevish and Cross to his Schollars. in Company he was Merry and a sensible conversant. his favorite [p. 46] Song was Plato. the School was the Middle tenement and a little before his Death he built a parlour &c at the South part of his house. the upper tenement was occupied by John Norris and the tenement next the Lane by John Harris. this House belongs to the Widow Aldridge, Wife of the late Jo Aldridge, father and Mother to the School Master and lives at a public House in Baydon.[3] My little Schoolmaster died from a fall of a Horse as he was going to Penclose Wood[4] to measuring for Timothy Bew, now a farmer at Hill Green Aug[u]st 1st 1783[.] the Corpse was carried to the Boar at North Heath[5] where the Coronor & Jury Attended and brought in their Verdict Accidental Death[.] he was interrd in Brightwaltham Church Yard Aged 38 Years.[6] this Richd Aldridge used to keep the parish Accompts and soon after his Death he was succeeded by his Nephew Sam[ue]l Mitchel & now by Henry Mitchel his Brother.[7]

[p. 47] On my School Masters Tomb Stone is Written the following Verse:

Certain and Uncertain is the State of Man
Certain to Die and yet uncertain when
An instance here we have before our Eyes
How soon the Strongest Man falls sick & dies.

In the Autumn after my father died which was in the Year 1772 I was inoculated wth the Small Pox by Dr Samson of Wantage wth my three Sisters, Mr Church John Church Ann Church, Thomas Stanbrook, Thos Taylor at the Marquis of Grandby Brightwaltham Holt, Jacob Pounds Junr

---

1. For the Barratt family, see section iii of the introduction.
2. Richard Aldridge (1744-1783), the son of John Aldrige and his wife Ann, née Richards, was baptised in Brightwalton on 29 November 1744. He was succeeded as Brightwalton's schoolmaster by his nephews, Samuel and then Henry Mitchell.
3. Baydon in Wiltshire, situated between Lambourn, Berkshire and Aldbourne, Wiltshire.
4. Penclose Wood is near Winterbourne, Berkshire.
5. This is the Blue Boar Inn, North Heath on the outskirts of the parish of Chieveley, high on the Downs with a magnificent, uncluttered view of Newbury. The pub itself, an attractive thatched building, had a life-size stone Blue Boar stood outside, supposedly brought from Yorkshire by Cromwell's men and left at the inn as they camped on North Heath. The pub dates back to before the Civil War and currently (2023) operates as a fish restaurant called the Crab and Boar.
6. Brightwalton's burial register records the date as 4 August 1783. Aldridge was in fact aged 39.
7. Given that Savory claims earlier that his father and uncle kept the 'parish accompts' in Brightwalton [20-21], this presumably refers to a different parish.

and Ann Hind Niece to Mrs Church[:] in all 11 persons. Mr Samson had 2
Guineas each of us Medicines included except my Sister Mary[,] she being
his God Daughter was Inoculated Gratis[.] we had the SmallPox [*sic*] all of
us very favorable at a House calld Collins or Sparrow Bill[,] the House where
my father died.

[*p. 48*] This Dr Samson who Inoculated Us was a particular acquaintance
of my fathers & who my father dealt with for most of his Drugs. he was a
very little Man & used to wear three or four pair of Stockings at a time. he
was a very merry Companion, a good Songster and died two or three Years
after my father.[1] at my Sister Marys Christening some of the Women put him
in the Cradle and almost killd him for being so Rachetty. After I was
Inoculated I kept to my School very diligent and began to make use of the
Geeses feathers in the Year 1775 before I was 7 years of Age[,] and in
Feb[rua]ry 1776 begun Arithmetic the Numeration Table[.] My Sister Mary
at that time was learning the Multiplication Table & Jenny in the Rule of
Three[,] and by the Year 1779 I was the first Schoolar in the Schoold and so
remaind till I left School.[2]

[*p. 49*]

[1780]

On 14th Feb[rua]ry 1780 Died Mr Richd Bew Schoolmaster at North
Heath[.][3] he was a good kind of a Man and went rather lame[.] He was father
to this present Rd Bew Surgeon at Thatcham.[4] In this Year the Well in the
upper street at Brightwaltham was dug by John Dolton of Leckhamstead
Egypt at voluntary contribution[.] my Uncle made the Well Carb [*sic*] &c. it
measured 82 Yards at 4/ pr Yard[.][5] this Year I began playing on the tenor
Vial at Church and Joseph Norris the Bass Vial and one Jo. Fisher a native of

1. Cooper Sampson was buried at St Peter & St Paul's Church, Wantage, on 19 February 1776.
   For more on Sampson, see section v of the introduction.
2. Savory's 'the first Schoolar in the Schoold' is curiously erroneous but there is no indication
   that he meant it ironically. A horizontal line drawn free-hand marks a section-break at the end
   of the page.
3. Richard Bew Snr was buried at St Mary the Virgin's Church, Chieveley, on 14 February 1780.
   He had been schoolmaster at North Heath since 1772: see *Berkshire Schools in the
   Eighteenth Century*, ed. S. Clifford (Berkshire Record Society, xxvi, 2019), 43.
4. The *Medical Registers* and RAI record that Richard Bew Jnr was apprenticed for five years to
   the surgeon Stephen Hemsted, at Hermitage, in May 1780, and took his own apprentice, Abel
   Bull, at Thatcham, in October 1804. An H. and S. Hemsted of the Newbury Union are
   discussed in M. Railton, *Early Medical Services: Berkshire and South Oxfordshire from 1740*
   (Cranbrook, 1994), 71.
5. RBA D/EW/O8, 234: 'The Well in the Upper Street was made in the Year 1779 by John
   Dolton of Leckhamstead which measured 84 Yards at 4/ pr. Yard & agreed to find [*sic*] the
   Well with Water for 12 Month, £16. 16. 0. The Well Curb made by John Savory 2. 12. 16.
   [Total] £19. 8. 6. Subscribers[:] Mr Herbert for Baileys, Deacons & Oakleys, 6. 6. 0.; Mr
   Stanbrook, 4. 4. 0.; Mr Blackneys for Heaths, Coopers and Rivers, 3. 13. 6.; Mr Holmes, 3. 3.
   0.; Mr Whiter, 2. 12. 6.; Mr. John Taylor, 2. 12. 6.; Revd. Mr Boucher, 2. 2. 0.; Mr Thos
   Taylor, 1. 11. 6.; Thos Henshaw Esqr for Toomlins, 1. 1. 0; [Subtotal] £27. 6. 0; Ballance, £7.
   17. 6. Fifteen Posts with Arms made and Erected in the Upper Street by John Savory at 3/9
   Each, £2. 16. 3.; Messrs Herberts & Whiter at that time Surveying of the Roads (viz)
   Oct[obe]r 10 1783. Richd Pain dug the Holes at 3d. Each, £0. 3. 9.'

Wellford and used to live wth Henry Horton[,] Blacksmith of Brightwaltham playd the Hoboy [*i.e. Oboe*]. the 14th of Dec[embe]r 1780 Was Married at Chaddleworth Mr Thos Horne[,] farmer at Brightwaltham[,] to Miss Eliz. Nelstone[,] daughter of the Old Schoolmaster[,] and gave Brightwaltham Ringers four Shillings.[1] [*p. 50*] Mr Boucher Rector of Brightwaltham[:] his first Visit was April 12th 1778[2] & Mr Herbert came to Brightwaltham to Occupy the Manor Farm in the Year 1779.[3] In April 1780 my Uncle John Savory was Inoculated for the Small Pox at farmbro'[:] at that time the whole parish of farmbro' was Inoculated by Mrs Samson & Mr Cooper of Wantage.[4] Mrs Sampson Inoculated my Uncle[.] she was the Wife of the late Mr Samson who inoculated myself and others.[5] the latter end of June 1780 I went to Oxford with Jas: Norris & Miss Sheppard, Miss Tyrrell who is since dead & my present Wife[.] we went to most of the Colleges[,] went to the printing Office and had our Names printed and gave them 6d each. I stood upon the Clapper of Great Tom & saw the two old Eagles.[6] Jos[ep]h Norris at this time had the Ague.

[*p. 51*] Soon after the Revd Mr Boucher came to Brightwaltham to reside he had a large Yew Tree cut down in the Church Yard which stood very near my families Tombs toward the South Wall.[7] it was a very pretty Tree of near 60 Years growing. Mr Boucher has made more alterations both at parsonage and Church[,] for when he became Rector of Brightwaltham he had the Commandments written in the Chancill which was before on the North Side of the Church near the Gallery[.] in the Room of the Commandments he has had some Verses written taken out of the Colossians Respecting Wives & Husbands behaviour to each other by Tarlton of Ilsley.[8] at the parsonage he hath taken down a great many Tree's [*sic*] in the Gardens & opposite the House was 4 Chestnut Trees.

---

1. In fact, the marriage took place on *12* December. Elizabeth Nelson, the daughter of John and Mary Nelson, was baptised at St Andrew's Church, Chaddleworth, on 12 June 1739.
2. RBA D/EW/O8, 234: 'The Revd Rich Boucher took possession of the Church at Brightwalton & did all the Duty himself April 12 1778.'
3. This is John Harbert (d. 1796). For more on Harbert, see [52].
4. Gilbert Cowper (1755-1799), son of the more eminent Wantage surgeon, Gilbert Cowper (1713-1779).
5. On the death of her husband, Lucy Sampson, née Spicer (1741-1821), publicly declared her intention of 'carrying on the Grocery, Stationary, and Drug Trade in all its branches, as usual, and has now laid in an entire fresh Stock of every Article, so that the Public may depend on being served with the best Commodities on the lowest Terms, and their favours will be most gratefully acknowledged': see *OJ* (30 March 1776). Mrs Sampson is listed as the sole Druggist in Wantage in the *UD*. She long outlived her husband, and was buried at St Peter & St Paul's Church, Wantage, on 26 September 1821.
6. *Old* Tom is the bell in Tom Tower, the imposing Wren-designed gateway to Christ Church College, Oxford, built in 1681-1682. The bell is still struck 101 times every evening at five past nine to recall the traditional closure of the gates to the original 101 scholars of the college.
7. RBA D/EW/O8 [*not paginated*] notes: 'The Yew Tree was Cutt Down March 15th 1779.'
8. This is Col. 3: 18-19, 'Wives, submit yourselves unto your own husbands, as it is fit in the Lord. Husbands, love your wives, and be not bitter against them.' RBA D/EW/O8, 236 notes that in 1801, 'the Verses in the Church new written & some of the old Letters new Coloured by Josh. Norris' as part of more extensive Church repairs.

[*p. 52*] Mr Harbert soon after he came to reside at Brightwaltham Built a New Barn near the Church Yard also a new Granary. he had all the Land dews plowd up. a great many borders of Wood grubbed up which was opposite my fathers House. I remember the Building of Ballards Granary[:] it twas when I was quite little & Ballard put me on my head on one of the Stones saying Remember what Ballard done.

I remember seeing Richd Birds house on fire in pudding lane & it was the general opinion of the people that himself set it on fire. Our New Brewhouse was built in the Year 1781 by James Winter of Chievely[.][1] I shall now proceed regularly and begin with Memoirs during the Year 1781.

[*p. 53*]

1781

Jan[ua]ry 28th. John Cook servant boy to Mr Herbert was killd at the Chalk pit in Ash Close[,] some Chalk falling in the pit upon him[,] it being at the time the new Church road was making in Ash Close[.][2] this Spring Madam Nelstones new House in Chaddleworth Bottom Hungerford Road was built by Dan[ie]l Whistler[,] now Schoolmaster at Chadleworth[,] for the Occupation of her Tenant, Farmer Jo. Butter who used to live in the old House adjoining the Manor House at Chaddlewth.

Sept[embe]r 11th. Went with my Grandfather Savory to London and staied till the 15th being my first Visit to London[.] I made some Observations on our Journey: we first went to Wantage & slept that Night at Mrs Samsons[;] next Morning to [*p. 54*] Wallingford[;] we went to Cromarsh & Ewelm, North Stoke and Haily in Grandfathers business respecting my G. F. late Sister in Law Mrs Stiles[,] who used to live in the house adjoining the Church Yard at Cromarsh. the next day we went to Moreton to see Mr Tyrrel and the 11th in the morning we set off for London by the Wantage Stage & went thro' Nuffield, Nettlebed, Fair Mile, Henly, Hurly Bottom, Maidenhead &c. we went to park Street to my Sister Sarah who lived then with Lady Head but the family being from home she was at Board Wages & we made that house our home.[3] I went to St Pauls, the Tower, Westminster Abby &c.

[*p. 55*] In Oct[obe]r my Mother was Inoculated three or four times with the SmallPox but to no effect. Nov[embe]r 12th. My Uncle Savory B[ough]t a flute of Avery Hobbs cost 1 Guinea[.][4] this Avery Hobbs lives at Hendred[,] keeps a school & is likewise a pouche maker.[5] he had the misfortune to Cutt his finger and it was thro' necessity Amputatd which was the occasion of his selling his flute. he since plays on the Violin. I soon learnt to play on this flute but James Church sent a Bassoon cost 4 Guineas exclusive of the Reeds & Box which cost 5/ <then I playd on that at church>.

1. This is James Winter (1728-1796).
2. RBA D/EW/O8, 235: 'The New Church Way in Ash Close made in *1782* (from the asistance of every Farmer)' (my emphasis).
3. For more on Lady Head, see [40*n*].
4. Avery Hobbs, then a barber, married Mary Champ at St Augustine of Canterbury's Church, East Hendred, on 26 June 1755. See also [117, 227].
5. i.e. a pouch or purse maker.

Dec[embe]r 10th. Richd Rowe was Mar[rie]d to Martha Rivers and gave Brightwaltham Ringers 3/-.[1]

*   *   *

[p. 56]

1782

Jan[ua]ry 29th. Mr Thos Langford of Shefford was Married to Miss Mary Mitchel[,] daughter of Saml Mitchel[,] farmer at that place.[2] On the 19th Died one Benj[ami]n Froude of Chaddlewth.[3] A man both Deaf and Dumb he used to come twice or three times a Year to my mother to be let Blood[.] he knew all the news in the Country & was ready to Understand any thing by different motions. he rec[eive]d weekly pay from Chaddleworth parish & when he died had 20 or 30 Guineas conceald in his Coffer. April 22nd. Died Mr John Nelstone[4] of Chaddleworth. he resignd his school sometime before & Dan[ie]l Whister was his successor[.][5] his first school was at his fathers House at Nodmor Pond[.] soon after he built a school House in Chaddlewth[.] the form of it is Round & underneath is a large Cellar[.][6] April 29th was inserted in the [p. 57] Redding Paper: Last tuesday was married after a long and tedious Courtship of 14 days Mr Wm Steptoe Aged 30 to Mrs Horn an agreeable Widow Lady Aged 79 of West Ilsley.

this Steptoe was Bailiff to Mr Morland and Mrs Horn was my Grandfather Savorys Aunt.[7]

May 13th. Died Mr Thos Hughes, of Leckhamstead Thickett[,] Malster and Farmer[,] & Brother to this present Miss Hughes of Thickett. Sept[embe]r 30. Was Married at Brightwaltham Church James Pa[i]ty of Enborn to Miss Levinah [*i.e. Lavinia*] Bartholomew & gave the Ringers 5/-. Dec[embe]r 25th was married John Stroud[,] Sheppard to Mr Herbert[,] to Ann Deacon and gave Brightwaltham Ringers 5/-. they went to reside at

---

1. Richard Row in fact married Martha Rivers at Brightwalton, on 24 *March* 1781.
2. In fact, the marriage took place on *9* January. Savory's son would later marry the couple's niece, Martha Langford. For more, see the afterword.
3. This is probably the Benjamin Frood/Froad born to Joseph and Anne in Chaddleworth in 1709. 'Benjamin Froud' was buried at St Andrew's Church, Chaddleworth, on 22 *March* 1782.
4. John *Nelson* was buried at St Andrew's Church, Chaddleworth, on 22 April 1782.
5. Daniel Whistler Snr (d. 1794) and his son Daniel Whistler Jnr (1748-1816), were schoolmasters on a salary of £17, the latter remaining in post until 1804. See *Berkshire Schools in the Eighteenth Century*, ed. S. Clifford (Berkshire Record Society, xxvi, 2019), 41.
6. The round house survived. Whistler was reputedly worried about French invaders, in the context of Anglo-French hostilities, and asked his pupils to 'dig out huge cellars for the whole village to hide in'. See
<http://www.berkshirehistory.com/villages/chaddleworth.html> (accessed 15 December 2022).
7. The actual newspaper entry differs somewhat: the marriage is dated to Thursday rather than Tuesday, Steptoe is described as 'about 30', and Mrs Horn is described as possessing 'a genteel Fortune'. William Steptoe (c.1752-1796) married Martha *Taylor* at All Saints' Church, West Ilsley, on *Friday*, 22 March 1782. Savory implies a connection with Susannah Taylor, Grandfather Savory's second wife. If she was an aunt, it is notable that she was younger than Savory's grandfather. Mr Morland was a member of the well-known brewing family. John Morland, a farmer, founded his brewery in West Ilsley in 1711, and the business, much enlarged, remained there until 1897 when it relocated to Abingdon.

Reading[.[he is since dead and she is married again. Dec[embe]r 1st 82. Was parted a dividend between the members of the late Club at Boxford. I had 10/6 for doing it. My father and Uncle was in this Club but it broke since my father died.

[*p. 58*] My father and Uncle was likewise members of Shefford late Clubb[.] my father was Clerk, and when my father died Thos Mitchel of Shefford by trade a Taylor was chosen Clerk.

[1783]

In the beginning of the Year 1783 was Mr Pettitt Andrews Auction at Donnington Grove sold by Mr Knight. this Pettitt Andrews was a very troublesome man to the Country was a Justice of Peace.[1] I have nothing more worth Notice till the time I went apprentice which was on March 24th 1783.[2] four or five Years before I went to live at Newbury I learnt to Ring at Church & used to go with the Ringers at Christmas round the Village. we used to ring two or three peals and go to Mr Harbert to Breakfast and stay till 11 or 12 o'Clock[,] from there to Stanbrooks, Holmes, Whiters, Mrs Taylors & spent the Eve[nin]g at my Uncles. and to Blackneys, Trumplets, South End, Birds, Mitchels &c., the following Evenings. [*p. 59*] We used to go to Comb[3] on New Years day. the Rector gives a Crown every Christmas. on Christmas Eve we have a fire in one Corner of the Bellfree and Rang almost <all> Night.[4] Sheepshears and Harvest homes was very much in fashion[,] particularly at Blackneys, Churchs, Horns &c. Healths [*illegible deleted word*] <were> very much used as mums [*i.e. a masked festival*]. Jolly Bachus, Masters, Cuckolds, Burrying, John Cook,[5] Tantaras [*i.e. a flourish on the trumpet or horn*], &c. but now almost laid aside.
the following Verses was sent to my father.

---

1. James Pettit Andrews (1737-1797), Justice of the Peace for Berkshire, author, and a member of the Andrews family of Shaw House and Donnington Grove.
2. The RAI records that Savory was apprenticed principally as a surgeon, though most of his apprenticeship seems to have focused on apothecaries' work, the main focus of David Jones's career.
3. Presumably Combe or Coombe Farm, near Sparrow's Copse, Brightwalton, then occupied by Timothy Bartholomew, and not a reference to the village of Combe, then in Hampshire, located to the west of Newbury, on the River Kennet, near Inkpen.
4. Presumably at Brightwalton.
5. The reference to 'burrying, John Cook' seems to refer back to [53].

The Lords Prayer[1]
(in Verse)

Thou to thy mercies seat our souls doth <gather>
To do our duty unto thee – Our Father
To whom all praise, all honour should be gi<-ven>
For thou art the great God, Which art in Heaven
Thou by thy wisdom rulest the worlds whole <frame>
For ever therefore – Hallowed be thy Name
[*p. 60*]
Let never more delay divide us from
Thy glorious grace but let – thy Kingdom come
Let thy commands opposed be by same
But thy good pleasure and thy Will be done
And let our promptness to obey be even
The very same – in Earth as it is in Heaven
Then for our Souls O Lord we also pray
Thou woulst [*sic*] *be pleasd to –* give us this Day
The Lord of Life wherewith our Souls are <fed>
Sufficient raiment and Our Daily Bread
With every needfull thing do thou releive us
And of thy mercy pity And forgive us
All our misdeeds in him whom thou didst <please>
To make an offering for Our Tresspasses
And for as much O Lord as we beleive
That thou will pardon us As we forgive
Let that love teach us wherewith thou ac-<quaint us>
To pardon all – them that tresspass against us
<*And tho' sometimes thou finds we have forgot*>
This love or thee yet help And lead us not
Tho Souls or bodies want to desparration
Nor let earth gain drive us – into Temptation
[*p. 61*]
Let not the Soul of any hue beleive
Fall in the time of trial – But deliver –
Yea save them from the malice of the Devil
And both in life and death keep – us from evil
Thus pray we Lord for that of thee and whom
Can this be had – for thine is the Kingdom
The world is of thy works the wondrous story
To thee belongs The power and the Glory

---

1. This is written in classic blackletter calligraphy, of the same Old English Gothic (textura) script that characterises the opening words, 'Willm Savory', at the head of the first page of the MS. The verses that follow are mainly written in the same style, represented here by use of italics. The remainder is in Savory's customary handwriting, and is represented here in standard text. The poem is of uncertain provenance, but was certainly still in circulation 70 years later during the American Civil War, see *Jefferson County Republican* (22 March 1922).

And all thy wondrous works have ended never
But will remain for ever and for ever
Thus we poor creatures must confess again
Till us shall say eternally Amen.

*   *   *

In the Year 1324 Wheat sold for 1 Shilling pr Qr and not many Years after for 20 Shillings a Bushell.

*   *   *

[p. 62]
Hymens[1] Commission

O Hymen I invoke thy Aid
    To chuse for me some harmless maid
      To be a tender Wife
Consult not riches in thy Choice
    Nor pride nor yet a clamorous Voice
      The rudiments of strife
But let thy choice be thus confind
    To temper good to nature kind
      A true passage to bliss
To gracefull Air and shapefulll mein
    I reccommend the Centaur line
      With neat and simple dress
OEconomy must warrant her Ample
    In Cooking, Curing taste a sample
      The needles use must know
Let health & happiness her surround
    From blemish free from sole to crown
      Whence unsaid pleasures flow
[p. 63]
Let her delight at home be found
    In me and Children tatling round
      Uncommon comfort this is
Her breast must not with envy burn
    To see her neibours fortunes turn
      From poverty to riches
And if from Tea she can refrain
    The better I shall like the swain [*sic*]
      Of which I have no notion
From Brandy she must quite be free
    So foreign to this Country
      And to our constitution

---

1. The tail of the letter 'y' is continued to form a wavy line under the remainder of the word.

But Hark! one word I must recall
   A fortune I must have withall
     With what I earn sufficit
Independent us to keep
   In meat and drink & quiet sleep
     Until we make our exit
[*p. 64*]
From honest blood descend must she
   Then Children of the same will be
     An homefelt consolation
And unity would instantly, pass a degree
   Triumphantly that harmony should dwell <with we>
     In whatsoever station
 As to religion nought Ive said
    But from the virtues here displayd
     What sect they do consist in
Our Saviour Christ from heavin [*sic*] down brought
   His Blood has seald the same & wrought
     No doubt but she's a Christian
Theres nothing now but Age remains
   Precission there is fruitless gains
     But Thirty let not her exceed
       Nor less than twenty one
Lest the number of her seed
   Involve me in perpetual need
     And so remain undone.

*   *   *

[*p. 65*]
Compleately finishd then is thy Commission
To add is silly – Folly is division
   One Year One Month One Day I will outstake
To you to finish what you did undertake
   I wish you luck to find my Souls desire
   Which when you've done I nothing more require
   Your golden chain to bend your vocal line to play
   Dont let escape thy mind for mirth shall close the <day>
That long wish for day In which I will thee pay
For all thy trouble more than double
What thy conscience bids thee say
If Hymen chance to come your way
With his request comply I pray

Exhortation

Awake, Awake to genious haste away
    No longer dormant lay
Thro' pathless Oceans take
    Not fearing gulph or lake
        All for thy tempers sake
           I'll guard thee night & day
[*p. 66*]
And with shakespears pinions
    We'el [*sic*] pierce the fleeting Air
And thro' more distant regions
    Our Works shall claim the Chair
When life shall cease to be no more
    Our name shall grow as heretofore
Untill each branch reach every door
    Of high and low and rich & poor

Cautions

Let not her Head expanded be
        Beyond its natural size
Nor on it stand a pyramid
        For fear the wind should rise
So hideous and forlorn it makes me shudder
Of Beasts the Unicorns they are like no other

Reason

The allwise Architect of our frame
    Who on our Image stamp our name
       Must be confest supreme
When down on Earth he sent his Son
    With holy Spirit thus among
       His Cloathing was but mean
[*p. 67*]
Alass! how vain ye mortals how depraved
    On precepts trample sacred Blood engravd
        In Satans Chains how fetterd how inslavd
In Satans Vice so firm so close are held
 Christs name thy forfeit – Gods Image have dispelld
 Such renovations of his Work cant spare
His sword is drawn ye fair sex take care
On this remark kind love bids you beware
So self conceited what they deem a grace
Would blush a gentile & a brute disgrace

However absurd this may seem to you
Unbiasd Reason deins to prove it true
Tho' no less strange this may to others seem
Thy still pursue a course no less extreme
Pronounce a sentence on that very crime
Themselves committed both in place & time
 I hope with them your conduct ne'er will Chime
 Gods grace be with you so I end my Rhime
As hurry pleads excuse for blunders
So lightning flies before it thunders
If you please when at your ease A line or two
 Oblige me do, Nodmor Pond & none beyond

Dan[ie]l Whistler to my Sister Sarah[1]

[*p. 68*]

[**1783 continued**]

On Monday March 24. 1783 I went to live at Newbury with David Jones and was Apprenticed the 30th of April from March 25th for 5 Years[.][2] My Uncle John gave him £60[.] how I became acquainted with Dr Jones was he used to Visit Mrs Price at Brightwaltham who had a Cancer in her breast[.] On June 15th I first had my hair dressd at Walsh and was to pay him 3/ pr Q[uarte]r for once a Week. this Old Walshs shop was where Mr John Kings the Atorney New house is (the House adjoining the dwelling house). the first tooth I drew was for Joe Adams July 27th. On July 27th we began distilling of peppermint, 5½ Cz in three days had from it only vi Oz of Oil Mint and so much Water that most of it spoiled for want of using it. I belive [*sic*] Davids contrivance did not answer well for he had a Wooden head fixt in the great Copper & an Opening in the middle to receive the Still Head & I think this Wooden contrivance must receive a good deal of Oil[.] he has since [*p. 69*] got a Copper head to fix in the large Copper in the room of the wooden one.

July 22nd I was confirmd at Newbury by the Bishop of Sarum.[3] Dr Kennett of Ilsley preachd the Sermon.[4] Aug[u]st 9th Died Old Farmer Iremonger of Rowdown and buried the 12th at Boxford[.] this Mr Iremonger lived before he went to Row down farm at Brightwaltham [at] the farm where Mr Church now lives in the Green. He was a close saving man and got great property leaving one Son & daughter[.] his Son John Died soon after[5] and the whole of Iremongers property is enjoyd by James Wards family who lives now at Rowdown. this Old Iremonger used to Carry Victuals in his pockett to

---

1. This phrase is divided above and below by a single, horizontal line drawn free-hand.
2. For more on David Jones, see section vi of the introduction.
3. This was Shute Barrington (1734-1826). He was ordained Bishop of Salisbury on 14 August 1782, and resigned in 1791 to become Bishop of Durham.
4. This is Rev. Dr Brackley Kennett BA, MA, DD (1741-1795), educated at Eton and Corpus Christi College, Oxford, who served as Rector for the parish of East or Market Ilsley from 1771 to 1795. He was succeeded by his son, Brackley Charles Kennett.
5. For John Iremonger, see [100].

Markett and sometimes his heart would be open enough to spend a penny. he once cal[le]d for half a pint of Ale at the Chequer and having drank it, God says he I was a dry. He was a bone setter.[1]

[*p. 70*] Aug[i]st 17th made Syr Spin a [?Cow]. Dec[embe]r 4th. Was maried at Shefford Mr Thos Barrat [*sic*] of Henly Farm to Ann Gilman his Housekeeper[.] she is daughter to Gilman[,] a small farmer at Lamborn.[2] she has 3 Brothers one mar[rie]d Wemhouse eldest daughter of fawly & who now occupies Kintbury Mill[:] his name is Charles Gilman.[3] Dec[embe]r 26th. Was Baptized Jane[,] the daughter of David and Jane Jones.[4]

1784

The beginning of the Year I learnt Astrology of Dr Waters who lived then in Maryhill by the Star[.][5] I went to him once a Week and gave him 6d a Lecture. at the same time Bo[ugh]t of him the following Books:

Gadbury's Doctrine of Nativities & horary Quest		
with Waters Improvements	8s 0d	
Rhumsay on Astrology	2s 6d	
Salmons Soul of Astrology	2s 6d	
Coleys Key of Astrology	5s 0d	
Whartons Works & Long Planetts	5s 0d	
Salmons Sinopsis & Phy: Dictionary[1]	5s 0d	£1 8s 0d

---

1. Thomas Iremonger (1720-1783) married Sarah Taylor at St Mary's Church, Boxford, on 25 April 1740. Sarah died in 1774, and was buried in Boxford on 16 May. The couple had three children, all baptised at All Saints' Church, Brightwalton: Thomas (1742), John (1744) and Sarah (1746). Thomas and John were executors of their father's will (RBA D/A1/88/152), made on 4 March 1780. They were to share 'Rough Down' (Rowdown Farm), Peasemore, and in addition Thomas was to have a house and land in Blewbury and John to have a house and land in Pudding Lane, Brightwalton. Thomas Iremonger Jnr predeceased his father, and John, who proved his father's will on 3 June 1784, died a little over a year later, and was buried at Boxford on 19 August 1785. Sarah Iremonger Jnr married James Ward (1727-1801) at St Barnabas's Church, Peasemore, on 8 October 1768. Surviving her siblings, she inherited everything, though under the original provisions of her father's will, she had been due to receive only £60, and her two sons and three daughters had been due to receive legacies of £20 each. The Wards probably moved to Rowdown after John Iremonger's death in 1785, but did not officially inherit the property until 1796. Sarah Ward died in 1797 and was buried in Brightwalton. The Ward family faithfully recorded their indebtedness by adopting Iremonger as a middle name for several generations, e.g. Thomas Iremonger Ward (1817-1884), who inherited Rowdown Farm and retained it until his death. The reference to Chequer is probably to the Chequers, the eighteenth-century inn at Newbury.
2. Ann, the daughter of William and Ann Gilman, was baptised at St Michael's and All Angels' Church, Lambourn, on 27 July 1755. She was 28 and Thomas Barratt (Savory's maternal uncle) was 46 when they married by licence. Their bondsman was William Wise, a watchmaker in Wantage.
3. Kintbury had a silk mill and three water mills at this time. *Berkshire Overseers' Papers: Records of the Overseers of the Poor up to 1834* (published on CD by Berkshire Family History Society) (Reading, 2005) record that Gilman (d. 1809) employed one John Heath as a miller for two separate periods, and the same man worked as under carter at Upper Farm, Farnborough for John Reeves. For more on the Reeves family see [252].
4. David Jones had married Jenny Hughes at St Nicholas's Church, Newbury, on 18 September 1780.
5. The Star was a beer shop on St Mary's Hill, a continuation of Cheap Street, see [119*n*].

[*p. 71*] April 12th. Was Married my Sister Mary to Joseph Norris and there was spent in the Evening at the Holt 10/.[2] the Sunday following was Married Benjamin Taylor Son of Thomas Taylor who keeps the Marquis of Grandby to Eliz: Hopson Niece to Thos Stanbrook of Brightwaltham[:][3] they resides at Mortimer[.] he is by trade a Cooper[.] this morning I bled Charles Holder of Winterbourn the first of Bleeding. May 30th made Syrrup of Coltsfoot flowers.[4] in June David went into Wales[,] his mother lately died. July 7th. Was born Wm Savory Norris Son of Jos[ep]h and Mary Norris, at 6h40'PM. Mrs Weston of Bidden was midwife and at that time they was making the Hay Rick at Brightwaltham[.] Aug[u]st 17th distilld Horehound, Sage &c. Sept[embe]r 14th distilld Fumitory to send to London at 5/0 pr Galln.

In Oct[obe]r Jeremiah Grant who married [*p. 72*] Swains Sister in Speenhamland I became Acquainted with.[5] he was a Clock Maker by trade[,] very injenious. he gave me great instructions in Astrology. he was Lame & was obliged to wear an Iron to support his Leg[.] the following is a Letter he wrote to me:

Dear Fidelis

Whatever may have been the secret ways of Providence towards me, either for good or Ill I deem myself in All most highly favoured, as it has been productive of that friendly union which subsists between you and me: while it confirms my opinion as to the reality of an All Directing Power. For amidst the numerous herd of sensual beings which pester this part of the Creation: I have found one who is able to elevate my Ideas above this little scene of things.

---

1. These are seventeenth-century works of astrology, namely: John Gadbury (1628-1704), *Genethlialogia, or The Doctrine of Nativities Together with The Doctrine of Horarie Questions* (1658) (his first and most traditional work of judicial astrology – Waters's improvements were presumably annotations in the form of marginalia or supplementary notes by Savory's tutor); *Lux Veritatus, or, Christian Judicial Astrology Vindicated and Demonology Confused* (1650) by the Scottish physician and astrologer, William Ramesey or Ramsay (1627-1676); William Salmon (1644-1713), *Horae Mathematicae seu Urania: The Soul of Astrology, containing that Art in all its Parts, in Four Books, &c.* (1679), an astrological textbook. The second of Salmon's volumes mentioned here, *Synopsis Medicinae: or, A Compendium of Astrological, Galenical and Chymical Physick* (1671), was a popular medical handbook which encouraged the poor to embrace self-treatment, and provoked censure from an outraged Royal College of Physicians. Savory also lists: Henry Coley (1603-1707), *Clavis Astrologiae, or a Key to the Whole Art of Astrologie* (1669, enlarged 1676), a widely used textbook; George Wharton (1617-1681), *The Works of that late most Excellent Philosopher and Astronomer George Wharton*, ed. John Gadbury (1683). For a discussion of Savory and astrology, see section vii of the introduction.
2. The couple were married by licence. It was noted that Joseph Norris was a minor, the son of Mary, of North Moreton. Their bondsman was John Hulcup, a clerk in Wantage.
3. Benjamin Taylor married Elizabeth *Hobson* at Brightwalton, on *Thursday*, 15 April 1784.
4. Coltsfoot or Coughwort, a yellow herb which acts as a diuretic, was often used to treat sore throats.
5. Jemy Grant of the parish of St Helen's, Abingdon, married Sarah Swain by licence at St Mary's Church, Speen, on 30 June 1784. The *Reading Mercury* reported, 'Last Wednesday was married at Speen, in the county, Mr Jeremiah Grant, of Abingdon, to Miss Sarah Swain, of Speenhamland; an amiable young lady, with a genteel fortune. – At the same time was married, Mr John Swain, to Miss Brown, of Maidenhead.' *RM* (5 July 1784).

The operation of chance could never effect this. Let Athiests and infidels say what they will. No my friend that being in whose hand we are hath found us for that social intercourse in [*p. 73*] which we live, and it is one of those Blessings for which I shall unfeignedly adore him. You will my dear Fidelis forgive this mode of xpression when you consider the xcellence of Friendship, fair in its form, pure in its intentions, and sacred as to its Original[.]

Indeed Fidelis in all my changefull Life I never knew one friend before who could find purity of Heart enough to support with propriety that inestimable character: for if we look thro' the World we shall find the friendship of Mankind more fickle than fortune & as wavering as the uncertain Wind. Some partial Motives to their own dear interest is the common spring of Action & thus the sacred fire of friendship is xtinguished by cold inconstancy[.]

Happy truly Happy therefore must that man be who can select from the knowing and discerning few, One Heaven born Friend! tis this in which I boast & this shall be my Solace and my Song. Perhaps Fidelis you may think my Judgments wrong, but if prescence [*sic*] is allowd to Man, your person & your genious prove me right.

[*p. 74*] The divine Plato was of opinion that nature without knowledge is blind, therefore much are you to be commended for seeking to adorn an amiable nature with the graces of Virtue & of Wisdom thro' the study of Celestial things. the more we cultivate, we are with Heavn more intimate. proceed therefore xcellent Youth! in so noble an attempt. continue to aspire after more of the Hyperion Fruit.

Afflict not thy Soul with the painfull View of Sickness or mortality, for things immortal are not fit subjects for affliction: Acquaint thyself with God! intreat the continuance of his light upon thy mind. implore his benediction upon all thy Works and ways and after contemplate the xuberance of this goodness with silent adoration. O my Friend as I now delight in thy instructive converse. I shall then gain more improvement from such an highly finish Copy[.]

but you may justly now call me to account for contradiction & indeed methinks I see you just ready to say "some partial selfish Motive is the Cause of your friendship["]. Yes it is [*p. 75*] Fidelis, I own it & Glory in it. I hope to gather some of your graces, to improve by your precepts, to be instructed by your understanding and to profess your lasting friendship which will ever be Dear Fidelis the Study & delight of your Avowed and Especial Friend[,]

Jemy Grant[.]

He left Newbury soon after he wrote this Letter which gave me great uneasiness for the loss of so sincere a Friend. as at this time I was very fond of studying Astrology. I shall insert the Nativities of my 3 Sisters Sarah, Jane and Mary. also of Sarah, David, Jane, Mary and Sarah Jones[,] Son & daughters of David and Jane Jones of Newbury[,] in all eight geniture which are as follows and first I shall draw a few observations on my Sister Sarahs Geniture who is now the Wife of Francis Fordham & who now keeps the Flying Horse Inn Lambeth Street, Goodmans Fields, London.

[*p. 76*]

Sarah Fordham
alias Savory Born
Oct[obe]r 26th 1756 at
3h. 10' PM. {Moon} a {Sextile} {Saturn} ad {Square} {Venus}[1]

Dignities & Debilities & Latt:

{Saturn}	19	9	0.47S
{Jupiter}	11	8	1.2N
{Mars}	15	7	0.11S
{Sun}	5	13	[*blank*]
{Venus}	17	8	0.13N
{Mercury}	17	5	2.42S
{Moon}	12	0	[*blank*]
{Lot}	12	0	[*blank*]

{Jupiter} Lord of the Ascendant angular but not free from combination. {Mars} who has likewise dignities in the Ascendant in his house yet [*p. 77*] near a {square} of {Saturn} – {Saturn} and {Sun} L[or]ds of the 11th 12th and 6th signifies the Native to receive trouble &c from things belonging to those houses as pretended friends, sickness, private Enemies, Servants &c. and as {Mercury} and {Venus} the opposite party is stronger than {Jupiter} or {Mars} she must expect to be ruld by her husband. {Moon} Lady 5th & {Cancer} a fruitfull sign gives her an Offspring. {Moon} in the house of {Jupiter} L[or]d Asc[endan]t and {Jupiter} Angular is a good token of a Natural Death. those planetts in the 8th denotes some Hott burning fever which may turn putrid. {Venus} Lady 2nd in 7th in {sextile} {Mercury} L[or]d 7th who is in the 8th denotes help from the Grandfather & persons deceasd. I shall draw a Speculum for the Nativity whereoff may be seen the good or bad directions Attending the Native thro' Life & the events of such directions may be seen in Gadbury, Coley, Lilly &c.

[*pp. 78-79*]

A Speculum for this Nativity

KEY

Ars	Ariies	My	Mercury	asc	Ascendant
Tau	Taurus	V	Venus	opp	Opposition
Gem	Gemini	Ms	Mars		
Can	Cancer	J	Jupiter	sq	Square
Leo	Leo	S	Saturn	tri	Tri
Vir	Virgo	Mn	Moon	an	ascending node
Lib	Libra	Sn	Sun	dn	descending node
Sco	Scorpio	Lt	Lot	con	conjunction

---

1. A typical horoscope, a geniture chart, see illustration in section vii of the introduction. Sarah and Francis Fordham are discussed in the introduction and afterword.

Sag	Sagittarius				Q	quintile
Cap	Capricorn				Sx	sextile
Aq	Aquarius				D	decile
Pis	Pisces					

[*N.B. Savory's own abbreviation, 't', probably signifies 'towards'; the significance of Savory's abbreviation, 'C', remains obscure. Doubtful transcriptions are indicated by a simple '?'.*]

D.M	0	30	60	90	120	150	180	210	240	270	300	330
0.0	Ars	Tau	Gem	Can	Leo	Vir	Lib	Sco	Sag	Cap	Aq	Pis
0.1	t J	t V	t My	tMs	t S	C J	t S	t Ms	t J	t V	t S	Q J
1.4												
2.0				D5		D7				D11		asc
28		opp		tri	sq	Sx		Sn		Sx	sq	
3.47	Sx	sq	tri		opp		tri	sq	Sx		S	
4.0			D3						D9			
			ocl									
5.0		D2	?					D8				
6.0	t V		Ald	t J	t My		t V	t J		t My	tMy	
7.0			t J			t V						
8.0		t My							t V			t J
9.0					C S							
10.0											Q.My	

D.M	0	30	60	90	120	150	180	210	240	270	300	330
	A7d						opp					
11.11	Lt		Sx	sq	tri		t J		tri	sq	Sx	
12.?	A J				CMa		C V				sqMs	
			Opp			Sq			Mn			sq
13.0	Tri			tMe	Tri		Sx			t J	tMy	
14.0			t V		t V	tJ						tMy
15.0		t J										
16.0												
17.11		Tri	Sq	Sx				Sx		Tru		
17.42		opp		CMn	Sq	V			Sq	QMn		opp
18.42				Tri		Sx		Ms		Sx	Sq	trt
19.0			D4		t J	QSu	tMy					CSu
						T S						
			t V						D10			
20.0			D6						t S	t Ms		
21.0	tMs	Hang	t S					tV				
22.0		t S								D12	t J	tMs
23.0						T						
24.2		opp		tri	sq	Ms	tMs	My		Sx	sq	tri
						Sx						
26.0												
26.13	t S	tMs			C Sn		Q S				Q Sn	t S
26.22		C S										
27.0			t S				t S					
28.0					Leo						sn	
29.9	opp		tri	sq	Sx				Sx		tri	

[*p. 80*]

The Ascendant to Promittors

[*N.B. Except in the first instance (see note), the pairs of numbers in the 4th and 5th, & 9th and 10th columns represent years and days. The capital letters 'T' and 'C' are Savory's, and their meaning is obscure.*]

To	tri	Sn	277d	23m	To	opp	Sn	27	113
	T	J	2	282		sq	S	27	167
	sq	Mn	4	324		D	2	28	51
	T	My	5	169		T	My	33	126
	opp	V	6	304		tri	V	34	242
	tri	Ms	7	37		opp	Ms	35	75
	T	Ms	8	18		T	S	37	209
	tri	My	9	283		opp	My	38	362
	T	S	10	226		T	Ms	10	52
	Sx	S	13	329		T	My	43	174
	T	V	14	291		D	3	45	301
	?H	?Angl	16	339		tri	S	45	233
	Lt		16	370		?Ocl	?Tau	46	208
	?Q	V	17	213		?Clde	b	47	127
	T	My	18	83		T	J	48	45
	T	My	21	122		Sx	Lt	51	191
	T	S	23	218		opp	Mn	53	23
	opp	J	25	189					

Mid Heavn to Promittors

To	Sx	J	12	39	To	Q	Mn	31	11
	T	V	13	80		Sx	Ms	31	239
	Sx	Sn	16	54		Sx	My	38	323
	T	My	18	251		sq	J	44	204
	sq	Lt	24	165		T	S	45	311
	T	J	25	140		sq	Sn	48	27
	tri	V	31	4		T	My	51	37

*   *   *

[*p. 81*]

{Sun} to Promittors

To	D	8	1	14	To	Q	S	22	334
	T	V	10	189		Sx	S	30	216
	Sx	V	13	267		tri	Lt	37	401
	con	Ms	14	99		con	Mn	39	277
	T	My	17	226		sq	V	44	62
	con	My	20	315		Sx	J	57	63

{Moon} to Promittors

To	sq	V	4	157	To	sq	Lt	28	285
	D	10	6	101		tri	V	34	311
	T	Ms	12	132		Q	Mn	34	316
	Sx	J	17	152		Sx	Ms	35	43
	T	V	18	168		D	12	37	266
	Sx	Sn	21	43		Sx	My	41	312

{Lot of Fortune} to Promittors

To	tri V	Opp Ms	15	172	To	opp	Mn	27	191
	Head	Arg	17	90		sq	V	29	191
	opp	My	22	351		tri	J	36	225
	Sx	V	48	169		tri	Sn	39	9

*　　*　　*

Asc[endant] to {trine} {Mars} at almost 9 Years of Age inclind the Native to be bold Witty and Stout hearted &c.

*　　*　　*

[p. 82]

Jane Savory alias
Eagles alias Brown
Born Oct[obe]r 10. 1760
11hs 25' A M

This Native is of a good disposition I am well assurd and may be seen by the above figures[.] {Sagittarius} and {Jupiter} in {Aquarius} declares her a chearfull Affable creature, hurtfull to none[,] delight in decency &c. {Mars} in {Sagittarius} in {sextile} {Jupiter} L[or]d Asc[endant] {Mercury} L[or]d 7 in {sextile} to the Cusp of the Asc[endan]t makes her an agreeable Companion, esteemd by people she converses or deals with. {Aries} in Asc[endant] gives her a hard pimpled Complexion[.] {Mercury} L[or]d 7 her Husband in {trine} {Jupiter} & {sextile} Asc[endant] signifies good agreement betwixt them also her husband {Venus} in {Scorpio} L[ad]y 5 {conjunction} {Moon} denotes a large offspring.

[p. 83] My Brother in law John Eagles is by trade a Carpenter[.][1] his proper Name is Sims (his Mothers name) who was the base born son of one Brown of Lockinge so as his Mother was not Maried. he must derive his name from his Mother which is Sims[,] that is John Sims not Brown. the

---

1. The RAI lists a John Eagles, apprenticed as a Carpenter & Joiner to Thomas Painter of East Challow, in December 1773 (having possibly been previously (and evidently unsuccessfully) apprenticed as a tailor to Thomas Chessell of East Lockinge, in August 1770. In turn, Eagles took on William Church as an apprentice carpenter at Brightwalton in November 1800.

reason of his name being calld Eagles, was he was put to Nurse when Young to one Eagles.

since he has been Married to my Sister he is got very religious and now frequents the Methodist Meetings &[c].[1]

I shall next treat on my Youngest Sisters Geniture who Mar[rie]d Jos[ep]h Norris my Uncle Savorys Apprentice.

* * *

[p. 84]

**Mary Savory or
Norris born Aug
2. 1765 9h.45'PM
{Moon} ad {square} {Saturn}**

{Mars} Lord of the first House in the sign {Leo} in {conjunction} {Sun} with the sign Ascending describe the Native as she is. Of a Middle Stature[,] lean and spare, Long Visage, light hair[.] for disposition very hasty and Choleric yet easily conquered or overcome by people she converses or deals with, the L[or]d Ascendant being so near the Sun. Or I may as well say she seems as a Mouse before a Catt who would get at the Cheese was she not under the paws of a ruling power.

[p. 85] {Moon} Lady 5th {Jupiter} in 5th sign of the 5th & sign of the {Moon} wld {Leo} old fruitfull gives sufficient Issue but {Moon} Lady 5th in 12 or 8th from 5th & L[or]d 9th or 4th from 5th in 5th some of them will be short lived & sickly. so many planetts in the 6th gives different diseases but most of it from affection of the Mind, small Cattle & Servants but principally from Religion {Jupiter} being L[or]d 9th. Yet I think it may comfort her mind but affect her substance. the Native and her husband cannot agree but middling as the Sun & Mercury is between them or by reason of Kindred, Religion, Servants &c. I shall next treat on the Geniture of Sarah Jones eldest Child of Dr Jones in Newbury.

---

1. John Eagles was one of five parishioners subsequently to apply to the Bishop of Salisbury for permission to hold Methodist meetings at the home of Richard Gibbins. The application, supported by William Franklin, Joseph Evans, Joseph Norris (like Eagles, one of Savory's brothers-in-law) and James Bew, was made on 4 June 1792. A further application, dated 25 January 1799, was signed by John Eagles, his wife Jane (Savory's sister), John May, Charles Hatley, Thomas Benham and Joseph Norris (in whose home permission for the meetings to take place was sought). See *Berkshire Nonconformist Meeting House Regulations 1689-1852, Part I*, ed. L. Spurrier (Berkshire Record Society, ix, 2005), 28, 41-42, citing WSA D1/2/29 f. 1v. reversed, and D1/2/29, f. 53v.

[*p. 86*]

Sarah Jones
Born April 21. 1781
8hs AM.

That this Native could not be of long Life is evident in the above scheme for Saturn L[or]d of the house of Death Afflicting the sign Ascending disposing of {Jupiter} who is possited in the 6th. L[or]d 6th in 8th L[or]d 4th in 12th {Moon} to {square} {Mars} in the 8th &c. she lived but six Weeks.[1] The {Moon} coming to her own opposition from the 12th and 6th house. {Saturn} by a retrograde motion to the degree ascending. The {Sun} gives of Life to {Lunar Eclipse} {Saturn} L[or]d of Death. {Moon} in 6th to {square} {Mars} in 8th are Sufficient testimonies of Short life.

[*p. 87*]

David Jones[2]
Born May 28th
1782 9hs 42' AM[3]

First. May the Natives Life be Long or <short> Regulus & Cor Leonis being in the Ascendant and being Stars of the nature of {Mars} is the worst configuration that I can foresee, which endangers fevers and sudden sickness in the Natives infancy. Yet given him a great and noble spirit of mind. {Sun} L[or]d Asc[endant] in [?plato's] {sextile} to Asc[endant] & {Venus} the lesser fortune in {trine} to Asc[endant] & {Moon} & {Jupiter} in {trine} to [*p. 88*] Asc[endan]t & both within Orbs of a {sextile} {Venus} likewise & no {square} Or {opposition} to Asc[endan]t {Sun} or {Moon} I should conclude the Native according to Natural Causes to be designd for a long Life and consequently may live till some very bad directions to the giver of Life.

2ndly <by> the birth being by Day and {Sun} in 10th I conclude to be giver of Life.

3rdly {Mercury} having most dignities in the place of Hyleg[4] and moderately fortified & in a succedent house.[5] I conclude {Mercury} to be giver of Years now the mean Year of {Mercury} signifies 48 therefore if no very bad directions to {Sun} & {Mercury} the Native may live to those

---

1. She was buried at St Mary's Church, Boxford, on 8 June 1781.
2. For more on David Jones and his family, see section vi of the introduction.
3. This geniture is drawn differently to the standard charts in Savory's MS. It is comprised of two intersecting ovals, one in a vertical orientation, the other horizontal, crossing at the central point, and the whole contained in a circle. Four sections lie outside the intersecting ovals and are each divided in half, creating a total of 13 sections. This chart is of the same type used by Savory for King George III [133] (see illustration).
4. The Hyleg is the planet (i.e. Mercury, in this case) with the highest essential dignity in five positions of the geniture: the degree of the Sun, the degree of the Moon, the Ascendant, the Lot of Fortune, and the pre-natal New Moon or Full Moon (whichever occurred nearest the subject's birth).
5. In astrological charts, the succedent [*sic*] house or houses follow (i.e. succeed) the angular houses.

Years or perhaps longer if at that time any benevolent directions should intervene: But the dangerous Years are but discovered by directions.

4thly. The Almuten or L[or]d of the Nativity is next to be considered. the strongest [*p. 89*] planetts are {Mars} & {Jupiter}. Mars has most dignities as by the collection of dignities & debilities. Yet Jupiter having essential dignities in the Ascendant & within Orbs of a {trine} thents [*i.e. thence*] I conclude {Jupiter} L[or]d of the Nativity.

5thly. The Stature and form of the Body {Leo} Asc[endanc]y & a fixed Star of the nature of {Mars} describes a full Body, strong and well set. broad shoulders, light coloured hair & Curling, rather low & short of stature, a bold stout hearted person, fearing Nothing.

6thly. Colour of the Face[.] {Sun} & {Mars}[:] both sig[ns] desclares a round full face, high forehead, the Visage fair. Yet of a Sun burnt Colour.

7thly. The Temperature Hott and Dry.

8thly. The Manners of the Native. Regulus & Cor Leonis in Asc[endant] with {Sun} {Saturn} {Jupiter} [*p. 90*] and they moderately fortified. gives ~~greats~~ greatness of Spirits joined with Majestic Gravity. Humane & Courtious.

9thly. The Understanding {Mercury} in {Gemini} gives a good understanding & being stronger than the Moon denotes that reason shall Overcome sensual Appetite.

10thly. L[or]d As[endan]t in 10th and falling in the 11th shews he shall be eminant in the Art or profession he shall follow and thereby gain many good and powerfull friends to help him.

Observations of the 2nd House

The Antis[c]ion of {Venus} falls exactly on the Cusp of the 2nd & {Venus} being Lady of the 10th. I should think the Native to have some profit by his own business. {Mars} likewise who disposes of {Venus} is in {sextile} to the Cusp of the 2nd & {trine} to {Lot of Fortune} will give help by [*p. 91*] Physic and Surgery. the {Lot of Fortune} being locally posited in the 8th gives Wealth by Wills &c of the Dead as also by his Wifes fortune but {Lot of Fortune} in {opposion} to 2nd and {Mercury} in {square} to them denotes difficulty in pursuit of these things.

Remarks on the 3rd House

{Venus} Lady 3rd in a masculine sign but {Venus} beholding {Jupiter} & {Moon} denotes more Sisters than Brothers. {Aries} so near to the Cusp of the 3rd betokens short Life to some of them & that their power and situation will be mean for the most part. also shews the Native to undertake many short Journeys wth some trouble and disatisfaction at the 1st setting out[,] and meets with many Crosses but in the end may be crowned wth pleasure and Content but {Venus} being rather Weak & in her detriment sig[nifies] the end to be toilsome for the most part.

[*p. 92*]

Hints on the 4th House

L[or]d Asc[endan]t an Enemy to the L[or]d 4th nor in no aspect to each other. {Jupiter} {Saturn} or {Moon} in no aspect or configuration with the L[or]d 4th but Yet disposes of {Mars} L[or]d 4th in {conjunction} {Jupiter} & {Saturn} denotes the native and his father will be sometimes at Variance. no great things to be expected from things signified by the 4th House as Lands, Houses &c.

Considerations on the 5th House

Notwithstanding the Asc[endan]t is a barren sign. Yet so many planetts being in the 5th in {trine} to {Venus}. the Native if he should live will have many Children and these prosperous and long lived. Will have more Boys than Girls. Will be fortunate in Gaming and all things represented by the 5th House. L[or]d 5th in 5th propends the Native to many Voluptuous & Vain Courses.

[*p. 93*]

Answers from the 6th House

The {Moon} overpowering {Saturn} L[or]d 6th denotes some dangerous fluxes & Cold Rhumes or Colds perhaps by being too great a friend to Bacchus, but these disorders are easily Cured, the Body being more robust & strong and of a different Nature to the signification of the 6th House. As the {Moon} is in {conjunction} {Saturn} in the Milky Way and within Orbs of an {Lunar Eclipse} with {Mars} I should be fearfull of some defect in the left Eye in particular. however the L[or]d 6th in 5th denotes diseases occasioned by Drinking.

Notes on the 7th House

{Saturn} L[or]d 7th in a double bodied sign in {conjunction} {Moon} in the 5th house very likely the Native may Marry more than once. also {Venus} applying to {Saturn} {Jupiter} & {Moon} in the 5th Argues [*p. 94*] more than one Wife. But this is best discovered by Directions. It denotes a person of a well set and strong able Body that the Native shall Marry. shes not very Tall[,] yet descently [*sic*] enough composed, a clear skin, a sanguine complexion. Yet more lovely than curious or beautifull, a fleshy face inclinable to an Oval form & sometimes a pale & whitely countenance, but rather slovenly inclined. {Saturn} {conjunction} {Moon} shews the Native and his Wife to disagree.

Judgments on the 8th House

{Jupiter} L[or]d 8th strong & {Lot of Fortune} on the Cusp are arguments of a Natural Death.

Predictions from the 9th House

The Native will reap small gains by Travelling & yet I cannot advise the Native to Travell long Journeys {Mars} casting a {square} to the Cusp of the 9th.

[*p. 95*]

Prognostications from the 10th House

{Venus} Lady 10th with {Leo} in {trine} to {Jupiter} {Moon} & {Saturn} denotes he will be of moderate honor & esteem by reason of {Venus} in her detriment. L[or]d 10th in 9th he may end his days in a far Country

Opinions from the 11th House

L[or]d 11th strong but separating from the L[or]d Asc[endant] argues but few friends and those he seldom agrees with.

Lastly Conclusions on the 12th House

{Mars} in 12th & L[or]d 4th and 9 denotes his own parents and his Wifes brethren to be private Enemies, but they can do him but little harm.

Next follows a Revolutional figure for the Year 1784 for this Nativity.

*   *   *

[*p. 96*]

**Revolution
1784
May 27th**

See Gadbury, page 211

The Radix serves for the 1st Year therefore under {Gemini} for the 2nd Year

you find	11.36
add time of	21.42 Birth
	———
	33 18
	24
	———
	9.18
	———

At which time set your figure for[1]

[*p. 97*]

Jane Jones Born Nov[embe]r 22nd 1783 at 9hs 23' A M but as I have no Ephemeris for that year so I shall proceed on the Geniture of Mary Jones.

---

1. Several pages have been cut from the MS here. Whilst the narrative is apparently interrupted, the page numbering continues in sequence. It is almost certain, therefore, that the pages were cut out by Savory himself at the time of composition.

Mary Jones
Born Ap[ri]l 29. 1785
7hs. A M.

The Native lived to be near 6 Years of Age[.] she was a very Cross sickly Child[.] {Jupiter} L[or]d Asc[emdamt] in {square} {Moon} L[or]d 8th {Sun} In the house of Sickness &c are testimonies of a Short Life & lastly the Geniture of Sarah Jones the Youngest daughter of Dr Jones.

[*p. 98*]

Sarah Jones
Born Dec[embe]r 25th 1786
15 [*sic*] P M

We see {Mars} seems to claim L[or]d of the Horoscope in {trine} thereto in {sextile} {Saturn} L[or]d 10. 11. and 12th houses declares the Native to be fortunate in those things signified by them houses. but {Moon} casting a {square} to the Cusp 2nd & from {conjunction} {Saturn} shews many Losses from her own Sex & people she puts confidence in. {Moon} a {sextile} {Mars} and {sextile} {Jupiter} she will be of a sharp Quick Apprehension addicted to Learning &c.

Next Memoirs &c on the Year 1785 the 17th Year of my Age & 3rd of my Apprentiship.

[*p. 99*]

1785

Jan[ua]ry 3rd. this day there was Cockfighting at the Jack of Newbury. My Master at that time was very fond of Cockfighting[.] he won 2 Guineas which inclined him to follow that sport some time but at last he grew tired by reason of bad Luck.[1] Mr Goatly of Marlbro' came with a Cancer near his Eye[.] the Wound when he first came was about the bigness of half a Crown but he could not Cure it[,] Mr Goatly being near 15 Years afflicted with it, he was upwards of 70 Years of Age & thro' which disease of died[.] he got to be worth 10 or £12000 by dealing in Wood[.] he descended from very mean parents and was a poor Boy. used to go to plow[.] he was a person of a stout heart & free Spirit.[2]

*   *   *

---

1. Although cock-fighting was still a relatively common so-called sport at this time, the *Bath Chronicle and Weekly Gazette* referred to it in 1789 as a 'cruel pastime' (7 May 1789). The pub Savory refers to was named after Jack O' Newbury, i.e. John Winchcombe, who as a boy in poverty ran away from home and became an apprentice clothier in the market town of Newbury. He eventually married his employer's widow. He successfully built up a substantial business and achieved such a prodigious output that it has sometimes been claimed that he established England's first factory, though no dependable evidence to support this has been found.
2. This is Edmund Goatley (1713-1789), wood dealer of Marlborough, Wiltshire. He was born on 8 March 1713 and baptised at Preshute, Wiltshire, the son of George and Mary.

[*p. 100*] March 15th was Born my Sister Fordham's first Child whose name was Jane. she died when quite Young.[1] July 23rd. I went to London by Newbury Coach Bo[ugh]t the 3 <1st> books of Cornelius Agrippa, some Old Ephemeris & Surgeons instruments.[2] Aug[us]t 9th. Bo[ugh]t of Esqr Pages Gardner ½ Cz of peppermint for 4/[.] Bo[ugh]t pennyroyal for 1d pr lb and Savin at 8d Pr lb. this Esqr Page livd on Speen Hill on the left hand going to Speen & died about this time[.][3] he was Justice for Newbury and father to this present Page who lives in the Wharff[.][4] Aug[us]t 15 died Mr John Iremonger of Row down farm Brother to Mrs Ward of Rowdown who when her Brother died went to live & family at Row down farm.[5] Sept[embe]r 3rd I drove Mrs Trulock in the Chaise to Brightwaltham. [*p. 101*] Mrs Trulock then lived at Thatcham wth one Mr Reeves who was a Surgeon[.][6] I had the Chaise at the 3 Tuns & drove her from Thatcham to Henwick by fair Cross pond thro' Chieveley & peasemore but mistaking the right road from Peasemore to Brightwalton I drove into Yeastly Copse and could not get backwards or forwards. however we got up the Banks and got off without doing any damage to the Chaise, but spoiled the old Ladys White Shoes. this Mrs Trulock is a very particular Old Lady of a Tall slender shape – a proud, Conceited, fancifull Queen. she lives now at Newbury and noticed by every one but respected by none.[7] the 18th Aug[us]t was Married one Dredge, a particular acquaintance of mine[,] to Sally Woods they lives now at Reading. [*p. 102*] he is by trade a Taylor.

Oct[obe]r 25th. Payd Richd Wilder 2/ for a pack of Cards which is divided from Corner to Corner [/][8] for a deception, and the following Words used to deceive the Company: –

---

1. For Jane Fordham's geniture, see [262]. She was buried in St Mary's Church, Whitechapel, on 27 December 1787, aged two-and-a-half years.
2. [Henricus] Cornelius Agrippa of Nettesheim (1486-1535), a scholar and writer on the occult, argued against the persecution of witches. Notable publications include *De Occulta Philosophia libri tres* (1529) and *De Vanitate Scientiarum* (1530). An ephemeris provides tables detailing the trajectory of astronomical objects which Savory would have used to draw up horoscopes.
3. Francis Page (1719-1785) of Coldwell House, on the Old Bath Road, was buried at St Mary's Church, Speen, on 10 September 1785. He was elected to Newbury Council in 1749 and served as Mayor in 1754, following his father who had been Mayor in 1719. Page ran a successful coal business. In 1768 he gained control of the Kennet Navigation Company and invested in the development of the Kennet and Avon Canal.
4. This is Francis Page Jnr (1757-1814). The *Reading Mercury* notes his proprietorship of Newbury and Aldermaston Wharfs, having taken over from Richard Baily as a coal-merchant and barge-master at Newbury (30 March 1789).
5. For the connection between the Iremonger and Ward families, see [69*n*].
6. Margaret Railton writes: 'In 1785 the Thatcham overseers advertised for a surgeon, apothecary and midwife to attend the poor of the parish for a salary of £27 10s a year. It was noted that the position had only been advertised as Mr Yates, the former surgeon, had left the parish. Mr Thomas Reeves, surgeon and man-midwife was appointed; the parish vestry was undeterred by the fact that he also "made, sold and prepared horse medicines of all kinds"', Railton, *Early Medical Services*, 11.
7. Probably Joan Trulock, who died in Newbury in 1797. For her will see RBA D/A1/131/17. For more on Mrs Trulock, see [103-105].
8. Savory has drawn a portrait-style rectangle (the shape of a playing card) with a dividing line running from the top right to the bottom left.

1st. Dioblem, Vengoblem, preste de fenum into Cocolorum change Quick & be gone.

2nd. Montorus, Mandibus, Grandibus change into operas Quick & be gone.

3rd. Ricktum, Sticktum, Starry Vatum Alzee, Bralzee foxe fonco change &c.

In December one John King used to come from Donnington with a Wound on his Leg[.] he was <a> Tanner and a very merry Joking man, and could play a great many funny tricks. says he: I can push a Quart Cup thro' the handle [*p. 103*] of a pint; put your finger thro' the handle of a pint and push the Quart[.]

Its no harm says he to Swear, lie or take advantage[:] first its no harm to swear to the truth, its no harm to lie with your Wife, & its no harm to take advantage of a Horse to get upon it.

This Mrs Trulock as I was just before observing came about this time to live at Newbury[.] her first lodgings was at Whites at the Bakehouse by the Monument. one Messetter of Thatcham used to make his addresses to this Old Ewe and after a while they had Writings drawn betwixt them but Messetter proving false some injenious person made the following Song.

*   *   *

[*p. 104*]

Song

An Elderly Bull much admired an old Cow
But how to get at her he could not tell how
For she was so wary so deep & so keen
So many droll fancys & Riggs she had seen
Yet nevertheless as he mett her one day
He made a low Bow and thus to her did say
How long will you make me to bellow & groan
How long will you make me to Wander alone
For <your sake> each Cow in the field do I slight
And hold my tail for me whenever I shite
Because you no fault with my Buttocks <find> should [*sic*]
Nor have an excuse for your being unkind
This cautious old Cow interrupted him here
And said I am sure you can[']t make it appear
That I have ungenerous been or unkind
For on all occasions I have told you <mind> my [*sic*]
Which is you shall never familiarly feel
Untill with a Lawyer you sign & do seal
Or if I perhaps must speak plainly sais she
With me you shall Article – wth me agree
[*p. 105*]
Ne'er to kiss nor to ride any other but me
The Bull was obliged to give his consent
So a nimble brisk Calf for a lawyer was <sent>

A Son of the Quill in a few minutes came
Soon drew up a Bond where ye Bull signd his <name>
For which every Calf did the poor Noodle blame
No matter for that he obtain his desire
And quickly he Quenched his Amorous fire
But would you beleive it this Wandring Bull
At another Cows Tail was for having a pull
When his subtle old mate came upon him quite <quick>
Upbraided him said he had served he[r] a trick
For which she would certainly make him quite <sick>
You want sais the Bull you may certainly <try>
But your Bond is as nothing between you & I
Because I can prove you are not fit for my Bed
Disabled you are in your Tail not your head
I will not expose you if you will be quiet
But I swear by my Horns if you make the <least riot>
I['ll go to the Lawyers your case he shall handle
And prove you can[']t – nor yet hold <the Candle>.

[*p. 106*] The following is a Chapter on Wm Pit prime Minister, L[or]d high treasurer &c.[1]

1st

And it came to pass in the Days of Georgius that a stripling of the house of Chatham found favour in the Kings sight and walked uprightly, so that all the people loved him.

2nd

And the King raised him above the elders among the people and cloathed him with purple and fine linen and put a Ring on his finger and the people reproved him not.

3rd

Moreover the dealers in spices who sat upon the high places beheld the virtues of this Youth and he found favour in their sight.

4th

And they gave him Meat and Drink in Abundance and stuffed him even as though he was an Alderman & they appointed him Ruler of the great City.

---

1. British statesman William Pitt the Younger (1759-1806) was Prime Minister (1783-1801 and 1804-1806), and was the dominant political figure of the period. His father, William Pitt (1708-1778), was appointed the 1st Earl of Chatham, and served as Prime Minister from 1766 to 1768.

[*p. 107*]

5th

And the dealers in Gold even of pure Gold Assembled themselves together & communed with each other and they sent Messengers to the Young Man and besought his presence in the City.

6th

And he hearkened to the Messenger and straightway Journeyed into the City & he was accompanied with Chariots and Horsemen.

7th

And fared sumptuously and fed out of Vessels of Silver and Vessels of Gold and he eat and drank abundantly, he was also cloathed in a City Garment.

8th

But he turned his back upon the people, even the people who had fed him and Cloathed him and he regarded them not.

9th

And he taxed them with heavy taxes & demanded a tribute for their Gold & for their Silver, he laid hands on the Vessels of Gold & on their Vessels of Silver wch had ministered unto him saying:

[*p. 108*]

10th

These are a chosen people of the City and their inheritance is very great, their riches who is able to account! Verrily I will make them tributary to the King. Tho' peradventure they may vex wroth, and turn away their countenance from me

11th

And he did so

12th

And he ceased to do what is righteous in the Eyes of the Multitude and wrought evil in their sight. The light which the Lord have given them hath he taken away and withheld from them

13th

He taxed also their Young Men & Maidens

14th

And the Maidens gathered themselves together and threw themselves at the feet of the Young Man and they besought him to have pity on them, but he hearkened not unto them

[*p. 109*]

15th

Then a Woman named Mary who was a sojourner in the City lift up her Voice and said unto him

16th

Once thou wast the Idol of the people but now thou art despised among them. thou hast deprived the poor of Bread & Rayment. Even the light of the Sun hast thou robbed them off.

17th

Therefore will I trundle my Mop in thy face, and blind thee with the Water of impurity, Moreover the Napkin shall be far from thee, that the filth may remain upon thy countenance for thou has dealt wickedly unto me.

18th

The Glazier shall smite thee wth his Hammer. And the Butcher with a portion of his Sheep. Yea every shopkeeper shall reach forth his hand against thee, [*p. 110*] because thou makest them poor & Needy. they have Cried unto thee, and thou hast not heard them.

19th

Woe be unto thee thou backslider. Woe be unto thee Chathamite for thou settest thy face against the poor & bestoweth thy good things on the rich and ungodly.

20th

The people cry out against thee in the Streets, thy name stinketh in the Nostrils of the upright, thy Effigy they have placed on a Gibbett and they mock thee when thou passes by them

21st

Turn thou then from thy evil ways, and thy sins shall be forgiven thee, neither shall thy countenance be any more defiled by the Waters issuing from the Mop[1]

---

1. This satirical chapter separates diary entries from the years 1785 and 1786, but may date from as late as 1791 when Savory compiled this volume as a digest of scattered sources. The second and seventh verses provide the key to this satirical critique of Pitt the Younger's policies. Both the reference to 'purple and fine linen' and to sumptuous fare hint at the Biblical story of the Rich Man (exemplified here by Pitt) and Lazarus (a symbol of the people/the poor) (see Luke 16:19-31). This is reinforced by references to conspicuous consumption and allusions to Pitt's general over-indulgence in food and drink, and unnecessary luxuries such as spice. Such greed and excess contrasts sharply with the impoverishment of the people who have allegedly been punitively taxed to pay for such extravagance. Pitt's selfishness (verse 8) parallels the rich man's rejection of the needy Lazarus which condemns the rich man to Hell, whilst Lazarus's essential goodness commends him to Abraham in Heaven. The expense of war, and Pitt's determination to base his Government on sound finance (running balanced budgets), demanded increasingly high levels of taxation. Verse 9 highlights the popular discontent that resulted. The reference to the gathering maidens in verse 14 refers to Pitt's unpopular tax on servants, for which he was

*   *   *

[pp. 111-114 missing, cut from the MS[1]]

[p. 115] forliten thaem the Scyldegat with us and ne gelaet, us gelude, in costnins gae Ah gelefe us of Yfle.[2]

To buy a Spirit

Give the condemn person something for his Spirit and make an agreement that he do serve you at all times and upon all occasions and it must be signd with 3 Drops of his Blood and 3 hairs of his head[.] this I was told off by Dr Jones who I think is supersitious [*sic*] enough to beleive it.

To appear Invisible

Take a Catt that is all over Black and put him instantly in a pott of boiling water. when its cold stand wth your back towards the pott looking in [*p. 116*] a Glass and pick out every bone seperately one by one looking at them in a Glass. there is a certain bone when you take it out of the Water you cannot see in the Glass then its done. keep that Bone for your use[.] with this bone any person may appear invisible – this is another of Dr Jones repartis [*i.e. repartees*] who when he was in Wales it was told him and that it was experienced on Board a Ship.

Over the Fire place at the George in Speenhamland[3] is the following Verse
Stand aside 'tis every ones desire
As well as you to see and feel the fire
At that time one Ventrice was LandLord[.][1] he used to Cure wounds &c. since the Rooms has been all altered[.]

---

persistently criticised and mocked, whilst both the references to light (in verses 12 and 16) and the glazier (in verse 18) target the controversial window tax (and in the case of the first two references, possibly also the tax on candles). The shopkeeper, also referred to in verse 18, contests the tax on rents for retail premises introduced in 1785 but reformed in 1789. Other references, to the filth and squalor of the mob and the mop appear to respond to (or otherwise anticipate) Pitt's taxes on soap and starch which were introduced in 1792. The satire hints that popular opposition to these taxes could threaten Pitt's continued electoral success and, if not remedied, might even result in popular riots.

1. Savory gives a hint of the missing material in his list of Contents at the end of the volume: 'Letter Inocent 3rd p. 111' and 'Lords Prayer, p. 114', see [(270)].
2. This would appear to be a passage from the Lord's Prayer in Old English, probably of the ninth century; the contents list on [(270)] indicates that it began on the previous page [114] which is missing.
3. This is the George and Pelican Inn, Speenhamland, one of the area's largest and most popular coaching inns. It was here, in 1795, that the Berkshire magistrates would devise the so-called 'Speenhamland System' of poor relief, which set the scale of payments made to subsidise the wages of the labouring poor according to the price of bread and the size of the labourer's family. For another reference to this inn, see [157].

*　　　*　　　*

[*p. 117*]

1786

Jan[ua]ry. this month the Shop and Bottles was new painted by one Powell,[2] he taught me to Etch and Engrave but in return he borrowd my flute as Uncle B[ough]t of Avery Hobbs, an incission knife and the 4 Books of Cornelius Agrippa[,] so thats a reward by putting to great confidence in a stranger. On Feb[rua]ry 1st I won a curious piece of Shell Work at Rafling. the 5th. Died my Grandfather Wm Savory at a ¼ past 3 o'Clock in the afternoon and on the 10th he was interrd in Brightwaltham Church Yard in the 90th Year of his Age. Mr Barns of Wantage was undertaker[.] every tradesman and farmer had Hatt bands & Gloves. My Grandfather left Uncle John Savory executor[:] to my 3 Sisters £60 each & to myself £100{;} to my Mother £150 & to [*p. 118*] the poor of the parish Bread.[3]

the 19th was the first time of going to Nathaniel Winters[4] to have my hair dressd. Old Walsh lately died[5] and his Grandson John (Son of the present Walsh in Northbrook Street) not minding the business as he ought to do for his Grand Mother, she declind business.[6] this said John Walsh left Newbury 4/ in my debt. Feb[rua]ry 20th. Died Mrs Waters wife of Dr Waters[.] Bo[ugh]t of Dr Waters Ambrose Parcy[7] for 10/6 & a Book of his own hand writing containing Receits for diseases &c.[8] this Wm Waters was very well versd in Astrology & casting Urine, he left Newbury about this time and went to live at Reading where he soon paid the last debt of Nature. he was very much addicted to drinking & Women which was his utter ruin.

---

1. John Ventrice (1744-1790) was buried at St Nicholas's Church, Newbury, on 12 January 1790.
2. Possibly Robert Powell, a bookbinder, listed in the *UD*. He appears to have owned a paper mill in Bagnor but was declared bankrupt in 1792: see *RM* (6 February 1792).
3. As Savory correctly states, his grandfather's will was proved on 2 October 1786 (TNA PCC ROB 11/1147/2). The will was made on 5 May 1784. It provided that £60 should be paid to each of his granddaughters: to be paid to Sarah within one year of his death, to Jane within two, and Mary within three. Savory himself was to receive £100 within four years. The testator's widowed daughter-in-law, Jane (Savory's mother), would receive £150 within five years. In none of these cases would interest be paid. He bequeathed 'a gallon loaf' to 'every poor family in the parish of Brightwalton', and 'a half gallon' loaf to a single (unmarried) poor person, to be distributed in the parish church by his son, John Savory. John Savory would inherit the remainder of the estate, except for the house in which Jane Savory and her children lived, which would remain in the joint ownership of Jane Savory and her brother-in-law, John Savory, and after their deaths, would be inherited by Savory. See also [125].
4. No Walsh is listed in the *UD*, but Nathaniel Winter, hair-dresser, is listed under Newbury
5. Thomas Walsh, buried at St Nicholas's Church, Newbury, on 3 April 1785.
6. Elizabeth Walsh, buried at St Nicholas's Church, Newbury, on 6 December 1791.
7. Ambrose Parcy, properly called Ambroise Paré (c.1510-1590), was a celebrated barber-surgeon in the French court whose works, translated into English in the seventeenth century, were still in use at this time.
8. Peachey, who reproduces this list of books, comments, 'it surely must have been exceptional to find a lad of that age [17] who would by choice expend so considerable sum on books of this description', Peachey, *Life of William Savory*, 7.

[*p. 119*] May 15th. We had a New Still Tub measurd 84 Galln at 4½d pr Galln. the 20th. One Jones a Britches Maker made me a pair of Blue Leather britches[.] he was a Methodist preacher[,] used to travel and had a Crooked Leg but a very false Lying fellow &c.

April 12th. My Sister Sarah sent me the 4th Book of Cornelius Agrippa[.] Bo[ugh]t of Toomer an Incission knife wth Gum Lancet, at 3/.[1]

May 8th. Mr Moore Druggist in London sent me 2 Lancetts and Case as a present.[2] the 16th. My Curiosity led me to Newtown Church[.] One Verse on a Tomb Stone I particularly noticed which was for Mr Geo[rge] Vokins a person of great genious –
"Injenious Friendship did thy Soul possess
"In science great thy works do well express
"Such wast thee George few could thee excell
"Alass: thourt [*i.e. thou art*] gone in hopes in heav'n to dwell.["][3]

[*p. 120*] June 21st. I sent the following lines to Reading & was inserted in the paper: –
Last Sunday was married Mr George Fuse Carpenter and Joiner of Brightwalton in this County to Miss Mary Coxhead of <Chaddleworth eldest daughter of Mr Anthony Coxhead> of Leckhamstead[,] a beautifull Young Lady of a considerable fortune & every accomplishment to render the marriage state happy.

The above caused great disquietness to George and his Wife as I did not know her parents I thought Anthony was a name as would do for her father, for she was a very disagreeable Woman both in her personal & mental accomplishments.[4]

27th. B[ough]t 3 Carboys of OC Turpentine for my Uncle at the rate of 36/ per [?CwZ].

[*p. 121*] I had a misfortune about this time to break a pane of Glass in the Shop Window owing <to> the highness of the Wind in putting up the Shutters[,] but it not being known to my Master or Mrs the next day – I went out the next evening & did my business as quick as possible. I made great haste back and seeing a good opportunity being a dark Ev[enin]g I broke the Glass again & ran off & came back again quite unconcerned and so I got rid of Censure from my Mas[te]r or Mrs.

About this time one Dame Harding an elderly woman of Shaw used frequently to visit our Shop[.] she was computed a Witch. used to tell fortunes by Tea Leaves &c. [*p. 122*] this Dame Harding used to say if any person carry a knife at 11 o'Clock at Night to a Cross Way on Midsummer

1. Joseph Toomer (1760-1853) was a well-known ironmonger with a shop on Northbrook Street, Newbury. Four times Mayor of Newbury, he organised a census of the town, 20 May-9 June 1815.
2. Peachey considered that this reference suggests a connection between Savory and the drugs firm of Savory and Moore, see Peachey, *Life of William Saory*, 7n. No connection has been uncovered and seems unlikely. The company was founded in 1794 and dissolved in 1992.
3. This is George Vokins, a clockmaker aged 34, who was buried at Holy Trinity Church, Newtown, Hampshire, on 10 February 1786, merely two months before this inscription was apparently read and recorded by Savory.
4. Mary Coxhead married George Fuse or Fuce at St Nicholas's Church, Newbury, on 11 June 1786.

Eve and say he (or She) that is my true Love come and fit a sheath to this knife & they will come.

And if you break an Egg at 12 o'Clock on Midsummer Day & put it in a Glass of Water till 1 o'Clock you will see comical things. if you rake the Ashes over on Midsummer Eve when you go to Bed, the next morning you will see the print of a Coffin in the Ashes if this will any friend or relation dies that Year.

July 18th. Begun learning of French Bo[ugh]t the following Books: –
[*p. 123*]

French Grammar	3/-
[?Thames]	2/6
Prayer Book	2/6
Dictionary	12/-
Entrance	10/6

Monsier used to lodge with Mr Attkins[1] in Batholomew street[.] he came to me twice a week for 1 Month but Monsier left Newbury without delivering the sentiments of his mind to any one I beleive by reason of his Debts. Aug[us]t 7th. Bo[ugh]t of Old Mr Whitewood a large Book title Riveruos on Physic for 5/-. the 17th & 18th of this Month distilld 3 Cz w[or]th of pepperm[in]t had only iv oz of Oil from it owing to Davids Wooden contrivance. the 21st. Mary Walker our Servant Maid was [*p. 124*] conducted to Newbury prison for Larciny. the time she was to be with Mr Jones was almost expired to a few days when she collected a few Articles together & packd it up with the cloathes[.] in the Morning prior to her parting with Mr Jones she carried down stairs two or three bundles privately & took it to a faggot pile in the Yard but fortunately it was observed by Mr Jones who was from Bed earlier that Morning than in general. in these bundles was found with her cloathes: Hankerchiefs, Silver Spoon, Blue &c; the property of Mr Jones[.] she was tryed at Sessions and received 1 Months imprisonment.

Sept[embe]r 13th. Was Married at Brightwaltham John Eagles to my sister Jane. the 20th. Bo[ugh]t Buckthorn berries at 10d pr Gall[o]n. Oct[obe]r 1st. Went with my Uncle Jo[h]n Savory to London by Newbury Coach & my curiosity[2] [*p. 125*] led me to Number the public Houses that we passd by from Speenhamland to Hide Park Corner which was 222 as also the distance of the places from Speenhamland to Hide Park Corner: –

from Speenhamland	Miles	from Speenhamland	Miles
to Thatcham	3	to Slow [*i.e. Slough*]	35
to Woolhampton	6 ½	to Colnbrook	38
to Theale	12	to Cranford Bridge	43
to Reading	17	to Hounslow	46
to twiford	22	New Brentford	49
to Harehatch	24	Turnham Green	51
to Maidenhead	30	Hide Park Corner	56
to Salt Hill	34	* * *	

1. Probably John Atkins, ironmonger, Newbury, listed in the *UD*.
2. The word 'curiosity' is split across the two pages.

We went the next day to Doctors Commons and Uncle administered to Grandfather's Will[.]¹ it cost him £10. 7s. 6d in all that was for transferring his name &c at the Bank instead of Grandfathers. Bo[ugh]t a Flute cost £2. 12s. 6d.

[*p. 126*] The Sunday we went to a Jews Burying. there was a Hearse to convey the Corpse to the burying ground)as² is customary for the poorest person that is). and two Mourning Coaches and upwards of 20 Hackney Coaches followed. the Corpse is never caried on Shoulders as is customary with us but when they get to the burying Ground the Corpse is taken out of the hearse and as many as can asist conveys the Corpse into the Meeting House upon their Arms and then the Corpse is putt on Stools, the Lead of the Coffin is unhapsed (as they seldom use Nails or Screws) and something done to the deceased then the relations Garment is rented by Cutting the Coat with a knife[,] afterwards a few prayers &c. spoke in Hebrew, the Lead of the Coffin is hapsed on again and conveyd to the Grave. when I went into the burying ground I was astonished to see so many relations & friends of Deceasd [*p. 127*] persons weaping and praying over the Graves for the good of the departed Souls. The Tomb stones were very numerous, mostly laid Horizontal most of the inscriptions was in Hebrew. its a very common custom with them to put Lime in the Graves and when the body is putt in throws in some water to burn the Body, sometimes there is holes at the bottom of the Coffin for the heat of the Lime to get at the body and sometimes the body is put in the ground & the Coffin broke to pieces and thrown in afterwards. they generally interr the Body in the Earth so soon as it has resignd its breath if it before Sun sett.

I remember being in London once when my Brother in law was sent for & several other Coachmen to attend with their Coaches a Corpse whom the relations thought Dead. When they came to [*p. 128*] the House to their mortification he had not quite resignd his breath and a person of the House told them he was not quite Dead.

Nov[embe]r 15th. My Uncle had some fruit trees from Reading and made an Orchard at Brightwaltham[;] before it was a Garden.

Nov[embe]r 16th. Mr Spanswick of Eastbury sent Mr Jones a Letter as follows:

Mr Jones, sir i hope your wife and family are well as we are at present. please to send me a little parsel of the true brown salt of phylosophers[,] the true salt you know is all they seek. White, Brown or Red it matters not so it be brought to the fire seven times, purified from all it's [*sic*] filth. Coagulated or Calsinated up to its true perfection. my Body is Dead and past fermentation & is ready for putrifacttion so next i intend by divine help to quicken [*p. 129*] the Dead, and revive the living into a pure transparent copus [*i.e. corpus*] or Body. though a few grains of the true Magnett being sprinkled upon and of borne again of pure water or transmutated into a pure spirit[,]

Thos Spanswick.

---

1. For details of the will, see [117-118 and *n*].
2. Oddly Savory has written this opening bracket as a closing bracket.

his Body being dead is meant the Liquor he has fermented and ready for Distillation, and the thing sent for was Grays Salts. This Spanswick is Dr Jones Landlord & is a Methodist preacher.[1]

Nov 25 I had the Misfortune of burning my hand by mixing together Oil Vitriol and Sp[iri]t Turpentine in a Vial by moving the Vial to Cork it and made as loud report as a Gun. Dec[embe]r 12th was born Wm, Son of John and Jane Eagles[.] he died in his infancy[.] the 20th. Th[oma]s Taylor at the Marquis of Grandby fractured the fibula.

[p. 130]

Mrs Andrews
Child born June
24th 1786 6h. 15' PM[2]

This Mrs Andrews was delivered of twins and one of them which the above Scheme is drawn for died when 6 Weeks old.[3] The testimonies of Short Life is very evident in the above Scheme for the degree Ascending is afflicted by the {Moon} Lady of the House of Death. {Jupiter} L[or]d Asc[endant] is afflicted in the house of sickness by {Mars} L[or]d 4 & 12th. the {Sun} Locally posited in the house of Death and {Venus} Lady 6th afflicted by Mala in the 8th are all testimonies of Short Life.

*　　　*　　　*

[p. 131][4]

1st experiment
of a Woman
dying in Child
Bed at 32 years
of Age

The terms of the infortunes being upon Angles of this Geniture above discover a Violent death but by dying in Child Bed is not thereby discovered. Yet in this Nativity its plain for not only {Aries} in 8 in dignities of {Mercury} but {Saturn} & {Mars} in 4th cast a {square} thither with {Mercury} his almost Cardinal {sqaure} {Saturn} {Jupiter} L[or]d 5th doth sufficiently demonstrate the very kind thereoff. Algol sais {Venus} afflicts in duo decim denotes danger in Child Bed.

---

1. Thomas Spanswick's applications to hold Methodist meetings are reproduced in *Berkshire Nonconformist Meeting House Regulations 1689-1852, Part I*, ed. L. Spurrier (Berkshire Record Society, ix, 2005), 28, 33-34. He was buried at St Michael's and All Angels' Church, Lambourn, on 2 January 1817, aged 72.
2. This is a standard geniture, Savory's preferred form of horoscope.
3. Lucy, daughter of Richard and Lucy Andrews, was buried at St Nicholas's Church, Newbury, on 13 August 1786.
4. This page and the next are divided vertically into two columns, each dedicated to a single geniture.

**2nd experiment
of a Woman
dying In Child
Bed at 22 Years**

The L[or]d Asc[endant] in {square} {Mars} & in {oppostion} {Mercury} &
the {Moon} in a Violent part of heaven in the times of a Malevolent denotes
a Violent Death & why may not the position of {Saturn} in 5 with {Aries} in
ill aspect of {Mars} & in warn of {Mercury} L[or]d 8 & 5 in a feral part of
the Zodiac declares the very kind thereoff, also adding the {Sun} in 12
disposing of {Moon} {Jupiter} L[or]d [?14] in 8th &c.

*   *   *

[p. 132]

**1st experiment
of a stinking
Breath.**

{Jupiter} in 6th in Dark and pitted degrees in the terms of {Mars} in
{square} of [?him] also. {Mercury} L[or]d of the Sp[iri]ts so {Jupiter} of the
Lungs is in pitted & Void degrees & {square} of {Saturn} L[or]d 1. all which
are arguments of a Corrupted & stinking Breath.

*   *   *

**2nd experiment
of a stinking
Breath.**

{Jupiter} L[or]d 6th in the degrees termed Void. {Venus} Lady 1st in
{conjunction} {Mercury} Combusts & in {opposition} to {Saturn} in Azimi
degrees also {Moon} in the dignity of {Saturn} in degrees termed dark and
pitted.

*   *   *

[*p. 133*]

Geo: 3rd King of
Great Britain &c.
Born May 24th
1738
7h. 51'. 40" AM[1]

God Bless great Geo: our K[in]g
Long live our Noble K[in]g
God save the King.[2]

*   *   *

[*p. 134*] The following is a Letter I received from Mr Ebenezer Sibley student in Astrology &c.[3]

Sir,

This moment your letter came to hand, and according to your desire I ~~have~~[4] insert the planetts places for June 28th 1768[5] they are at Noon: –

{Sun}	7.. 8	{Cancer}	Declination	23. 17
{Moon}	17.. 34	{Sagittarius}	Latt. South	2. 17
{Saturn}	7.23	{Cancer}	Latt. S	0. 27
{Jupiter}	13.34	{Libra}	Latt. N	1. 12.
{Mars]	6.40	{Aries}	Latt. S	2. 33
{Venus}	24.34	{Gemini}	Latt. S	2. 0
{Mercury}	0..9	{Leo}	Latt. N	1. 23
{Leo}	12.9	{Capticorn}	_____	
{Aries}	12.9	{Capticorn}	_____	

Thus Sir as you are a lover of Science I have complied with your Request. wishing you all the success [*p. 135*] as possible to be desired from being a Son of the divine Urania & remain your friend,

E Sibley

P.S If you want any Ephemeris you may have them by directing the parcell with Money to me No. 39 Castle Street Bristol[:] the price of them is 1/ each.

---

1. In fact, George III was born on 4 June 1738, and his successors, George IV and William IV, both officially marked their birthdays on 4 June in order to minimise disruption to the court calendar of public celebrations.
2. These words were first publicly performed as a song in 1745 in the reign of George II, but did not become the National Anthem of Great Britain until the early nineteenth century.
3. The Sibly brothers were the most famous contemporary astrologers in Britain at this time. Ebenezer Sibly (1751-1799), who was also a physician, published a large textbook on astrology, the most complete study of the subject since Partridge's time. He sought to incorporate astrology into the scientifically informed world-view of Copernicus and Newton, blending medieval and modern views.
4. Savory has struck through the word 'have' with a heavy curling line.
5. i.e. Savory's date of birth.

To conclude this Year I shall insert the Geniture of my nephew Wm Savory Norris Son of Joseph and Mary Norris in Brightwaltham.

*   *   *

[*p. 136*]

Wm Savory Norris
Born July 7th 1784
6hs. 46' PM

The general testimonies that declare the shortness of this Natives Life are many. {Saturn} in Asc[endan]t In {opposition} to {Venus}[1] who hath great dignities in the 8th.{Mercury} who hath dominion in the 8th afflict the degree Ascending but I take {Saturn} to be principal L[or]d Asc[endan]t who is in his own house must asist the Native in his infancy & in {sextile} {Moon} and {Moon} from {trine} {Sun} who as I call giver of Life is in {sextile} to {Saturn}[,] however the {opposition} {Sun} and {Saturn} & {Mercury} L[or]d 6 in {opposition} Asc[endant] denotes dangerous [*p. 137*] sickness in the Natives infancy. {Jupiter} also L[or]d Asc[endan]t in his own house with {Leo} in {trine} {Venus} Lady 4th & {Mars} in 8th in friendly aspect to the Asc[endan]t signifies the Native to live past his infancy to some malignant direction which may be seen by a Speculum for this Geniture. {Saturn} {Jupiter} and {Mercury} seems to surmount the rest in essential dignities and accidental fortitudes denotes the Native will be inclind to a changeable disposition sometimes Witty & Merry mixt with Melancholy and grave. will be given to study and reading & delight in Religion. nevertheless subject to Slanders saying of him such things has been committed by him he never thought off [*sic*] and Vice Versa.

 [*p. 138*] {Saturn} and {Jupiter} Accidental gives him a mean Stature inclinable to Brevity[,] well set and shall obtain substance by his own Labour and Industry.

 {Saturn} L[or]d 2nd of Substance & well dignified. {Jupiter} {Moon} & {Leo} near the 2nd House in {sextile} to {Saturn} gives a very good fortune and that which is durable[,] but {Mercury} in {opposition} to {Saturn} denotes that by Sickness, Success or Curiositys, people he deal with, adversarys shall afflict his substance. {Mercury} in {square} to {Moon} & Cusp of the 3rd & L[or]d 4th from the 3rd denotes short Life or great sickness to some of his Brothers or Sisters. if the Native should live to Years of maturity he will marry & perhaps more than once as {Mercury} L[or]d 7th is in {Gemini} {Moon} in {Pisces} &c. the significations respecting the 9th House signifies him to be an Hypocrite in Religion.

---

1. The sign for Venus appears to be encircled.

[*p. 139*]

1787

Jan[ua]ry 4th. Uncle John Savory went to London and on the 17th he returned[.] My Sister Fordham was at that time very dangerous Ill.[1] A Verse told me by Mrs Goddard who was nurse to my mistress at that time to be said St Agnes Eve[:][2]

"St Agnes good pray, do me right
And send my true Love here this Night
That I may behold his face
And he in my kind Arms embrace[."]

28th. Was inserted in the Reading paper:
Lately was married Mr Dan[ie]l Whister of Chaddleworth to Miss Grace Goodluck.[3]

this Dan[ie]l Whister is scooldmaster at Chaddleworth and his wife was the daughter of Rob[er]t Goodluck who keeps the turnpike at Shefford cal[le]d Sr Rob[er]t.

[*p. 140*] The 12th of Jan[ua]ry was Buried at Speen Mr Thos Phillips[4] Brandy merchant at Speenhamland[.] he left behind him 1 Daughter who was married to Mr Hicks at Skinners Green but is since dead[.] when I was in London I br[ough]t home the following Verses that I took off of Tomb Stones: –

My Time is spent in time repent
In living learn to Die
Old and Young defer not long
For Death comes suddenly

Grieve not for me for why my Race is <Run>
It is the Lords so let his Will be done
I change this present Life but for a new
Then with a Groan he bid the World adiue [*sic*]
He presently submitted unto Death
And like a Lamb resigned up his breath

[*p. 141*]
Since none excepted are from Death
Pray serve the Lord while you have <breath>
Prepare to Die without delay

---

1. In August her daughter Miriam would die, followed in December by her eldest child, Jane.
2. i.e. 20 January.
3. In fact, the notice read, 'Lately was married, at Wantage, Mr Daniel Whistler, of Chaddleworth, to Miss Grace Goodluck, daughter of Mr Robert Goodluck, of Charlton.' See *RM* (29 January 1787). Daniel Whistler Jnr, schoolmaster of Chaddleworth, married Grace Good*lake* by licence at Wantage, on 3 January 1787. See *Berkshire Schools in the Eighteenth Century*, ed. S Clifford (Berkshire Record Society, xxvi, 2019) 41. For references to the Whistlers, see [53, 56, 67].
4. 'Thos Philips' was buried at St Mary's Church, Speen, on 12 *February* 1787.

For in my prime I was cal[le]d away

The World is nothing Heavens all
Death have not wronged me by this fall
My time is spent my Glass is Run
And now Lord Jesus I am come

March 1st. Died Wm Savory Eagles, my sister Janes 1st Child[;] at this
time the Measels was very prevalent and my Sisters Jane and Mary was
infected with it – people young and Old – but I escaped it at this time.

Mr Falshaw Druggist in London told me his private marks which I [*p.
142*] have used ever since.[1]

> B u y   a n d   s e l x
> 1 2 3   4 5 6   7 8 9 10

<April> 17th. Rec[eive]d a Letter from my sister Sarah that her Youngest
Child Miriam was Dead.[2] May 26th. was buried at Boxford Church Farmer
Rd Nalder who married Sarah Hughes of Westbrook & Brother in law to Mrs
Jones[.] they used to live at a lone farm near Huntsgreen[.] since his Death
Mrs Nalder keeps a grocery Shop at Westbrook.[3] June 1st. Bo[ugh]t 9lbs of
Adderstongue at 4d pr lb[.] the 7th had my hair tied the first time[.] the 9th.
The Revd Richd Boucher Rector of Brightwaltham came from London with
his new Wife and gave Brightwaltham Ringers two Guineas[.] her name was
[*p. 143*] Rebecca Coney.[4] the 25th. Died Mr John Blackney farmer at
Brightwaltham. he was a particular acquaintance of my fathers & Uncle[;]
had a good estate of his Own one time in Brightwaltham but when he died his
Son John sold it to Mr Herbart [*sic*] it being mortgaged for nearly what it was
worth.[5] July 7th. at 2 o'Clock this Morning we was alarmd by fire in Mr
Jones Bed Room occasioned by Mary Jones a Child of two Years of Age
setting fire to the Bed Curtains with a Rush Light that was then burning in the
Room, but fortunately it was prevented from doing any further damage than
burning the Bedding &c. in that Room being computed about £10 damage.
    this summer we had the players in Newbury.

---

1. Falshaw and Horner, 'druggists and chymists', based at 11 Old Fish Street, London (*Kent's
   Directory for the Year 1794. Cities of London and Westminster, & Borough of Southwark*).
2. Miriam Fordham, aged five months, had been buried at St Mary's Church, Whitechapel, on 15
   April 1787, having been baptised there on 7 March.
3. Richard Nalder married Sarah Hughes by licence at St Mary's Church, Boxford, on 24
   October 1781. The register confirms Richard's burial on 26 May 1787; Sarah was buried on
   27 April 1808.
4. The couple had married in Tottenham, on 7 June 1787, a date confirmed in RBA D/EW/O8,
   235, which also confirms the payment of 2 Guineas to Brightwalton's Ringers.
5. John Blackney (1720-1787) was one of the few freeholders of Brightwalton in the eighteenth
   century, see Osment, Sayers and Stephens, *Brightwaltron*, 12-13. He was buried on 28 June
   1787. His son, John Blackney (1759-1849), had a large family and moved to Hampshire.

[*p. 144*] 14th Aug[u]st Went to Paughly[1] tempis primus.[2]

22nd. Mr Richd Bird of Brightwaltham was presented with a Ride to Reading Goal[.] [*sic*] this Bird is since Dead[.] he was a Crafty roaguish person[,] was by trade a Taylor but not content with his business he occupied a farm[,] the farm where Fruin Wicks now lives[,] Ballards Farm[,] after that to Hungerford & kept the Red Lion[.] A little while from there back to Brightwaltham where <he> was taken and had to Reading[.] since that they went to Live at Langly Broom by Slow[3] & was a Master of a Workhouse and there he paid the last debt of Nature[.] he built the Barn at Brightwaltham cal[le]d Birds Folly was left near £2000 by his friends but died worse than nothing[.] has three Sons left and 4 Daught[e]rs (viz) R[ichar]d John & Luke, [*p. 145*] Phebe, Mary, Eliz[abe]th and the young one.

Bo[ugh]t of Charles Moore who was apprentice to Mr Thomson a Jeweller in Newbury some Engraving Tools[,] he was a particular companion of mine[,] also one James Hawthorn, Nephew of Padburys in Speenhamland.

The following Verse was written in a prayer book of a Young Ladies

Of on my knees at Church I've been
> One prayer my first & last
A Husband is the thing I mean
> Good Lord I am in haste

The following is a few Questions, Rebuses, Enigmas &c. I have taken from my fathers Books: –

Divide a Number by a line thats straight
The half is evidently Eight
Ans[we]r XIII[4]

[*p. 146*] I am twenty Years of Age yet never saw ten birth days
> Ans[we]r
Last 29th of Feb[rua]ry by the sages I am told being 20 Years of Age
He was but 6 birth days old.

What is less than Nothing ____ NO

Whence came the respectable name of Cuckold
The respectable name of Cuckold came from a Cuckow who lais her Eggs in the Nest of other birds as a Cuckold Maker who begets children on other mens Wifes. so contraryly we call the poor husband Cuckold when in fact he is only Cuckeld or Cuckood and therefore would in fact be cal[le]d Anticuckold.

---

1. Probably connected with the historic Poughley Priory in Chaddleworth; for a further reference, see Appendix A.
2. i.e. the first time.
3. i.e. Langley Broom, Slough, in east Berkshire.
4. i.e. 13, in Roman numerals: XIII is written with a horizontal line through the middle, so that above the line it effectively reads VIII (8), with its mirror image below.

[*p. 147*] What God never made, nor commanded not to be made & yet twas made & has a soul to be saved _____ Cuckold!

How near Kin is my Uncles, Wifes sister in law _____ My Mother

There is a Child born of my Mother,
is neither my sister nor my Brother,
But as other Children are _____ Myself

I am still in expectation but never in Fruition _____ to Morrow

Good Morrow Mr Miles pray how does your good Lady! O Farmer, very Ill with a great Noise in her head. I am sorry for that Sir. indeed, Farmer and so am I.

A Scold

[*p. 148*]

On a Time piece[1]

See how I strive with all my might
    To tell the Hour of Day and Night
My Moments pass and so do thine
    Pray do not slight thy precious time
But take example now by me
    As serve thy God as I serve thee.

On a Taylor

On a time Mr _____ an honest Taylor of _____ was ordered to measure the Rector of that place for a Doctors Gown. the Dr had 5 Y[ar]ds of pure Scarlet & withall desired him to save every thread to mend a hole in case the Moth should eat it. the Taylor having found that there was enough laid it by. nay quoth the Doctor let me see it Cut out before I go for tho' thou canst play the knave abroad I think you are honest at home and at your work. God forbid else. [*p. 149*] quoth the Taylor and that you shall find me. for give me but 20/ from you and I will owe you 40/ in the making of your Gown. that I will said the Dr, with all my heart. The Taylor having put the money in his pockett. The Dr desired to know how he would save him 40/. Why Sir let some other Taylor make it for if I take it in hand I shall utterly spoil it for I never in all my Life made any of this fashion.

There is a Barrell belonging to Mr Moses Kittier of Ringwood in Hants, made of Juniper Wood which came from Newfoundland[,] held 350

---

1. A version of the first and last couplets, but not the middle couplet, has been noted on many clocks, sun-dials etc, see, e.g. the inscription on a Shropshire clock c. 1745, recorded in G. F. Jackson, *Shropshire Folk-Lore: A Sheaf of Gleanings* (1886), 575.

Hogsheads now full of Strong Beer. The Staves 4 Inches thick 27 Iron hoops. 19Ft High. 11Ft Wide at top & bottom 15Ft wide in the middle cost £1000.[1]

[*pp. 150-151*][2]
The silent Language
(by motion of the hand)[3]

The top of the thumb is	A
1 finger on the left thumb is	b
2 fingers on the left thumb is	c
3 fingers on the left thumb is	d
The top of the forefinger is	e
Your 2 fingers together is	f
Clinch both your hands together is	g
Shake the palms of both hands is	h
The top of the middle finger is	j
Your forefinger upon the left rist is	k
One finger upon the back of the left hand	l
3 fingers on Do.	m
2 fingers on Do.	n
The top of the ring finger is	o
Clinch your left hand is	p
Clinch your right hand is	q
Link your little fingers together is	r
The back of your hands together is	s
The top of the forefinger to the middle joint of the other is	t
The top of the little finger	u

---

1. Moses Kittier, of Ringwood, Hampshire, a brewer and Presbyterian, was also a shipowner who traded out of Notre Dame Bay, Newfoundland, until he was declared bankrupt in 1789.
2. The list is split across the two pages: [150] ends with the letter 't', and [151] begins with the letter 'u'.
3. There can be no doubt that people communicated with sign language from the earliest times. In the eighth century monks used a system of gestures and 'manual spellings'. The first written evidence of sign language among the deaf dates from 1576 when a marriage register recorded signs and gestures used at the wedding of a deaf man. The first book on teaching sign language to deaf people that contained the manual alphabet was published in 1620 by Juan Pablo de Bonet. In 1755 the first school for the deaf was founded in Paris and institutions were quickly established around Britain teaching in sign-language. Regional variations in signs resulted, some of which remain in British Sign Language today. There are important commonalities between modern-day British fingerspelling and the system Savory's father recorded: the five vowels are identical. The description for fingerspelling the letter 'g' is too ambiguous to assess, but other letters are similar in modern BSL: 'f' is the first two fingers of each hand crossed; 'h' is signalled by crossing the palms of both hands across each other; 'l' is the forefinger on the palm rather than the back of the left hand; 'm' and 'n' are likewise as Savory describes but formed on the palm rather than the back of the hand; 't' is made by pointing the right forefinger to the middle of the bottom of the left hand itself and not simply the left forefinger. Other letters are significantly different: 'b', 'c', 'd', 'k', 'p', 'q' and 'w' are substantially different in BSL to the system Savory describes, whilst some signs are now differently assigned, e.g. Savory's sign for 'r' is now the sign for 's', and his sign for 'v' is now that for 'x'. Note that both 'j' and 'x' are missing from Savory's alphabetical list.

the right hand fingers put across the \<left\>	V
the forefingers across is	x \<w\>
the right hand Do. rub[be]d against the left \<hand\>	Y
the forefinger rub[be]d toward the top	Z

[*p. 151 continued*]

To Win at Whist

You and your partner must know that your 1st finger lift up of your left hand is to play a heart, the 2nd finger a Club, the 3rd a Diamond the 4th a Spade & to know whether you have the Ace King Queen or Knave the 1st finger of your Right hand let be Ace the 2nd K[in]g &c.

*   *   *

[*p. 152*]

1788

I am now got to the Year 1788 to the 20th Year of my Age and near the expiration of my Apprentiship which caused my Spirits to be elevated on the thought of Liberty. about this time Mr Charles Southby Miliner &c. left Newbury[.] he used to live opposite the Monument[.][1] I was a great plague to him sometimes[.] his Shop door was Sr Revg[.] one time a Q[uar]t of Soap Lees was thrown over his Shutters and the paint came off. Jan[ua]ry 8th. Died Sam[ue]l Mitchel[2] SchooldMaster at Brightwaltham Son of Jos[ep]h Mitchel[.] he was a clever young man, and generally beloved by all and Henry his Youngest Brother succeeded him.[3] the 13th was the general Inoculation in Newbury for the Small Pox.

[*p. 153*] the 28th I sent Miss H. Lovelock of Grange Farm a Love Letter written backwards in the name of Wm Rolfe for this Rolfe wanted to be in her Company.[4]

My Dearest Miss[5]

I put the letter in the post, the next Markett day Rolfe went as usual into the butter Markett very innocent of the matter but they was att him like so many Birds at an Owl. It was never found out.

March[6] 13th. Was Maried at Chaddleworth the Revd Mr Wroughton to Miss Musgrave Niece of Esqr Tipping of Wooley park.[7] During the time I was with Dr Jones we had a great many patients supposed to be under an Ill

---

1. The Monument is a public house at 57 Northbrook Street, dating to the turn of the seventeenth into the eighteenth century.
2. Samuel Mitchell (1769-1788) was buried 12 January.
3. This is Henry Mitchell (1771-1797).
4. There had been a large family of Lovelocks associated with Grange Farm, Shaw, since the 1750s.
5. This is mirror-written, from right to left, and sloping backwards.
6. RBA D/EW/O8, 235 notes that in the parish of Brightwalton, 'In March 1788 was Bo[ugh]t a new set of Standard Measures Weights, and Scales for £3 9s 8d.'
7. For Rev. Philip Wroughton and Mary Anne Musgrave, see [3*n*].

tongue and used the means laid down for Witchcraft. many Boys we cured with dislocated Ancles &c. [*p. 154*] We had a great many come to us to know the event of their future Life, things lost &c. We used to distill a great many sorts of Herbs for simple Waters & Oil. We made Cordial such as Sp[iri]t Mint &c, Sp[iri]t Wine, Gin mostly from Molasses sometimes from fruit. We had Grounds from L[or]d Craven used to give 2d Gall[o]n to [?Britok] – for Beer.[1] March 25th. I left Mr Jones my Apprentiship being expired. My Uncle invited all the farmers and tradesmen in Brightwaltham[.] after dinner a half pint bumper went round

> Heres a health to he that is now set free
> That once was a 'prentice bound
> Now for his sake this holliday we'el [*sic*] make
>   So let his health go round

the beginning of April Jos[ep]h Norris painted the Draws & bottles.

[*p. 155*] April 24th. Was Maried at Brightwaltham John Tomlin to Miss Church.[2] My 1st. patient was Mills boy[3] of farmbro' whose metatarsel bones was very much disformed so that he could not walk for near 6 Months. I Cured him in 7 Weeks[.][4] I stood Godfather to Mr Hills first Child at Hill-Green[.] he was named Thos. the Godmothers was Miss Ward of Paughly and Miss Alley in Bidden Common & Hill himself was the other Godfather[.] we staid till about 3 o'Clock in the Morning. this Hill was a Mallster [*i.e. Maltster*] at Hill-Green & Married Mackrils daughter of peasemore[.] they are since gone to Whitchurch near Reading.[5] I staied at Brightwaltham after I was out of my apprentiship till Oct[obe]r 2nd and then I went to the Hospital.

[*p. 156*] During the time I was at my Uncles which was from Mar[ch] 25 to Sept[embe]r 28, I Bled 62 people and drawed 17 teeth. I got myself a little in disgrace at this time when Wm Dance was Married[6] (who is since dead)[7] being with the ringers at Lilly coming home with Joe Taylor & Joe Mitchel we must needs have a frolic[.] our first exploit was throwing Wood in the Well at White Lands and breaking all the gates to Sargeant Taylors. we then went to Wm Janaways who lives in the Corner of the Holt Common, and threw down his Hay Ricks & broke a new wickett gate to pieces[.][8] we then broke what gates we could all the Way to Trumpletts[.] we was taken up [*p. 157*] and appeared before the Justices at the pelican at Speenhamland upon

---

1. William Craven (1738-1791), 6th Baron Craven, a major landowner, and from 1786 Lord Lieutenant of Berkshire, and Colonel in the Berkshire Militia. See [257*n*].
2. John Tomlin married Ann Church, on *21* April 1788.
3. One of the six children of Benjamin (d. 1781) and Ann Mills (d. 1811).
4. Peachey comments caustically, 'His surgery was happily of a higher quality than his English', see Peachey, *Life of William Savory*, 10.
5. This is Thomas Hill, baptised at St James's Church, Leckhampstead, on 20 September 1787, the son of Francis Hill and his wife Elizabeth, née Mackrill, who married at Peasemore, on 12 July 1786.
6. This was 10 July 1788, when William Dance married Dinah Dance at All Saints' Church, Brightwalton.
7. William Dance was buried at Brightwalton on 12 July 1791.
8. This is William Janaway (d. 1811).

susspission & likewise Jos[ep]h Mitchel Sen[io]r, but they could <do>
nothing with us. Another time we pushed down a high pile of fellies that
stood in Painters Y[ar]d. Also put Old Arthur Whiters Cow Racks in the
Middle of the pond in the upper street. Francis New[1] and myself and one
Norris that lived there car[rie]d Charles Whistlers plow from out of
Chaddleworth field by Whitings to Chaddleworth Common and hung it up
~~the~~ A tree. and wrote on it

The Man is bad and if you can
Take down the plow & hang the Man.

                    *   *   *

[*p. 158*] The following pleasant devise was what was done by my orders
at Mr Harberts Brightwaltham Farm.

Some of the Servants in the Harvest 1788 lost some of their Cloathes. I
ordered them to get a large Kettle or pott which was all over black and put a
Cock underneath and all the Servants to go in the room which was to be
made dark, and some one say, I command you to walk round three times
hand in hand and then touch each of you the Kettle and as hard as you can[,]
and that as is guilty the Cock will Crow when he touches.

now its being dark the Guilty person will not touch, so that they was all
let [*p. 159*] out of the room immediately[:] when examining the suspected
persons hand he had no black on it therefore pronounced him Guilty. I shall
now add all the Charms I have collected from Dr Waters and others and first
Charms for the Tooth Ach or Ague.

Write on a piece of paper (a quarter of a sheet) in large letters[2]

                    S A T O R
                    A R E P O
                    T E N E T
                    O P E R A
                    R O T A S

Rowl it up and hang it about the parties Neck that it may lay betwixt the
breast.

---

1. For Francis New, see [232*n*].
2. Peachey, who published this amulet, among other examples of witchcraft 'charms' in his
   selection from Savory, incorrectly transcribes the second and fourth lines 'A R E B O' and
   'O B E R A' respectively: see Peachey, *Life of William Savory*, 8.

[*p. 160*]

or

Abracadebra	
Abracadebr	
Abracadeb	Rowl this inscription
Abracade	
Abracad	and hang it on
Abraca	
Abrac	a string round the
Abra	
Abr	parties neck &
Ab	
A	a little Pulv Creta[1] in it

or

Take a part of a Hoop of a Barrell cut as many notches as the patient has had fitts and other piece of the same length and Write the patients name laying them a Cross the fire saying this Charm: –
Abracadebra
with the blessings of God I comm[an]d this away <from thee>
Abracadebr
with &c.

[*p. 161*]

A Charm for the Ague[2]

Kalendenta	
Kalendent	This never fails
Kalenden	any kind of Ague
Kalende	write down on a piece
Kalend	of bread these characters
Kalen	then Cutt off the top
Kale	line and give to the patient
Kal	to eat and so every day
Ka	for 9 days and the last
K	piece give to the Dog

A Charm for Warts

Set down as many dotts as the person has got Warts supposing 8 makes a {X}[1] touching the warts with your middle finger wrapping up a Snail or Spider wth this inscription[:]

---

1. i.e. chalk.
2. See T. R. Forbes, 'Verbal Charms in British Folk Medicine', in *Proceedings of the American Philosophical Society*, cxv:iv (20 August 1971), 293-316.

[*p. 162*]
[?Sun is] Steady
{X}[2] bury it in the Earth & say with the blessings of the 4 Apostles I command these Warts away from thee.

Against the Falling Evil[3]

Gasper [*i.e. Gaspar*] wth his mirth [*sic*] began
These presents to unfold
Then Melchior bro[ugh]t in frankincense
And Balthasar bro[ugh]t in Gold
Now he that of these holy things
These names about shall bear
The Fall[in]g Ill by grace of Xt [*i.e. Christ*]
Shall never need to fear.[4]

*   *   *

[*p. 163*]

The Charm of Charms

Against Witchcraft taken from the 6 Chapter Epesians [*i.e. Ephesians*] beginning at the 10th Verse to 14th.[5]

Whoso beareth this sign about them, all Sp[iri]ts shall do them homage	Whoso beareth this Sign about them let him fear no foe but God.[6]

*   *   *

---

1. A cross, in the form of an 'X', with two dots written in each quarter.
2. As above, a cross, in the form of an 'X', with two dots written in each quarter.
3. Immediately below this heading, on the right-hand side of the page, Savory has drawn a cross in the form of a '+', the centre of which is encircled. Each quarter of the cross contains numerous dots which together form the outline of a diamond; each quarter also contains one small x-shaped cross, these four crosses marking the corners of a square within the diamond.
4. Alongside this verse, Savory has drawn a complex pattern of 25 crosses and circles, each surrounded by a series of dots, and the whole is arranged in a diamond pattern.
5. 'Finally, my brethren, be strong in the Lord, and in the power of his might. Put on the whole armour of God, that ye may be able to stand against the wiles of the devil. For we wrestle not against flesh and blood, but against principalities, against powers, against the rulers of the darkness of this world, against spiritual wickedness in high places. Wherefore take unto you the whole armour of God, that ye may be able to withstand in the evil day, and having done all, to stand. Stand therefore, having your loins girt about with truth, and having on the breastplate of righteousness' (Ephesians 6:10-14). What follows are two double-lined circles drawn side-by-side, each divided by lines into eight segments (see illustration).
6. Each of these incantations is enclosed in a separate rectangle with similar but not identical asymmetric decorated borders, resembling the appearance of plaques (see illustration).

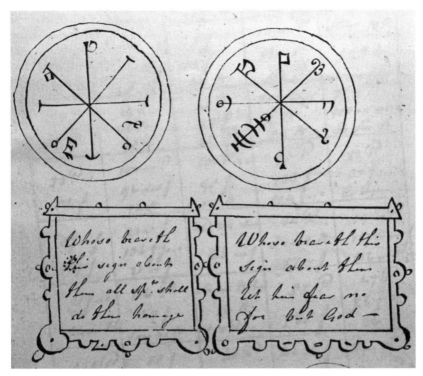

4. 'The Charm of Charms': an example of Savory's keen interest in witchcraft [163].

[*p. 164*]

Magi

By these two Characters some of the Israelites & Negromancers of Judeae obtained many things & they are now esteemed of great price amongst very many and held as great secret for they are of so great price, Virtue & power that whatsoever is possible to be done by Characters & Words the same may be affected by y[ou]rs or one of them.

[*Here Savory has drawn a pentagram and hexagram side-by-side. In the five outer sections of the pentagram (clockwise from top left) Savory has written*] Te-tra-gram-ma-ton [*i.e. Tetragrammaton*[1]]

[*and in the six outer sections of the hexagram (clockwise from top left)*] a-d-o-n-a-i [*i.e. adonai*[2]]

– on the Works of thy own hands O Grant our petitions O Sweet Jesu hear great & glorius name & the good of my fillow [*sic*] [*p. 165*] Lord I beleive – help thou my Unbe-lief [*i.e. Unbelief*[1]]

---

1. i.e. the four Hebrew letters (*Yod*, *He*, *Waw* and *He*), the Tetragrammaton. The four characters correspond to Y H W H, transliterated I A U E or *Yahweh*. *Yahweh* is the name of the Almighty Father in Heaven, commonly called the Lord, or God.
2. i.e. the Hebrew word for Lords or Masters.

[Here Savory has drawn (apparently free-hand) two double-lined circles, one inside the other. Inside the smaller circle he has reproduced, upside down, the pentagram from the previous page, with the word Tetragrammaton split as before, but written clockwise from bottom left. Inside the pentagram (and slightly overlapping it) he has copied the hexagram, with the word adonai split as before but also written clockwise from bottom left. Around the inner edge of the smaller circle he has written (clockwise from bottom)]

Defend this thy Servant from all Evil & heal her disease of Witchcraft & Sorcery Amen sweet

[and below this, in the five segments of the circle created by the pentagram (written clockwise from bottom left)]

Jesus Amen sweet Jehovah Amen[.]

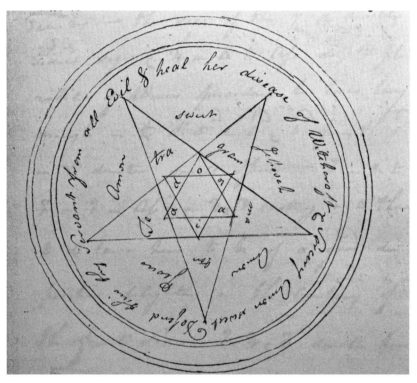

5. 'Magi': an example of Savory's keen interest in witchcraft [165].

[Below the diagram he continues]
O the Debts of the riches & Wisdom of God how unsearchable are his Works and his ways past finding out[.]
O Great God shower down thy Gifts – most mighty Jehovah Tetragrammaton me & my petitions for the honour of thy Creatures fiat Amen.

---

1. The word 'Unbelief' is split in half and written above either side of the diagram below it.

[*p. 166*]

Dedication of the Church

I Conjure thee thou creature of Water in the name of the Fa+ther of the So+n[1] & of the Holy +[2] Ghost that thou drive away the Devil from the bounds of the Just that he remain not in the dark corners of this Church & Alter [*sic*]. NB. At the hallowing of Churches there must be a Cross of Ashes made on the pavement from one end of the Church to the other one handfull bread & one of the priests must write on one side there the greek Alphabet and on the other side the Laten [*sic*] Alphabet. it represents the union of faith of the Jews & Gentiles and the Cross reaching from one end of the Church to the other do signify that the people which was the head shall be made the tail.

[*p. 167*] The Epistle of <St Saviour which> Pope Leo sent to King Charles saying that whosoever carieth the same about him or in what day soever he read it. he shall not be killed with an Iron Tool nor be burned with Fire. nor be drowned with Water neither any evil Man or beast shall hurt him.

The Cross of Christ is a wonderfull defence + The Cross of Christ is true health + The Cross of Christ be always with me + The Cross of Christ is it which I always do Worship + The Cross of Christ do love the bands of Death + The Cross of Christ is the truth and the way + I take my Journey upon the Cross of the Lord + The Cross of Christ beateth down every evil + The Cross of Xt [*i.e. Christ*] giveth all good things + The Cross of [*p. 168a*] Christ taketh away pains everlasting + The Cross of Christ save me + O Cross of Christ be upon me, before me & behind me + because the antient enemy cannot abide the sight of thee + The Cross of Christ save me, help me, keep me, govern me & direct me[.] Thomas bearing this Not of thy divine Majesty + Alpha + Omega + first + and last + Middest + and end + beginning + and first begotten + Wisdom + Virtue +

Falling Evil

Take the sick person by the hand & whisper in his ear these words softly: I conjure the [*sic*] by the {Sun}, {Moon} & by the Gosple for this day delivered unto by God to Hubert, Giles, Cornelius & John that thou Arise and fall no more.

* * *

---

1. 'Father' is written with a cross between 'Fa' and 'ther', and 'Son' between 'So' and 'n'.
2. i.e. a cross resembling a Crucifix.

[*p. 169a*]

To Drive away Spirits that
Haunt the House

Hang in 4 Corners of the House this somtime [*sic*] written upon virgin parchment
Omnis Spiritus laud et dominus Mosen hubert & prophetis. Exurget Deus & Dissipantur inimici ejus.[1]

For any thing that sticketh in the Bones: say 3 several times kneeling[:]
Orenus praeceptis solutaribus manite pater noster Ave Mari[2] Thus make a Cross saying[:] The Hebrew Knight shake our Lord Jesus Christ + by the same Iron Blood and Water to pull out this Iron &c. In Nomine Patris + Filis + & Sp[iri]t[us] Sancta.[3]

* * *

[*p. 168b*[4]] This is a true Copy of the holy Writing that was brought down from heaven by an Angel to St Leo Pope of Rome and he did bid him take it to K[in]g Charles when he went to the battle [?Ranneval]. And the Angel said that what Man or Woman beareth this Writing about them with good devotion and say every day 3 paternosters 3 Aves and 1 Creed shall not on that day be overcome of his enemies. neither shall be robbed or Slain of theves, pestilence, thunder, lightning[.] neither be hurt by fire or Water. Neither shall have displeasure of Lords or Ladies. he shall not be condemnd by false Witnesses nor be taken with the falling Evil. if a Woman be in travel [*sic*] lay this [*p. 169b*[5]] Writing upon her belly she shall have easy deliverance, the Child right shapd & Christendom & thro' Virtue of the following Words:

+ Jesus + Christ + Messias + Soter
+ Emmanuel + Sabbaoth + Adonai
+ Uniginitus + Majister + Paracletus
+ Salvatornoster + Agros is kros[6] +
Agios + Adonatos + Gasper + Melchior
+ and Balthasar + Mattheus + Ma-
rcus + Lucas + Johannas.[7]

---

1. i.e. All praise to the Spirit and the Lord Moses and the prophets. God will arise and His enemies will be scattered.
2. i.e. Let us pray, warned by saving commands, Our Father, Hail Mary.
3. i.e. In the name of the Father, the Son, and the Holy Ghost.
4. Savory mistakenly numbers this page 168 again.
5. Savory mistakenly numbers this page 169 again.
6. Peachey suggests this should be 'Agios Yschyrios', see Peachey, *Life of William Savory*, 9.
7. Peachey writes that this is 'somewhat similar to an old formula used "against the pest"', see Peachey, *Life of William Savory*, 9*n*.

A Charm which must never be said but caried about against Thieves.
I do go & I do come unto you with the love of God, wth the humility of Christ, with the holiness of our blessed Lady, with the [*p. 170*] faith of Abraham, with the Justice of Isaac, with the Virtue of David, with the might of Peter, wth the constancy of Paul, wth the Authority of Gregory, Wth the prayer of Clement, Wth the flood of Jordan, p p p
c ge g a q q est pts h a b g l h 2 a
Oc t g t b a m g 2 4 2 l g : p x e g
h q a g g p o q q r O onely Father +
O only Lord + And Jesus + passing
thro' the midst of them + Went in +
the name + the name of the Father
+ & of the Son + & of the holy Ghost +[1]

Amulet

Joseph of Ari<ma>thea did find this Writing upon the wounds of the side of Jesus Christ written by Gods finger [*p. 171*] when the body was taken away from the Croos. Whosoever shall carry this Writing about him shall not die any evil Death if he beleive in Christ & in all perplexities he shall soon be delivered neither let him fear any danger at all.[2]

Eons Alpha & Omega + Figa + Figalis +
Sabaoth + Emmanuel + Adonai + O +
Neray + Saha + Pangitus + Commen + a
+ g + a + Matheus + Marcus + Lucas
+ Johannes +++ tytulus triumphalis +
Jesus Naserum rex Judeorum + ecce
dominicae crusis signum + fagita partis adversa vicit leo de tribu Judae radix
David alleluijah Kirie Eluson
Christi eluson paternoster Ave Maria
& ne nos & Venial supernos Salutare tuum Orenus.[3]

---

1. Although this looks like gibberish, it has nevertheless been transcribed exactly as written in the MS, with individual letters separated by single spaces without punctuation.
2. These charms and amulets are typical of the witchcraft and quackery which persisted into the eighteenth century. Words written on paper, and worn around the neck or otherwise near the skin, were believed to beguile would-be lovers or protect against disease: e.g the word 'Abracadabra' (see [160]), familiar from its continued use by magicians today, dates to the second century, when it was engraved and used as a charm against illness.
3. Presumably 'Fons Alpha Et Omega, Figa, Figalis, Sabaoth, Emmanuel, Adonai, O, Neray, Sahe, Pangeton, Commen, Agla, Matheus, Marcus, Lucas, Johannes, titulus triunphalis, Jesus Nazarenos Rex Iudaeorum, ecce dominicae crucis signum Fugite partes adverse, vicit Leo de tribu Judae, radix David aleluyah, Kyrie Eleison, Christie Eleison, Paternoster, Ave Maria, et ne vos, et venia super nos Salutare tuum, Oremus'. See T. R. Forbes, 'Verbal Charms', 307.

[*p. 172*]

[1788 continued]

Oct[obe]r 3rd 1788 I went to attend at St Thos and Guys Hospitals in London[.] I went on Newbury Coach and the next Morning I went over the City &c. and seen during the day most all off my acquaintance: John Davenport Surgeons Instrument maker & West Draper in White Chapple, Crawly and Adcock Bishopsgate St Druggists &c.[1] the 5th. I breakfasted with Mr Hurlock Surgeon in St Pauls Church Yard & went with <him> to see his patients.[2]

Monday Morning Oct[obe]r 6th. I went to Mr Cline in St Mary Axe who is first Surgeon & Lecturer on Anatomy at St Thos Hospital[.][3] I paid him 7 Guineas for attending as a perpetual pupil to his Lectures on Anatomy and Surgery and 5 Guineas for [*p. 173*] Dissections[.] at 11 o'Clock I went to St Thos Hospital and payd at the Office (for seeing the practice of both Hospitals (viz) St Thos and Guys) [*sic*] 18 Guineas for half a Year[.] I also payd £1 2s 0d fees at the said Office of St Thos.

The Terms of the Hospital

For Attend[in]g Lectures on Anatomy and Surgery as perpetual pupil £7 7s 0d.

 For Phycis [*i.e. Physic*] two Courses £5 5s 0d.

For 1 Course £3 3s 0d.

For 2 Courses in Midwifery £5 5s 0d.

A Physitians pupil 6 Months £22 1s 0d.

A Surgeons pupil 6 Months £18 18s 0d.

D[itt]o for 12 Months £25 4s 0d

Dresser for 6 Months £31 10s 0d.

   _____ for 12 Months £50 0s 0d.

[*p. 174*] Mr Clines Lecture this day was the 4th and on the Absorbent Vessells I paid 2/6 for a Tickett on my entrance into the Theatre. The Surgeons at St Thos are Messrs Cline, Chandler & Burch.[4] Phycitians at St Thos are Drs Fordyce, Crawford, and Blane.[5] Surgeons at Guys are Messrs Warner, Lucas and Cooper.[6] Physicians Drs Sanders, Skeete and Harvey.[7]

---

1. John Davenport, surgeon's instrument maker, 17, Whitechapel Road; Samuel West, linen-draper, 16, Whitechapel Road; Adcock and Crawley, Chymists and Druggists, 187, Bishopsgate Without (*UD*). Savory returned to Davenport and Adcock & Crawley in May 1791 as a fully qualified surgeon, apothecary and man-midwife, see [253].
2. Probably Joseph Hurlock (1754-1845), whose father Philip Hurlock (1713-1801) was already established as a surgeon in St Paul's Churchyard by 1769. Joseph Hurlock of St Paul's Churchyard was a Fellow of the Medical Society at Bolt Court by 1791 and was a respected and eminent surgeon.
3. For Henry Cline (1750-1827) see section xvi of the introduction, and for Savory's notes on Cline's lectures on anatomy and surgery given at St Thomas's Hospital in 1788-1789, see Appendix D.
4. George Chandler (d. 1822); John Birch (c.1745-1815) (see [184*n*] and introduction).
5. George Fordyce (1736-1802); Adair Crawford (1748-1795); Sir Gilbert Blane (1749-1834).
6. Joseph Warner (1717-1801); William Lucas Snr (?1734-1818, see [190*n*]); William Cooper, uncle to Sir Astley Cooper.
7. William Saunders (1743-1817) (see section xvi of the introduction and Appendix D); Thomas Skeete (1757-1789); James Hervey (1751-1824).

every Surgeon has a phycitian particularly as Mr Chandler and Dr Fordyce, Mr Cline and Dr Crawford, Mr Birch and Dr Blane &c.

There are 18 Wards in St Thos Hospital: 12 Mens Wards & ~~7~~ 6 Womens Wards including 3 Wards calld fowl Wards for patients with the Venereal disease[.] the names of 'em are: [*p. 175*] Abrahams, Isaacs, Jacobs, Georges, Henrys, Williams, Edwards, Cuttings, Kings, Anns, Marys, Elizabeth, Lidias, Queens, Dorcas. Fowl Wards are Jobs, Naples & Magdalens.

I shall next write what Mr Clines Lectures consisted off during 1 Course.

Oct[obe]r 1st. Introductory Lecture

2nd. Lecture 1st. On the Blood

3rd. 2nd. On the structure of <the Arteries>

4th. 3rd. On the diseases of the arte<ries>

6th. 4th. On the Absorbent Vessells

Lecture 5th. On the Cellular Membrane

   6th. On the Nerves

   7th. On the Muscles

   8th. On the Glands

   9th. On the Bones

   10th & 11th. On the Appendages

[*p. 176*] Lectures

   12th ~~to~~ 23rd.[1] on the Bones – 11 Lectures

   23rd to 30th. 8 Lectures on the Muscles

   31st & 32nd. Lectures on the Ligaments

   33rd & 34th. On the Male Organs of Generation

   35th &c. 4 Lectures on the Urinary Organs

   39th, 40th, 41st. on the Visera

   42nd, 43rd. On the female Organs of Generation

   44th. On the structure of the Liver

   45th. On the pancreas & female breast

   46th. On the Lungs

   47th. On the Heart

   48th. On the Alimentary Canal & diseases <thereoff>

   49th. On the Teeth

   50th. On the Compages[2]

   51st to 55th. On the Arteries

   55th. On the Veins

   56th. On the Absorbent System

   57th. On the Circulation of the Blood

   58. 59. On the Nerves

[*p. 177*]

Lectures

   60. 61. On the Brain

   62. 63. 64. On the Organs of Vission

   65. On the Organs of Taste

---

1. It is not obvious why Savory crossed through the word 'to', but he evidently meant to write '22nd' not '23rd'.

2. i.e. the system or structure of linked vessels.

66. On Anatomical preparations
67. On the Organs of Smelling
68. 69 On the Organs of Hearing
70 On the diseases of the Heart
71st. On the Hystory of Anatomy[1]

These Lectures was read again the 2nd Course which began in Jan[us]ry & On April 22nd 1789 began the Lectures on Surgery which is always immediately after the Spring Course: –

first 3 Lectures on the Disease of the Bones

4th & 5th. On the Sutures & Bronchome<try>

Gastrorophy, Hare Lip. Wry Neck, Fistula Lacrymalis, Couching, Cutting the Iris, Remov[in]g the Eye, [*p. 178*] Castration, Empyemae, of Calculi Searching, Amputation, Removing the Tonsills & piles, polypus Uteri Usulae, Nasal polypus, Schirrus Breast, Fistula in Ano, Paracentasis, Aneurism, Phymosis, Paraphymosis, Amputation of the penis, Remov[in]g Stones, Suppression of Urine, Stone in Woman, Hydrocele, Operation of the Trephine, Hernias, Trepanning the Sternum, Carbuncles, Erysepilas, Fracture Patella, Bandages, in all 21 Lectures[2] & immediately after these Surgical Lectures Dr Louder reads 6 or 7 Lectures on the Gravid Uterus at the Theatre at St Thos & begins at ½ past 7 o'Clock in the Morn[in]g.

[*p. 179*] The Surgeons goes 'round the Wards every day at 11 o'Clock by turns[:] Mr Cline Mondays, Chandler Tuesdays and Birch Wednesdays. Thursdays is the days for taking in patients which is by turns and on Saturday all go round both physitians and Surgeons. this Mr Cline is an excellent Surgeon & is near sighted.

In the Operation Theatre at St Thos is a very fine drawing of Chiselden[3] & are also these Words:

Theatrum Hoc Chirurgicum
De Nova conformandum ac decorandum
Sempter [*i.e. Symptu*] suo ceravit [*i.e. curavit*]
Georgius Arnold Armiger
Senatur Londinensis et Huss [*i.e. Hujus*]

---

1. Peachey, a notable medical historian himself, and Savory's successor as the resident medical practitioner in Brightwalton, commented, 'A hundred and twenty years have passed. There is no professional chair of medical history at any of our universities; it is included neither in the schedules of education nor examination – even as an optional subject – in any medical school, and there is no existing society which makes it a speciality!' Peachey, *Life of William Savory*, 11*n*. Fortunately, the history of medicine is now an established and respected scholarly discipline, though the extent to which medical students study the subject varies significantly between institutions.
2. Savory's student notes, which he refers to below (see [187]) have survived and are now preserved in the archives of King's College, London. See Appendix D for the list of contents covering Henry Cline's lectures.
3. William Cheselden (1688-1752) was the most celebrated surgeon of his generation. He specialised in ophthalmic work and lithotomy (an operation for removing calculi, or 'the stone'). For most of his career he was associated with St Thomas's Hospital and became Head Surgeon there.

[p. 180]

Nosocomii praesis meritissimo Colondus
Ann Dom Mdccli

Miseratione non penede[1]

There is also in the same Theatre the figure of one Sam[ue]l Wood a Miller whose Arm with the Scapula was torn off from his Body by a Rope winding round it[,] the other end being fastened to the Coggs of the Mill[;] this happened in 1737.[2] The Vessels being stretchd it bled very little[;] the Arteries and Nerves was drawn out of his Arm[.] he was Cured by Mr Ferne Surgeon at St Thos,[3] by superficial dressings, the Natural Skin being left almost sufficient to cover it.[4]

[p. 181] In the large Theatre at St Thos where Clines Lectures are given is a Table in the Middle & seats round it one above another. opposite is a little Room containing an immense Number of Anatomical preperations which are shewn every day at the time of Lecture relating to what the subject was upon[,] and on the other side of the Stair Case is the disecting Room.[5] Oct[obe]r 15th. payd Dr Lowder five guineas to attend two Courses of his Lectures on Midwifery[.][6] I went to to his Lectures every Morning at ½ past

---

1. In fact 'Miseratione non mercede', according to Benjamin Golding, who gives the complete and correct transcription, see B. Golding, *An Historical Account of St Thomas's Hospital* (1819), 125.
2. Samuel Wood, a native of Worcestershire, suffered his accident aged 26 on 15 August 1737, while working at Felton's Windmill on the Isle of Dogs.
3. The surgeon James Ferne (1672-1741) was the master of Cheselden (see [179n]), and was himself lithotomist at St Thomas's, having been specially licensed to cut for 'the stone', an operation described in notorious and excruciating detail by diarist Samuel Pepys.
4. Savory is referring to a large colour print, formerly in the St Thomas's Medical School Archive, and removed to King's College, London, ref. TH/ILL1/21 [1737]. A copy at St John's College, Cambridge, is inscribed, 'Samuel Wood whose arm with the shoulder blade was torn off by a mill the 15th of Aug: 1737. He was brought to St: Thomas's Hospital the next day where he was cured by Mr Ferne. Publish'd by Samuel Wood according to Act of Parliament Nov: 1st 1737.' For more, see John Belchier's contemporary account in *Philosophical Transcripts*, cdxlix (1737). Wood recovered within two months, Ferne having stitched the wound with a needle and suture bandages.
5. A new theatre was built in 1813-1814, above St Thomas's Church, and is now preserved as a museum. John Flint South's description agrees with Savory's but adds considerable detail: see J. F. South, *Memorials of John Flint South: Twice President of the Royal College of Surgeons, and Surgeon to St Thomas's Hospital (1841-63)* ed. C. L. Feltoe (1884), 29-30. For further context, see section xvi of the introduction.
6. William Lowder (1732-1801), who had an MD from Aberdeen, lectured on midwifery from 1775, variously at the theatre at St Saviour's Churchyard, Southwark, and later at the theatre at Guy's Hospital, assisted first by David Orme (1727-1812), and later by John Haighton (see [191n]). He does not appear to have occupied any official hospital post, and was an army surgeon before becoming a lecturer. He is mentioned in the description of the United or Borough Hospitals of St Thomas's and Guy's written by the surgeon Joseph Warner in 1792 (see [205n]). Lowder is also alluded to in the preface to J. Blunt, *Man-Midwifery Dissected; or, the Obstetric Family Instructor* (1793), x-xi, and is remembered in the title, *A syllabus of the Lectures on Midwifery delivered at Guy's Hospital and at Dr Lowder's and Dr Haighton's Theatre in ... Southwark* (1799). Savory describes his experiences under Lowder in more detail below [191-195], and lists midwifery instruments purchased from Davenport [196]. For more on Lowder, see section xvi of the introduction.

7 o'Clock till 9. his Theatre is at his own home in St Saviours Church Yard near St Thos & Guys Hospitals[,] and on the other side of [*p. 182*] of [*sic*] St Saviours Church is his Labour house[.] Oct[obe]r 21st begun disecting and the 29th came from my Sisters in White-Chapple to a Lodging in Joiner Street at No. 32 with one Mrs Meakin[.]¹ I paid 2/ pr Week[.] the reason of my coming from my sisters it was so inconvenient in attending Labours & accidents[.] the prices for an

	£. s. d.
Adult Subject is	2. 2. 0.
Foetus	0. 7. 6
Extremity	0. 7. 6
Head	0. 7. 6
Injecting a Head	0. 3. 0
placenta	0. 2. 0

The first Week I was at the Hospital my head was greatly affected by going in the fowl Wards & dissecting Room [*p. 183*] but afterwards it did not hurt me.

Oct[obe]r 9th. two patients were bro[ugh]t in one a fractured Elbow[,] the other a wound on the Scalp but no fracture[,] also I see this day two Amputations.

11th. I saw two operations performd at Bartholomews Hospital[.] one was on a Spaniard by Mr Pitt² who extrac[te]d a Stone from the Bladder weighed 6 Ounces[:] it was very ragged[;] the patient recovered[.] the other operation was an Amputation of the Thigh. the 15th. Mr Cline performd the operation of Castration[.] he was about 15' [*i.e. minutes*] in doing it and after taking out the diseased testicle the lips of the Wound were closed & a sticking plaster applyd. the 16th. was an Operation by Mr Birch. [*p. 184*] the patient was upwards of 60 Years of Age & had an Inguinal Hernia[.] the intestines were very difficult to be reduced and the patient next day died.³

Oct[obe]r 17th. Mr Birch performd two operations. one the Hydrocele which was by Incission two Inches or more in length & more than 1 p[in]t of Water discharged[.] the Wound was not quite closed but dry-lint put between the edges. the other was a seperation of the preputium.⁴ 24th. two

---

1. Joiner Street formed the eastern boundary of St Thomas's Hospital, running from Tooley Street to St Thomas's Street, towards the entrance to Guy's. St Saviour's Churchyard, where Savory attended midwifery lectures under Lowder, also the location of the labour-house, was on the western side of Borough High Street, with which Joiner Street ran parallel (though it was on the opposite side to St Saviour's, in the east). Joiner Street is now incorporated into the railway and underground stations at London Bridge, which sits on the site of the bulk of the old Borough Hospitals.
2. Edmund Pitts (c.1710-1791) had been an Assistant Surgeon at St Bartholmew's Hospital from 1760 until his election as full surgeon in 1784, a position in which he served until his death in 1791. He was also a Warden of the Company of Surgeons.
3. John Birch was appointed a surgeon at St Thomas's Hospital in 1784. See section xvi of the introduction.
4. i.e. prepuce: an operation to separate the foreskin from the penis to allow retraction.

operations[:] the one was an Amputation of the Leg by Mr Chandler;[1] and the extract of a Cataract by Mr Cline. Nov[embe]r 1st. I saw an Operation performd at Bartholomews w[hi]ch was on a schirrus breast[2] & it weighed upwards of a pound Weight & afterwards [*p. 185*] a soft plaster was applyd[.] the 19th. Was a Man tap[pe]d for the Ascites[3] by Birch & I suppose 4 Gall[o]ns was evacuated, there were during the time I was there several operations for the Hare lip,[4] Stone, Fistulas,[5] Trepanning,[6] &c. two or three times a Week.

One of the Nurses in the Hospital died before any asistance could be got soon enough from an obstruction of the Air tube as she was eating Beef[.] she fell down & immediately expired[.] on opening the Air tube it was found obstructed by a bit of Beef. there was likewise during my attendance at the hospital three or four patients with [*p. 186*] the Lock Jaw[7] and all died.

Mr Caw late Surgeon at St Thos extracted a stone weighed 13 Ounces from the bladder of a man & in the form of the Bladder. Mr Sharp[8] late surgeon of Guys Hospital extracted a great number of small Calculi from a patient[.] he gave him Soap Lees[9] qt x in Aq[ua] pura[.] the patient grew weaker and weaker till he died. Mr Sharp examind the Urinary Bladder and found a vast number of Calculi with which came away before his Death was 214[.] I saw them in St Thos Theatre[.] they was of a whitish Colour some as large as a hasel Nutt some smaller.[10] Calculi may be known from Pebble or Stone by [*p. 187*] making a Section where he may see the different Laminae[11] in the Calculi, see Clines Anatomy, page 167.[12]

There was a Lad about 14 Years Old had his Leg Amputated by Mr Burch when he astonished us all by being so chearfull during the time of the operation & did not express <pain> any time 'till tying the Blood Vessells & then but little. the most frequent operations as was performd was

---

1. For George Chandler, see section xvi of the introduction.
2. i.e. scirrhous breast: a breast covered in hard excrescences, swellings or tumours, often cancerous.
3. i.e. a collection of serous fluid in the peritoneal cavity; dropsy of the abdomen.
4. i.e. cleft lip, a fissure of the upper lip, caused by developmental abnormalities in the upper lip or jaw; so-called from its perceived similarity to the cleft lip of a hare.
5. A long, narrow, suppurating canal of morbid origin in some part of the body; a long, sinuous pipe-like ulcer with a narrow orifice.
6. i.e. an operation with a trepan, a surgical instrument in the form of a crown-saw, for cutting out small pieces of bone, often used on the skull.
7. i.e. trismus, or tonic spasm of the muscles of mastication, causing the jaws to remain rigidly closed; usually a synonym for a variety of tetanus.
8. Samuel Sharp (1700-1778), who served at Guy's Hospital from 1733 to 1757, had been apprenticed to the celebrated Cheselden at St Thomas's. He dedicated to his eminent master his influential work, *Treatise on the Operations of Surgery* (1739). This, and his study, *Critical Inquiry into the Present State of Surgery* (1750), received appreciative critical attention. He retired in 1759 after a lifetime's struggle with asthma. A Fellow of the Royal Society, he was a cultured and scholarly man who travelled widely. His *Letters from Italy* (1767) were praised by Samuel Johnson.
9. Soap lees were recognised for their power as a solvent.
10. i.e. vesical calculi (stones in the bladder).
11. i.e. the thin layers of bone, membranes, or other structures.
12. See Appendix D. The section on 'Calculi' begins on p. 164, searching for calculi on p. 169, and the performance of the operation, p. 174.

Amputations and Hernias. I wrote from Mr Cline during two Courses of his Lectures which may be seen in two Volumes title Clines Anatomy.[1]

Bone put in Sp[iri]t Turpentine renders it transparent.

[p. 188] When a Bubo[2] is opened they apply dry Lint and upon it a plaster but never use tents. There was a Case in Jobs Ward[,] an ulcerated penis as large as the top of a pint Cup & even to the pubes[.] was ordered by Mr Birch an Hemlock poultice.[3] Mr Cline divided a Nerve in a Dogs Leg and in about 6 Weeks after the Dog was killd & the Nerve was found united again[,] so that union takes place in a tendon if Cutt & separated at some distance.[4]

A Young Woman was brought to the Hospital burnt all over as black as a Coal[:] she died in a few days after. also a Girl of 12 Years of Age came to be under Mr Birch with the Venereal disease [p. 189] contracted from a Young Chimney Sweep.[5] One patient at 18 Years of Age of a Cancerated Uterus[.] her Cries ~~was~~ and pain was very great.

I see an Operation at Bartholomews on the Hydrocele tap[pe]d with a Trocar[6] & an injection thrown in for a few Minutes, also a Woman with the fistula Lachrymalis[.][7]

I shall next give a general description of the Hospitals & first of St Thomas which hath 4 Squares[.] the 1st next the Borough was built by Guy and contains the Womens Wards. the 2nd Square is offices & Rooms for the Stewards, Butler, Cooks, the Ministers residence & Chapple. the other Squares has Wards for the Men[.] at the lower side of the 3rd Sqr [p. 190] is the Surgery then kept by one Lucas.[8] on the south side is the Apothecarys Shop &c.

Guys Hospital has two very large Squares[.] this Hospital was built by Guy and has much better Wards than what is at St Thos. the 1st square on the West side is the Chapple &c. the other square has Wards all round. the Apothecary was Mr Babington.[9] it has an excellent Theatre and is where Dr Sanders gives his Lectures on Physic, Chymistry &c.[1]

---

1. See Appendix D.
2. i.e. an inflamed swelling or abscess in glandular parts of the body, especially the groin or arm-pits.
3. Highly toxic, hemlock was used as a powerful sedative. This reference to an ulcerated penis was omitted by Peachey, presumably for reasons of taste.
4. Cline's experimental discovery thus predates that of his colleague, John Haighton, (on whom, see [191n]) whose thesis, 'An Experimental Inquiry Concerning the Reproduction of Nerves' (1795), details other instances of this phenomenon. Medical and other scientific discoveries made in the course of experimentation necessarily predate their official documentation and were often shared in lectures long before they appeared in print.
5. As with the reference to the case of ulcerated penis, this reference to the venereal disease was also omitted by Peachey.
6. i.e. a surgical instrument consisting of a perforator or stylet enclosed in a metal tube or cannula, used for drawing off fluid from a cavity.
7. i.e. in the canal between the eye and the nose.
8. This was presumably William Lucas Snr (?1734-1818), an eminent surgeon associated mostly with Guy's Hospital, and Master of the Corporation of Surgeons in 1791.
9. William Babington (1756-1833) was appointed Apothecary at Guy's in 1781. His extensive knowledge of chemistry led to his assisting William Saunders in his medical lectures. Elevated to Assistant Physician in 1795, Babington remained at Guy's until 1811. He was respected as hardworking and dedicated to scientific enquiry. A distinguished physician, he became a Fellow of the Royal Society, and was a founder of the Geological Society which he

Bartholomews Hospital is one large Square, is on the east side of Smithfield.

The London Hospital is very large and Spacious, but several Wards are empty[.][2] this [*p. 191*] Hospital is supported by voluntary Contributions but its very poor at present owing to the Quakers who used to contribute very largely, but the occasion they dont now so much was some time ago there was a Surgeons place vacated and a Gentleman of their sect was a Candidate but was not admitted by reason of fewer Votes, by which the Aminadabs were offended.[3]

I Bo[ugh]t of Davenport a Case of dissecting Instruments cost 19/ containing 6 knives, Nippers, Hook & blow pipe[.] Mr Heighton was master of the disecting.[4]

I shall next leave the Hospital 8 Cline and return to Dr Louder Man-Midwife in St Saviours Church Yard. [*p. 192*] Dr Louder begins his Lectures on the bones of the pelvis and then a description of the female organs of generation and the difficulties & diseases in general. next signs to distinguish pregnancy and diseases of pregnant Woman and then on Labours: Natural, lingring and laborious, and preternatural[,] and how to manage before and after delivery, how to use the instruments &c. Of twins, Miscarriages, Diseases of the Mother and Child &c.

the Dr will not take a pupil for 1 Course only except he has attended somewhere else before. two or three times a Week was labours at the lying in house[.] we was all cal[le]d & used to take them by turns. the 1st [*p. 193*] Labour I attended was at Redriff[,][5] a Natural Labour[.] gave the Woman 2/6.

---

served as President in 1827. He also played a significant role in the formation of the Hunterian Society. The esteem and affection of his colleagues, and his widespread popularity, is evident from the tributes paid on his death. For a reference to Savory's student notes, see Appendix D.

1. This theatre was built at the time Saunders was appointed in 1777. For Savory's student notes on Saunders's lectures, see Appendix D.
2. Founded in Whitechapel in 1740, the London Hospital (now the Royal London) had eighteen wards, but some of them were empty in Savory's time, as he observed.
3. Amminadab, from the Hebrew, 'my people are noble', was a pejorative term for members of the Society of Friends (the Quakers). Peachey writes, 'This refers to the case of John Whitehead M.D., Leydon, who, at first a Wesleyan, afterwards became a member of the Society of Friends, and by their influence successfully contested the vacant post of physician − not surgeon − to the London Hospital in 1784. The election was afterwards declared invalid, and he then seceded from the Quakers and rejoined Wesley whom he attended in his last illness. He was more famous as a preacher than as a physician'. Peachey, *Life of William Savory*, 14*n*.
4. John Haighton (1755-1823) was an anatomist of great distinction, and was assistant to Henry Cline before the appointment of Sir Astley Cooper. Later he became the first lecturer in Physiology at Guy's. Like Lowder, he also lectured on midwifery at St Saviour's Churchyard. Argumentative and irritable, he was nevertheless a fine lecturer and teacher, and he became a Fellow of the Royal Society.
5. i.e. east of Southwark Park, in the area now occupied by Surrey and Canada Water.

[1789]

Jan[ua]ry 29th. I experiencd the use of the Catheter on old Dame Penny[,] gave her 1/-. Feb[rua]ry 2nd. I was at a Labour 9 hours[.] it was a Young Woman and her first Labour[.] they were Irish people and I delivered her kneeling which is their Country way. they told me 'twas always customary with them to give the Child Rue or Black Cherry Water and not to give them the breast till 3 or 4 days after they are born[.] so much for Labours.

The Doctor had a figure in the form of a Woman and a little leathern Child to experience difficult Labours & preternatural Cases. about the time he was lecturing on using the [*p. 194*] Instruments[.] we had two cases each[,] a Natural presentation and a face presentation[.] when he was treating on preternatural Cases we had two Cases[:] a breech presentation & a back presentation. also when he was Lecturing on searching there was 8 or 9 Woman at the Lying in house to be examined by us.

I was at a Labour with a fellow pupil Scammell[1] and our old Midwife was with us[.] the Woman had very slight pains[.] on examining the Membrane was not broke[.] I felt the Head like so many Oyster Shells, the Child being Dead for near 1 Month.[2]

the 20th of Feb[rua]ry. I got my Certificate for Midwifery and gave Mrs Gibson 5/, and the Nurse 2/6[.] I often used to frequent the Labour House[.] I Bo[ugh]t of Mrs Gibson a placenta to inject[;] gave her 1/.

[*p. 195*] I wrote out the pharmacopeae of St Thomas[,] also a Book I wrote out of Clinical Cases at Guys Hospital. I wrote Dr Louders Lectures during two Courses which see Louders Midwifery.[3]

After Clines 1st Course of Lectures was ended I came in the Country[.] I car[rie]d down with me two hearts injected, two Arms, penis[4] & foetal Skeleton.[5] I went to Moreton staid all Night & came home to Brightwaltham the next day. the 25th of Feb[rua]ry. after I finishd Midwifery I left my lodgings in Joiner Street and went again to my Sisters. Bo[ugh]t the Medical pockett Book[,] had him bound, and interleaved[.] I did not give any money for my Certificate at the Hospital,[6] gave Lucas the Surgery Man 2/6.

[*p. 196*] I wrote out the Lectures on Chymistry by Dr Saunders and Wm Babington, which see Book title Chymistry.[7] Bo[ugh]t of Davenport Midwifery Instruments <&c.>

---

1. This is Edward Scammell, who first appeared – on the same page as Savory – in the lists of *Examined and Approved Surgeons, of the Corporation of Surgeons* (July 1789), 48.
2. This whole paragraph was omitted by Peachey, presumably for reasons of taste.
3. None of these three volumes appears to have survived (see Appendix D). The Royal College of Physicians in Edinburgh has two volumes of notes on Lowder's midwifery lectures, one dating from 1778-1779, the other from 1790. Other volumes of notes on his lectures can be found, among other places, at the Wellcome Library for the History and Understanding of Medicine, Glasgow University, and King's College, London.
4. Peachey omitted the single word 'penis' from this list.
5. John Ford notes how shocked the father of a medical student was to receive a prepared penis sent home by his son in 1802, see J. M. T. Ford, *A Medical Student at St Thomas's Hospital, 1801-1802. The Weekes Family Letters* (1987) 27, 138-140.
6. This suggests he would not have received the ostentatious certificate of attendance proving he had heard Cline's lectures.
7. This volume has not survived.

	s. d.		s. d.
Forceps	15.0	Caustic Case	1/
Blunt Hook	1.9	Abscess Lancet	2/6
Womans Catheter	5.6	3 Crooked Needles	1/3
Mans Do.	5.0	two trusses	24/
Forceps	2.0	Pou[c]h	10/6

Feb[rua]ry 6th. 1789 gave Dr Saunders 3 Guineas for attending one Course of his Lectures[.] I wrote after him which see Saunders on Physic & at the end of the Spring Course was given two Lectures on Electricity & how far it should be used in Diseases.[1] he is an excellent Lecturer & fine Orator.

[*p. 197*] My Sister and self tryd our Luck in the Lottery but proved all Blanks.

Khuns who kept the flying Horse before my Sister had half the £30-000 prise in the Lottery (viz) £15-000 amongst some poor German Sugar Bakers, about £700 each.[2] One Morning in feb[rua]ry I went to Newgate to see 7 Men and 1 Woman hangd opposite the door at Newgate. the Woman received her reward in this life opposite the 7 men & was afterwards burnt.[3]

Easter Monday[4] I went with three or four of my Acquaintances to Greenwich fair[.][5] there is a very fine hospital and is at the edge of the water side.[6]

I Bo[ugh]t Smellies Midwifery 3 Books 18/ in the Strand.[7] the Electrifying Machine I Bo[ugh]t of Simson[8] [*p. 198*] a book binder in Lombard Street cost 12/[9] I used to go to the Medical Society at Guys and to the Medical Society in Bolt Court fleet Street.[10]

After the Kings recovery the principal streets in London was illuminated two Nights: the Bank, Royal Exchange, Sun fire Office, India House &c. was very elegantly illuminated, on the India House were large letters of Lamps May the King live for Ever, and over it a beautifull Star set with different coloured Lamps[.] we travelled all Night to see the fire Works[.] we was 7 hours going on a Coach from Aldgate Church to the Royal Exchange on

---

1. This volume has been preserved, see Appendix D.
2. For details of this lottery, see section ix of the introduction.
3. The date was Wednesday, 18 *March* 1789. For details, see section xiv of the introduction.
4. i.e. 13 April 1789.
5. Greenwich Fair, on *Whit* Monday, was very popular among Londoners, but notoriously riotous. Dickens's account in *Sketches By Boz* (1836) is particularly evocative.
6. The Royal Greenwich Hospital was founded by Queen Mary II who gave over the royal estate at Greenwich in 1694 for the use of pensioned seamen and mariners. The hospital was generally admired for its architectural grandeur and elaborate interior decoration.
7. William Smellie (1697-1763), a member of the Faculty of Physicians and Surgeons of Glasgow, had been the leading authority on midwifery, and helped to develop the modern science of obstetrics. His *Treatise on the Theory and Practice of Midwifery* was published in 1752 and was still widely consulted in Savory's time.
8. The name 'Simpson' is split 'Sim'-'pson' between the two pages.
9. Probably Thomas Simpson, of 16, Rolls Buildings, Fetter Lane.
10. For the Physical Society of Guy's Hospital, see section xvi of the introduction.

account of so many Coaches.[1] When the King was very Ill reports spread about one Morning [*p. 199*] that he was dead and almost all the black Cloth was bo[ugh]t even old Black Cloth at Rag fair.

I displaced 3 large teeth for Josh. Cullum at Stratford. Went to Guild Hall to see the drawing of the Lottery ticketts. there are two Wheels one on each side of Guild Hall[,] one containing the Ticketts the other Blanks & prises. the Blue Coated Boys change every hour. they have one Arm tyed behind them.[2]

I went to a burying at White Chappel Church but the Curate read none of the service in the Church nor was the Corpse carried into the Church but the customary prayers said at the Grave. they will not admit the Corpse to be carried into Church to read the Lessons &c without paying 17/.

[*p. 200*] The day before Valentines day I sent a Letter to Miss Tyrrell my Wife as is now & another soon after.[3]

Dear Miss

> It is now 6 Weeks ago since I sent to you and having received no answer makes me very uneasy. I presume the freedom to send to you and as absense exempts me from flattery, give me leave to assure you that none of your sex ever attracted my sincere regard to this moment but yourself, and if fortune would favour me with an equal return, I would then look upon myself to be one of the happiest persons upon Earth especially as I have seen so much of the agreeable Companion shine in your behaviour and Conversation which I hope to enjoy when [*p. 201*] I come in the Country at Whitsuntide. if you'll favour me with a letter I shall esteem it as a particular favour. I therefore conclude with the hopes of a mutual return and beg leave to stile myself Yoars Affec[tionate]ly. _____

I rec[eive]d a letter from her about a Week after & soon after I sent the following:

Dear Miss

> The favour of your letter I received which gave me pleasure I want words to express. very sorry to hear of your indisposition, glad to hear You are better conscious to the pureness of my heart and the Rectitude of my intentions imbolden me to write being truly sensible that flattery is so susceptable a crime is the grossest affront. there- [*p. 202*] fore will avoid even the appearance of it and as all females claim our attention men of our profession especially, being the softer part of the Creation, and out of respect to she that brought me forth into the World, and has discharged the duty of a parent by me, I would wish to shew them all the respect and lend them all the asistance in my power when wanted. but dear Miss please to beleive I never

---

1. The King had fallen ill in November 1788. He did not recover until the following year. Celebrations were widespread throughout the country. Public buildings were illuminated throughout London. For more, see section xii of the introduction.
2. Prizes of £10,000 and even £20,000 in the lottery were not uncommon. Encouraged by the Government, it was phenomenally popular, with 49,000 tickets sold in one state lottery in 1779. The lotteries attracted criminals and corruption and were declared illegal in 1826. For more, see section ix of the introduction.
3. For more on Mary Tyrrell (1765-1844) of North Moreton, whom Savory married, see section xviii of the introduction and the afterword.

felt the power of female attraction till I saw you, as the perfections of your mind are such as can never fail to please; even in sickness or in Age, when Youth and beauty is no more. beleive me, I am truly ignorant as yet of the Art made use off by my Sex, for a sincerer passion never possessed the heart of Man, [*p. 203*] and if I shall be so happy as to meet with an equal return, the rest of my Life shall be devoted to make you happy, and study the good of my fellow creatures in regard to my business. Dear Miss the favour of a Letter as soon as possible & please to beleive I am with the greatest respect in sincerity your Affectionate Friend and Admirer till Death.

I inoculated John Savory Fordham wth the small Pox & put some Ear Rings in Khuns Childs Ears whilst I was in London. I also went to a Romish Meeting in Holborn[:] just agoing in is a pillow [*sic*] of Wood and a bason of Water fixd up on one side of this pillar, every Catholic as enters dips his finger [*p. 204*] in the bason of Water & Crosses their faces. I recollect hearing of a Story that some person black the Water and every person had black Crosses upon their faces.

I went also to a Jews Synagogue[.] there were 7 priests and all the people had branches of Trees in their hands & they beat them so much that at last all the leaves were off it – it was on the Account of Joshua's taking Jericho, see Joshua Chap 6th.[1] they went 7 times round the Meeting & the Rams Horn was blown each time in going round.

during my time in London I was never at leisure for at ½ past 7 o'Clock in the Morning I went to Dr Louders Lectures and staid till 9. then to breakfast[,] at 10 to Dr Saunders Lectures till 11 o'Clock[,] then to the Hospital [*p. 205*] till Clines Lectures which were from 1 o'Clock to 3. by this time I used to get a good appetite to my dinner, the remainder of my time was taken up in Writing Lectures, Clinical Cases, attending Labours & Accidents, dissecting &c.[2]

May 7th 1789

I was examined at Surgeons Hall and had the honour conferrd on me to be a member of their Body. this Hall is a large pile of building in the old Baily Street[.][3] we was calld in the Room & examined one at a time[.] about a fortnight before I was examined I went to the Hall & entered my name in a [*p. 206*] Book and payd 2/6. when I entered the Room I was a little timid by

1. Joshua, 6:4-6, 'And seven priests shall bear before the ark seven trumpets of rams' horns: and the seventh day ye shall compass the city seven times, and the priests shall blow with the trumpets. And it shall come to pass, that when they make a long blast with the ram's horn, and when ye hear the sound of the trumpet, all the people shall shout with a great shout; and the wall of the city shall fall down flat, and the people shall ascend up every man straight before him. And Joshua the son of Nun called the priests, and said unto them, Take up the ark of the covenant, and let seven priests bear seven trumpets of rams' horns before the ark of the LORD.' Savory is describing the festival of Sukkot (akin to harvest festival in the autumn) as celebrated at the synagogue for Sephardi Jews near Whitechapel, see section xi of the introduction.
2. Joseph Warner (1717-1801), surgeon at Guy's, wrote an account of student life in 1792, discussed in section xvi of the introduction.
3. The offices of the Corporation of Surgeons moved to Lincoln's Inn Fields in 1797.

seeing the Surgeons, however I recovered of that dread and answered every Question they askd me. the Table they sits round is in the form of a Semicircle[.] the Master sits in the middle and the two Wardens, each side and three or four Surgeons each side of the Wardens and the Surgeons examine the pupils by turns. the Master[1] asked me where I received my Instructions, I told him at St Thomas Hospital, and attended Lectures under Mr Cline[.] I was then ordered to Pile to be examined.[2]

[p. 207]

Q. What are the common integuments

A. The Cutis Cuticle & Retum Mucosum

Q. What are the Arteries

A. Vessells which carry the Blood from the heart

Q. What comes first to view after the common integuments is of the Abdomen

A. The Linea Alba

Q. How does the urine enter the Bladder

A. By the Ureters Obliquely

Q. What are the parts in the Thorax

A The Heart, Lungs, pluera &c.

"Now I have askd you a few Questions in Anatomy I shall ask you a few in Surgery["]:

[p. 208]

Q. Where would you Cutt off a persons Leg

A. If below the knee I would Amputate about 4 or 5 Inches below the extremity of the patella.

Q But where would you make your first incission

A. A little below to allow for the excess of Contraction

Q Where would you apply the Turniquit and how would you stop the Haemorhage after the Limb is amputated

A I would apply the Turniquit on the middle of the Thigh because there the Artery is nearer the Bone & I would stop the Blood with a Needle and ligature and after that [p. 209] I would keep the Skin forwards with a Bandage & apply dry Lint and Adhaesive plaster

Q Which side would you stand on to Amputate the Leg

A On the inside because of taking off the Fibula first

Q Supposing your patient is Weak & low after the operation what would you give him

A I would give him Bark

Q Suppose you have a Stone in the Urethra how would you extract it

---

1. Henry Watson (d. 1793), a member of the Court of Assistants (1791-1793), a member of the Court of Examiners (1784-1793), and surgeon at Westminster Hospital.

2. John Pyle (c.1723-c.1799), assistant surgeon at the Westminster Hospital from 1735, and full surgeon 1746-1788, was a well-established and long-serving officer of the Company/ Corporation of Surgeons. He served on the Court of Assistants, 1761-1793; was an Examiner, 1773-1791; a Governor, 1772-1774; and an anatomical officer, 1756-1758.

A   If it was impossible for me to get it out without making an incission I would pull the prepuce over the Glands & make an incission the length of the Stone through the teguments.[1]

[*p. 210*] It cost me £13 5s. the Diploma cost the 5/. we was all cal[le]d in afterwards and took our Oaths and received a little pamphlet containing Rules & Orders. the next day we received our diploma's [*sic*].

May 20 My Brother in law J. Norris came to London and I should came back with him had not I (the day before he left London) been attackd with the Measels[.] I was in Bed a Week and two or three days after I left London and came home to Brightwaltham[.] I sent my Anatomical preparations and Drugs by Clarks Waggon[2] (viz)

A Skeleton of a Girl about 8 Years old

Anatomy of a Boy about 2 Years

An Arm well injected and dissected

_____ of a Young Woman

[*p. 211*] A Foetal Anatomy shewing the Circulation of Blood from the Mother to the Child

A Placenta & Penis[3] &c.

I came from London to Brightwaltham June 3rd 1789[,] the Lectures being all ended. it cost me in all upwards of 100 pounds.[4]

at this time the Hooping Cough was very prevalent my Uncle Thos Barratts Children Was affected with this disease[.] I was sent for June 5th to see them and sent Emetics of Vin Ipecacuanha, a pectoral mixture & Aperient powders.

[*p. 212*] June 6th. I varnished my Anatomical preparations with White Spirit Varnish & put them in a little Closet in the parlour at Brightwaltham, indeed Anatomical preparations should be Varnishd once a Year. about this time I went to Moreton to see my Wife as is now for the first time and received such encouragement as every person ought who is sincere and behaves with Honour. I went to Abingdon fair and sold a little poney as was my Uncles for 8 Guineas and Bo[ugh]t a Black Mare for 12 Guineas but Altho' I had Mr John Holmes Opinion at the same time he was what is cal[le]d Wall Eyed[.][5] however I had him [*p. 213*] to Cromarsh fair and the dealer took to him again.

---

1. Peachey remarks, 'The coffers of the Company of Surgeons were in this year at a very low ebb, and it is scarcely to have been expected, under the circumstances, that the fees of candidates for the membership should have been refused. This may account for the ridiculous simplicity of the questions as a test of knowledge. Well might Savory say that he answered every question they asked him!'. Peachey, *Life of William Savory*, 18*n*.

2. John Clark & Co. operated a coach from Newbury to London in the eighteenth century. They pioneered a 'flying coach' in 1752 which travelled at four to five miles per hour. The journey would have taken about 12 hours. See W. Money, *A Popular History of Newbury* (1905), 17, 52.

3. Peachey omitted the reference to the penis.

4. Peachey's not quite 'verbatim' transcript of Savory's account of his medical training ends here.

5. i.e. exotropia, or divergent strabismus, in which the eyes turn outward away from the nose. Savory's use of the pronoun 'he' implies that he did not know the correct sex of his 'Black Mare'.

July 1st. I had a patient, one James Hasel son of John and Mary Hasel of Brightwaltham[1] who was driving plow for Mr Lanfear of Wooley farm[.] this Horse took fright [and] ran away by which accident he received a very extensive wound of 7 Inches long on the Scalp but no fracture. the Bone was visible from the nape of his Neck to the Crown of his head, and the Wound was entirely cicatrizd[2] by the 12th of Aug[u]st. Mr Lanfear[3] likewise received an Accident on his Sheep Shear day which was July 12th. [*p. 214*] As he was standing at his Barn Doors the Sheep struggled and kickd the Shears from the Shearers hands & Wounded his Leg which was very deep.

I went to Moreton feast and came home to Brightwaltham the next Morn[in]g.

The most remarkable Cases I had this Year was a dislocated Clavicle, a Servant man to Mr Auber of Chaddleworth;[4] a flint I cut out of Dances Eye at Brightwaltham with the Lancet;[5] Amputated Selwoods finger of Farmbro'.[6]

I went to farmbro' feast this Year upon the Wall Eyed Nag I bo[ugh]t at Abingdon fair my companion was Digweeds Evil Magnus {conjunction} at Oak [*p. 215*] furlong Gate.

Last Chrismas Mr John Holmes[,] Taylor at Brightwaltham left the Gallery at Brightwaltham Church who is a Ringer & Singer because my Uncle gave 2/6 to them instead of entertaining them at his own house. he spoke many Oaths that he would not sing any more in the Gallery being in the heat of Liquor. My Uncle & him sung together upwards of 40 Years. this John Holmes used to peal the PSalms and sing the tenor parts.[7]

I shall conclude this Year with some mixt medlies as usual.

*   *   *

1. James Hazell, son of 'Jo Hazell' and Mary Turner, was baptised at All Saints' Church, Brightwalton, on 20 April 1777, so that the lad was 12 years old by this time. Although banns were read on 19 January 1777, John Hazel [*sic*] married Mary Turner at Brightwalton, on 29 July 1777.
2. i.e. healed by scarring-over.
3. Ambrose Lanfear (1717-1759) was the first of the family to settle in Chaddleworth, having moved from Wiltshire. Several Lanfear family graves are preserved in the churchyard.
4. John Auber BA (1764-1798), educated at Trinity College, Cambridge, and at that time curate of St Andrew's Church, Chaddleworth.
5. Probably William Dance (d. 1791). Savory describes his own antics following Dance's wedding in 1788 [156].
6. Probably John Selwood or Sellwood (c. 1740-1812), whose wife Elizabeth bore him seven children in Farnborough between 1767 and 1786.
7. John Holmes (1729-1798) was a tailor and farmer. He had married Ann Hill of Hampstead Norris at St Nicholas's Church, Newbury, on 24 August 1749. For other references to Holmes, see [28, 49*n*, 58, and 212] and he is listed in Appendices B and C.

[*p. 216*]

Cascinomancy[1]

Is practised with a Sack or Sieve wherein a pair of tongs is put in the middle of a Circle & each side of the tongs is put upon the Nails of the thumb of two persons which look one upon another (some prefer the middle finger)[.] when they are so placed they call upon the name and surname of those who is suspected to be guilty of the Theft &c. then pronounce these words[:] Deis Meis Jestitt benedarfat devasema entemeas.[2] and then the sieve shakes, moves and falls upon him that hath pronounced the name of him that is guilty.

*   *   *

[*p. 217*]

Alectromancy[3]

He that desires to know any thing must in a good clean place make a Circle which must be divided for the 24 letters then put a Wheat Corn upon every letter continuing to say this Verse: Ecce enum veritatus &c.[4] do it {Moon} in {Aries} or {Leo} or {Sun} in {Aries} or {Leo} take a Young Cock all white Cut of [*sic*] his Claws and cause him to swallow them together with a little scrawl of Lamb ~~Wool~~ <Skin> wherein shall be these words written [*six obscure symbols follow, possibly of Hebrew origin*] and holding this little Cock he must say O Deus Creato omnium qui firmamentum pulchritudim, stellarum formesti constituens eas in signa & tempora infrendi virtutem tuam openribus nostris ut per opus in eib consequentur effectum Annen.[5]

    [*p. 218*] this prayer being ended in putting the said Cock into the Circle he must say these two Verses which are taken out of the PSalm of David Domine dilexi decorum domus tua & locum habitationis tua. 2 Domini deus virtutum converte nos & Ostende faciam tuam & salvi eremus.[6]

---

1. Coscinomancy, also known as coskiomancy, is a form of divination similar to cleidomancy (see below), but using a hanging sieve instead of a key. Another method also employed a pair of tongs or shears beside the sieve, which were supported upon the thumb nails of two persons facing each other (sometimes the nails of the middle finger may be used). This type of divination was usually used to discover thieves and criminals in general.
2. Flawed Latin presumably intended to implore God to bless the desolated soul.
3. Alectromancy, also alectryomancy and alectoromancy, is an ancient method of divination using a cock or hen which is placed in a circle of grain around which are placed letters of the alphabet. The letters closest to the place the bird pecks are interpreted to answer specific questions. Another method was to recite the letters of the alphabet, making note of those at which the cock crowed. In both cases, this was done when the Sun or the Moon was in Aries or Leo.
4. i.e. here is the truth.
5. This is a prayer, in flawed Latin, beseeching God, the Creator of the stars in the firmament, to bestow his powers on the person seeking knowledge.
6. i.e. Psalm 26: *Domine dilexi decorum domus tuae et locum habitationis gloriae tuae* (I have loved, O Lord, the beauty of thy house; and the place where thy glory dwelleth) and Psalm 79: *Domine Deus virtutum converte nos et ostende faciem tuam et salvi erimus* (O God of hosts, convert us. And reveal your face, and we will be saved).

Now the Cock being placed it must be observed from what letters he eat the grains & there put others instead of them.

Clidomancy[1]

Wherein <is> used a key about which was written the name of him that was suspected of the theft or other thing upon paper which key was tyed to a Bible &c.

[*p. 219*]

Botts in a Horse[2]

You must both say and do thus upon the diseased Horse 3 days together before Sun Rising.
In Nomine Pa+tris & fi+lia [*sic*] & Spiritus + Sanctii.[3] Exorcise to vermin per deum. Pa+trum & fi+lii & Spiritus + sanctum: that is in the name of God the father the Son and the Holy Ghost. I conjure thee O Worm by God the father the Son and the Holy Ghost that thou neither eat nor drink the flesh Blood or Bones of this Horse, and that thou hereby mayst be made as patient as Job and as good as St John the Baptist, when he baptized Christ in Jordan. In Nomine pa+tris &c. you say 3 paternosters & 3 Aves in the right Ear of the Horse.

[*p. 220*]

To find a person drowned

Take a White Leaf and cast it into the Water near the suspected place & it will rest on the Water over the Body.

To know if a sick person shall Live or Die

Take Nettles whilst green and put them in the patients Urine[:] if they remain green they will live – vice versa.

Observation on the 1st person you meet in the Morning

if their names begins with A E I O or U, it signifies a good Journey; if with L or B then shalt perform thy Journey with content[;] if with C or D or T shall be in danger[;] if with S, N or R then shall find great delays in thy Affairs.

---

1. Cleidomancy, also clidomancy, refers to a method of foretelling the future by use of a key.
2. i.e. bots, insects which attach their eggs to the horse's hairs and cause anxiety and irritation that can lead to injury.
3. i.e. In the name of the Father, the Son, and the Holy Ghost.

[p. 221]

How to Cure any Swelling, Sore, Wart

Aromart & Adderstongue gathered at the hour of {Mars}, the {Moon} increasing & let {Mars} be in {trine} to {Venus} or {Moon} applying from {Mars} to {Venus} or from {Venus} to {Mars}. steep the herbs 1st in fair Water & well moisten it then apply it unto the part affected untill it be Warm, after which bury it and as it perisheth In the Earth so the patient will recover.

The [?Ungns] Mirabilis[1]

Rj Moss of a Dead Mans Scull & Mans Grease aa ii oz Mummy & Mans Blood & Bol Armes aa i ounce Ol Lini & Roses aa ii oz mixt.

   The way to use it. Take the Blood or matter of the wound upon the Weapon or Instrument which made the wound, *[p. 222]* or otherways dry it on a piece of Wood, then put the Wood in the Ointment or else anoint the Blood being kept dry upon the Wood and keep it from Air. you must every day with a fresh linen Rag with the Urine of the patient & so bind up the Wound. its excellent for the Tooth Ach by pricking the tooth with a Tooth pick so as to make it Bleed & immediately put the tooth pick in the Ointment.

The Powder of Sympathy[2]

Rj Roman or Blue Vitriol [*i.e. copperas (cupric sulphate)*] vi oz or viii oz[,] reduce it into very fine powder, do it when {Sun} enters {Leo} then spread it finely upon an earthen glazen pan, set it dayly in the heat of the Sun during 40 days & keep it Warm at Night & be carefull it take no Wett nor Cold [*p. 223*] afterwards. get something that has the Blood or Matter of the Wound upon it and put it into a Bason of Water with some powder[,] in a moderate heat of the {Sun} & in a Closet, at Night in the Chimney Corner. for fitts let the persons Blood mix some of the powder with it[.] whilst it warm mix it together in a little bag, and let the patient wear it about his Neck. To cure any disease see what herbs are good for the disease, get a select Number and gathered at the right hour[,] dry & reduce it to a fine powder and take the quantity of i ounce & the same quantity of pulv Sympathy, mix with the patients blood[,] whilst warm make it up in a little Bag & let the patient wear it next the Skin.

---

1. The final letters, probably 'ns', are written in superscript in tiny writing, and might conceivably be 'us', 'uo' or even 'm'. Savory possibly meant '*unguen*' (fat or grease), or '*unguo*' (to anoint with oil), i.e. the wondrous grease, fat or oil.
2. Applying the Powder of Sympathy to a weapon by which a wound had been inflicted was reckoned to remedy the injury and was popular during the reigns of King James I and Charles I.

[p. 224]
How to lay the Spirits of Men & Woman that come again to trouble the Earth

Observations thereupon by Jacobus [de] Chusa a great Doctor of the Romish Church.[1]

1st he sais it is expedient to fast 3 days and to celebrate a certain number of Masses & to repeat the 7 penitential psalms. 4 or 5 priests must be called to the place where the haunt or Noise is then a Candle hallowed on Candlemas day, thats made of Virgins Wax must be lighted and in the lighting thereoff must be said the 7 PSalms and the Gosple of St John, then there must be a Cross and a Censor with frankincense & the place must be Censed or perfumed. Holy Water must be sprinkled & a holy stool must be used, & after other divers ceremonys a prayer *[p. 225]* to God as follows:

O Lord Jesus Chirst the knower of all secrets which allways revealest all wholesome and profitable things to thy faithfull Children & which sufferest a Spirit to shew himself in this place. We beseech thee for this bitter passion & Vouchsafe to command this spirit to reveal & signifie unto us thy servant without our terrour or hurt which is to thy honor and Glory and to his comfort. In Nomine Patris &c.

And then proceed in these Words. We beseech thee for Christs sake. Oh thou Spirit that if there be any of us or among us whom thou wouldst answer name him or else manifest him by some sign is it fryar P or &c., or any of us. Et sic de caeteris cir cum stanibus.[2] If *[p. 226]* the Spirit make any sound or Noise at the naming of any one – he is the master that must have the charge of this Conjuration. he must say to him Whose Soul art thou! Wherefore comest thou! What wouldst thou have?[3] wantest thou any suffrages, Masses or Alms. how many Masses will serve thy tune 3, 6, 10, 20, 30 &c. by what priest might he be religious or secular! Wilt thou have any fasts! what! how many! how great! and by what persons! Among Hospitals, Leprosy or Beggars! what shall be the sign of thy perfect deliverance! Wherefore was thou in purgatory! & such like. this must be done in the Night &c.

*   *   *

[p. 227]

1790

Jan[ua]ry 6th. Uncle bo[ugh]t of Avery Hobbs of Hendred a Spinnett[,][4] gave him 2½ Guineas. 12th. Died one Ventris who was Landlord at the George at Speenhamland[,][5] he used to practice Surgery. the 27th, Mr Stanbrook made his exit from Brightwaltham being very much in debt and

---

1. See R. Scott, *The Discoverie of Witchcraft* (1583), specifically chapter 22.
2. i.e. And so on for the rest of those around.
3. The question mark is reversed.
4. For Avery Hobbs, from whom Savory's uncle, John Savory, had previously purchased a flute, incision knife and four books, see [55, 55*n*, 117].
5. John Ventrice, see [116].

the Auction was March the 1st of all his household Goods. Mr Church and Thos [?Guilman] of Soal Farm was chief Constables for this County this Year[.] I asisted Mr Church in his office and wrote the following letter to the petty Constables

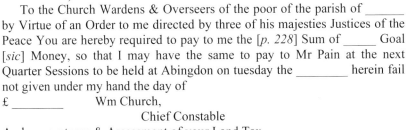

Berks to Wit}
   To the Church Wardens & Overseers of the poor of the parish of _____ by Virtue of an Order to me directed by three of his majesties Justices of the Peace You are hereby required to pay to me the [*p. 228*] Sum of ____ Goal [*sic*] Money, so that I may have the same to pay to Mr Pain at the next Quarter Sessions to be held at Abingdon on tuesday the _____ herein fail not given under my hand the day of
£ _____   Wm Church,
                    Chief Constable
And your returns & Assessment of your Land Tax.

   Feb[rua]ry 7th. Was Married at Brightwaltham Church Wm Butler to Anne Cooper and the Bells was rung backwards.[1] the 10th, the Prince of Wales came in these parts to Hunt with Lord Cravens Hounds.[2] 22nd. Fruin Wicks commenced Shopkeeping.[3]
   24th. Died Arthur Whiter of Brightwaltham a Butcher & uncle to this present Arthur Whiter[,] he was upwards of 70 Years of Age [and] was interrd in Brightwaltham Church under his pew.[4] James Major of Wantage mended [*p. 229*] the Measuring Wheel and I measured the following places.
   From the lower Corner of Mr Herberts Stable to the 1st holt gate is 1M 0F 18P.[5] To the farther holt gate by Thos Taylors is 1M 2F 38P. To Pointers at Egypt 2M 0F 20P. To the Cross way at Chapple 2M 4F 36P. To the Ivy House North Heath 3M 3F 34P. To the 1st gate at North Heath 3M 5F 21P. To the Boar at North Heath 3M 7F 0P. To the House beyond the Boar 4 Miles. To the Cross Way at Winterbourn is 4M 5F 0P. To the 1st. Gate at Snelsmore Heath 5M 1F 29P. To the farthest Gate at Do. 7 6M 5F 4P. To Donnington Cross Road 7M 2F 4P. To the Cross Way at Speenhamland this side Mr Baylys from Harberts stable is 8 Miles & 29 Poles. [*p. 230*] From my Uncles Kitchen Door to the Church Door is 3 Furlongs & 25 Poles. From the Church Door to the Holt is 1M 4F 14P. From the Marquis of Grandby Kitchen Door to the public House at Lilly is 1M 38P.
   March 1st. This day being Stanbrooks Auction. Faulkner was Auctioneer. 19th. Was Married Mr Giles Brickell of North Heath to Mrs Bew.[6] 31st.

---

1. The parish register gives the date of the marriage as *8* February 1790.
2. 'Tuesday last [9 February] his Royal Highness the Prince of Wales paid a visit to Lord Craven at his seat at Benham, near Newbury; and on Thursday his Highness took the diversion of fox-hunting with his Lordship at Shefford.' *Bath Chronicle and Weekly Gazette* (19 February 1790).
3. For Frewin Wicks, see [42].
4. He was aged 73, and was buried on 27 February. RBA D/EW/O8 shows that Whiter shared a pew in 1768 with R[ichard] Fulbrook and J[ohn] Deacon on the left-hand side of the aisle diagonally and rightwards across from the Church door.
5. KEY: M: Mile, F: Furlong, P: Pole (the abbreviations are Savory's, and the key inferred).
6. Giles Brickell married *Mary* Bew at St James's Church, Leckhampstead, on *18* March 1790.

Went to Abingdon as Witness on a Tryal between David Jones of Newbury Plaintiff and Thos Hasell of Benham Defendant, respecting a Bill the Plaintiff had on the defendant[.] April 21st. I attended Brooks Wife in Labour at Brightwalton & delivered her of a Son[,] this was the 1st Labour I had since I came from London. this John Brooks was a Taylor at Brightwaltham but since is gone to live in London.[1]

[*p. 231*] The beginning of May my Uncle putt up new posts and poles at the House at Brightwaltham. 13th. Went to Newbury Holy Thursday fair and coming back I first became acquainted With the Revd E[dwar]d Jones who lodgd at Mr Brickells at N[orth] Heath. this parson Jones was an excellent Minister in the Church but a person very much addicted to Drinking & Swearing. a few Weeks ago was Married Miss Charlotte Bew of North Heath.[2] June 3rd. was Married Mr Ebenezer Whitewood of Newbury Glazier &c.[3] 21st. planted Nightshade I had from Pryar of Steventon[:] he sais its good for Witchcraft given in powder or any other form, but he could not cure his Wife with it. he also sais the Urine of a person that is afflicted with Witchcraft will bubble in a Glass.

[*p. 232*] The Revd E[dwar]d Jones sais there is but one Rule without exception which is u after q in the English Language. July 4th. Was married Francis New Son of John New, farmer of Chaddleworth to Eliz[abe]th Buttler daughter of John Butter [*sic*] farmer in Chaddleworth.[4] Went to Fawly Church & playd the Bassoon[,] Sung the 21st A 133 A and 150 A[;] we met the Letcomb Singers. 17th. Died Ellen Taylor daughter of Thos Taylor in Brightwaltham Holt.[5]

Aug[u]st 1st. Went to farmbro' Church and playd the Bassoon[.] we met there the Letcomb Singers Sung 148 Bath & 47 A. 29th. Was Married Thos Sanders Carpenter to Esqr. Tipping to Ruth Taylor daughter of Thos Taylor at Brightwalton Holt.[6] Sept[embe]r 10th. This Morning as I was going along the lane at the lower end of a ground calld [?Juspisen] on a Visit to [*p. 233*] Mr Whiter who was then Ill, I met John Deacon Collar maker at Brightwalon with a firkin of Tar at his back & <a> head of the Firkin was out. he thought I meant to throw something at it, went to stoop to pick up a stone to throw at me, and great part of the Tar run over him. he was obliged to go back after more Tar & his Wife went after his Coat with a prong[.] Oct[obe]r 4th. was the Revd Mr Williams Auction at Farmbro' who left that Curacey at this

---

1. This is Richard Brookes, the son of John and Jane Brookes, baptised at Brightwalton, on 2 May 1790.
2. Charlotte Bew married William Eaves at St James's Church, Leckhampstead, on 11 May 1790.
3. Ebenezer Whitewood married Sarah Sims by licence at St Nicholas's Church, Newbury, on 3 April 1790. One Thomas Whitewood is listed as a plumber and glazier in Newbury in the *UD*.
4. Francis New, baptised at St Andrew's Church, Chaddleworth, on 27 August 1769, the first of ten children born to John New (1743-1802) and his wife Elizabeth, née Whiting (c.1744-1810). Francis married Elizabeth *Butler* by licence. He died in 1825 and was buried in Chaddleworth on 23 September. For more on New, and his friendship with Savory, see [157].
5. Buried 21 July.
6. The marriage of Thomas Saunders and Ruth Taylor took place at St Andrew's Church, Chaddleworth.

time[.] the 11th. Was Married at Brightwaltham Church Wm Digweed to Ann Pickett and gave the ringers 2/6[.] they went to live at Hamstead Norris. 15th. payd my last Visit to the Revd E[dwar]d Jones at N. Heath[.] he gave me two Books title Bayly on the Bath Waters[1] & Chinese Tales[.] he went to live at Shaftsbury.

[*p. 234*] Nov[embe]r 15th. Died Wm Clinch who drove the Newbury Coach.[2] 22nd. Was Married at Catmore John Clarke of Lilly.[3] Dec[embe]r 9th. Was Married Mr Dewe of Milton to Miss Han[na]h Mallam of the Heath.[4]

During this Year I bled 126 persons & before about 150 so that I have bled in all 276 persons to the end of this Year. during this Year I drawed 29 Teeth, divided the Frenum Lingua[5] of 3 Children. had many remarkable Cases this Year fractured Clavicle, Witchcraft, Scold Heads[6] &c. which may be seen in my Book of Clinical Cases.[7]

During this Year I playd the Bassoon at Brightwalton Church & never doubled one Tune & Psalm except the 55th Anthem which was when I was not there and for Memorandum I sett them all down which are as follows.

---

1. Probably William Baylis (d. 1787), *An Essay on the Bath Waters* (n.d.)
2. According to the *Reading Mercury* Clinch, who was a proprietor of the Newbury Coach, died at five o'clock on the morning of *Tuesday the 16th* 'after a few hours illness', *RM* (22 November 1790). William *Clynch* was buried at St Nicholas's Church, Newbury, on 20 November 1790. For Clinch and Kimber's coach service, the 'Newbury Machines', see section xiii of the introduction.
3. John Clarke married Hannah Cozens at St Margaret's Church, Catmore, on 22 November 1790.
4. *John* Dewe married Hannah Mallam at Milton, on 9 December 1790.
5. i.e. *frenulum linguae*, the skin between the floor of the mouth and the midline of the underside of the tongue.
6. A name popularly given to several diseases of the scalp characterised by pustules (the dried discharge of which forms scales) and hair-loss.
7. This volume has not survived. See Appendix D.

[*p. 235*]

3 ov f 42 A 132 ov f	66 ov '' 55A	116 f 128 A Hymn 22 times	new 2 f 132 A Old 81 f	2 P 30 f ?works
old 4th ov f 55A 68A	2 ov 122 f key 150 nv f	111 P 95 5th PS 51 P	new 23 f 148 ?Bell 105 Gay	Yeovil Moll 21 A
13 f 99 f 44 P	Good friday 89 & 111 times/Hymns	9 f 77 f 71 f old	5 f ?Sanside 118f 126 f	67P old 147 f
16 d f 95 nv f	Easter Hymn ov 90 Xm ser Pass 16 f ?single	8 f 15 f 67 A	33 nv P 124 ov P 89 P	?Stome 105 133 A
149 f 18 A	26 f 114 A 48 A	68 P 92 f 42 P	103 Gay 9 A 84 A	71 ov P 100 ov new Ev. Ser. A
33 P ov 84 f	150 ov P 96 Law f 96 A	100 P in c 98 f 55 A	98P 133 f 104 f nv	23 P 33 f Ev Hymn
57 ov f 119 f	23 ov f 104 f ?Jose 21 ov f	Olf 44 dem 66 nv f	34 P Isia 1 A 57 ov f	19 nv P 167 ov ns f 106 nv P ?
21 f nv 24 ?Lantle	116 P 47 f Isai 40 A	Straw Boly 16A 150 P in c	 85 P 128 f	47 P J. 6 7 A 26 A
136 P 102 A	88 f 21 A 145 f	40 P Car XI A 84 P	old 22 f 39 A old 122 P	Hym 81 in d Isai 9d A Lent 2d A
104 P old 1 ov A	10 f 100 nv f 150 A	Mitchels 106 Rev 19 A	old 106 ov P 118 ?Law f 16 P	37 P 100 A Hym Wt wds
100 P ov 108 f	Hym 42times 145 A 81 f in d	18 P 72 A New 4 ov f	19P ov ?Ched 103 f ns 40 f	_____

[*p. 236*]

Hints to a New Married Sister[1]

Let not my sister now a Wife
Bid all her Cares adiue [*sic*]
Contforts [*sic*] there are in a Maried life
And there are Crosses too
I do not wish to Mar your Mirth
With an ungratefull sound
But yet remember bliss on Earth
No mortal ever found
Your prospects and your hopes are great
May God those hopes fullfill
But you will find in every state
 Some difficulty still
The Rite which lately joind your hands
Cannot insure content
Religion forms the strongest bands
And Love the best Cement
A Friendship founded on esteem
Lifes battering blasts endure
It will not vanish as a dream
And such I hope is yours.
[*p. 237*]
But yet Gods daily blessings Crave
 Nor trust thy youthfull heart[2]
You must divine asistance have
 To act a prudent part
Tho' you have left a parents wing
 Nor longer ask his Care
Yet husbands very seldom bring
 A lighter Yoke to wear
For Husbands have humours & faults
 So Mutable is Man
Excuse his foibles in thy thoughts
 And hide them if you can
No longer no resentment keep
 Whatever is Amiss
Be reconciled before you sleep
 If 'eer [*sic*] you hope for bliss[3]
Or if theres Cause to reprehend
 Do it with mild address
Remember he's the dearest friend

---

1. This is often reproduced as a song, 'Hints to a new married sister, and it wont be my fault if I
 die an old maid': see, e.g. *Poems on Various Subjects, Chiefly Sacred, by the late Mr Thomas
 Greene, of Ware, Hertfordshire* (1780), 22-24.
2. Here Savory starts to indent alternate lines.
3. This line is the most different in Greene, which reads, 'And seal it with a kiss'.

And Love him near [*sic*] the less
[*p. 238*]
Tis not the Way to scold at Large
    Whate'er proud reason boasts
For those their duty best discharge
    Who condescend the most
Mutual attempts to serve and please
    Each other will endear
Thus you may draw the Yoke with ease
    Nor discord interfere
Thus give your passions tender[1] scope
    Yet better things pursue
Be Heavin the object of your hope
    And lead him thither too
Since you must both resign your breath
    And God alone knows when
So live that you may part at death
    To meet with Joy again
And may the Lord sit you above[2]
    And Grant you both a share
In his redeeming Sovereign Love[3]
    And providential Care.

*   *   *

[*p. 239*]

Pharmacopola Circumforaneus[4]

Gentlemen,

I waltho van Claturbank[,][5] High Gorman Doctor, Native of Arabia, Burgamaster of the City of Brandipolis, 7th Son of a 7th Son Unborn Doctor of above 60 Years experience, having studied over Galen, Hyppocrates,

---

1. Instead of 'passions tender', Greene reads 'tender passions'.
2. In Greene, the phrase 'sit you above' reads 'your ways approve'.
3. In Greene, 'Sovereign Love' reads 'saving love'.
4. i.e. a travelling hawker of medicines (a mountebank). The title is probably taken from Cicero. This burlesque on quackery originally bore the sub-title, 'the horse doctor's harangue to the credulous mob': see M. A. Katritzky, 'Marketing medicine: the image of the early modern mountebank', *Renaissance Studies*, xv: ii (June 2001), 121-153.
5. This pseudonym seems to date to the 1670s, but according to Robert Chambers's celebrated *Book of Days* (1864) (entry for 14 April), this burlesque was the work of the actor Joe Haines. Haines was associated with the Drury Lane Theatre at the beginning of the eighteenth century, part of the company assembled by Christopher Rich (1657-1714). The work was published as a broadside, with an engraving of Haines stood on a stage, medicine in hand and a harlequin by his side. The setting is Tower Hill, then a recognised rendezvous for mountebanks. The audience of tourists is called to attention with a trumpet blast. A gouty patient is seated in the operating chair, with boxes of medication in the background. There are patients with walking-sticks, and there is a young pickpocket in the crowd. For a full analysis of the burlesque, see <https://digitalis-dsp.uc.pt/bitstream/10316.2/32730/3/BiblosVII_artigo7.pdf> (accessed 10 December 2022).

Albumazar & paracelsus[1] am now become the Aesculapius of this Age,[2] having been educated at twelve Universities and traveld through 52 Kingdoms, and been Counsellor of Counsellors to several Monarchs. I have lately arived from the farthest part of Utopia, famous throughout all Asia, Africa, Europe & America from the Suns Oriental exaltation to his occidental declimation. out of mear [*sic*] pity to my own dear self & languishing [*p. 240*] Mortals have by desire of several Lords Earls, Dukes & honorable personages been at last prevaild upon to oblige the world with this Notice.

That all persons Young or Old, Blind or Lame, Deaf or Dumb, Curable or incurable, may know where to repair for Cure in all Cephalalgias, paralitic paroxysms, palpitations of the pericardium, Empyemas, Hysterical Effusions, the Hen Pox the Hug pox the small Pox and Whores Pox, the Acites, Anarsarca & the entire Legion of Lethiferous distempers.

Imprimis Gentleman, I have a never failing styptic Coroborating Anodynus, Odoriferous Balsam's Balsam of Balsams made of Dead mans fatt Resin & Goose-grease which infalible restores lost Maidenheads, Raises demolishd Noses & in fine preserves all superanuated Bawds from wrinkles.

[*p. 241*] Item I have the true Carthramophra of the triple kingdom never failing Heliogenus being the tincture of the Sun, deriving vigour, influence & dominion from the same lights. it causes all complexions to laugh and smile at the very time of taking it. its seven Years in preparing and being compleated secundum Artem[3] by fermentation, Cohobation, Calcination, Sublimation, fixation, Philtration, Circulation & Quidlibitification in Balneo Maria, its the only sovereign remedy in the World.

This is Natures palladium, Healths Magazine[;] it works seven manner of ways in order as nature herself requires, for it scorns to be confind to any particular way of Operation: so that it effecteth the Cure either Hypnotically, Hydrotically, Carthatically, poppismatically, Hydrogogically,[4][*p. 242*] Pneumatically or Senochdochically, it mundifies the Hypogastrium, Wipes of [*sic*] Abstersively those ternacious, conglomerated sedimental sordes that adhere to Oesophagus and Vicerae.

A Dram of it is worth a bushel of March Dust for if a man chance to have his brains beat out or his head chopt off, two drops I say two drops Gentleman seasonably applyd will recall the fleeting Spirits. Reinthro' the deposed Arteries cement the discontinuity of the parts and in 6 Minutes restore the lifeless trunk to all its pristine functions, Vital, Natural and Animal so that this, believe me Gentlemen is the only sovereign remedy in the World.

I have the Antepudenda Gragan Specific in Venus regalia which infallibly Cures [*p. 243*] the Venereal Disease with all its train of Gonnorrheas, Buboes & Shankers, Phymosis, Paraphymosis with as much pleasure as the same was

---

1. i.e. Galen (the second and third-century Greek physician, surgeon and philosopher), Hippocrates (the Greek physician of the classical period), Albumasar (the ninth-century Muslim astrologer), and Paracelsus (the German Renaissance physician, alchemist and theologian).
2. i.e. the Greek God of Medicine.
3. *Secundum artem*: according to practice.
4. The word is split across the two pages, 'Hydrogogi' - 'cally'.

contracted so that its worth any persons while to get into that modest distemper once a fortnight if it be to be had for Love or Money to enjoy the benefit of so diverting a Remedy.

I have the panchymagogan in Hermes trismegistus an incomparable spagyric Tincture of the Moons Horns which is the only infalible remedy against the Contagion of Cuckoldum.

Besides my Vermifugus pulvis or Antivermatical Worm Conquering powders so famous for destroying all the sorts of 'em incident to human bodies, breaking their complicated knots in the Duodenum & [*p. 244*] and [*sic*] disolving those phlegmatic Crudities that produce these Anthrophohogus [*sic*] Vermin it has brought away Worms by Urine as long as the Monument on Fish Street Hill[1] tho' I confess not so large.

Look ye Gentlemen I have it under the hands and seals of all the greatest Sultans, Sophas, Bashas, Viziers & Mufties in Christendom to verificate the truth of my operations that I have actually performd such Cures as are realy beyond human abilities.

I Cured the King of Spains Godmother to the admiration of all the Court of a stupendous dolar about the os Sacrum so that the good old Lady really feared the perdition of her huckle bone. I did it by fermenting her posteriors with a Mummy of Nature alias cal[le]d pilgrims salve [*p. 245*] mixt up with the Spirit of Mugwort tartagraphated thorough [*sic*] an Alembic of Cristaline transfluency.

Thence was I sent for to the Emperor of Morocca [*sic*] who was violently afflicted with the Rheumatism. he came to meet me 300 Leagues in a go Cart but I gave him so speedy an acquittance of his Dolar that the next Night I caused him to dance a saraband with flipflops & somersetts.

I Cured the Dutchess of Barsanolpha of a Cramp in her tongue.

I also Cured the Count de Rodomontado who was corrupt with an Iliac passion contracted by eating buttered parsnips.

Now Gentlemen you that are willing to render yourselves immortal by a packett of me, or repair to the sign of the prancers in Vico Vulgo Rattle Cliffero, S.E. of the templum danicum in the Square of profound Close.

Re enfacta.[2]

[*p. 246*]

1791

Jan[ua]ry 11th. had 2 Stocks of Bees of Mrs Jones of Lilly. 21st. Was Maried at Letcomb Mr F. Pigott to Miss Lintell a Young Lady who went there to lodge.[3] at this time I had some bad Cases. one Wm Pain at Court Oak[4] who had a large Wound on his Ancle bone also another such a Case at

---

1. i.e. 1677, when the Monument (to the Great Fire of London of 1666) was completed.
2. i.e. in reality. Savory has omitted several lines towards the end of the burlesque, as published, and his writing appears increasingly cramped presumably because he was trying to contain the burlesque and not continue on a fresh page.
3. Mary Lenthall married Francis Pigott by licence at St Andrew's Church, Letcombe Regis, on *16* January 1791.
4. Court Oak, a farm to the south of Leckhampstead.

fawly. Zachariah Hind with an extensive burn on his Leg. James Kingham of Farmbro' who by accident shot his hand with a Gun.[1] Allens Daughter who had the Dropsy of Hamstead Norris. Thos Duck of Chaddleworth who had the Small Pox & Died.[2]

March 17th. Mr Wm Adnam of Leckhamstead[3] & I agreed for the House situated in Bartholomew Street Newbury for the Sum of £252. We had an agreement [*p. 247*] made by John Blagrave[4] & I paid down 1 Guinea[.][5] 23rd. I gave Charles Hamblin orders to do the Carpentering &c[,] Whitewood the Glazing & George Brown the Bricklaying & Dan[ie]l Brown the inside painting the Shop excluded.[6] the 27th. John Jarvis came upon tryal.[7] April 10th was buried Mr Pratt of South Moreton. he used to play the Bass Vial.[8] Mr Green preachd the funeral Sermon from 7 Ch[apter] Eclesiastes & latter part of the 2 Verse.[9] 12th. Died Mr Thomas Whiting of Chaddleworth[10] & left the poor of Chaddleworth £100 to be laid out for them in Linen which was bought at Mr Vincents. I beleive 1500 Ells of Doughles.[11] I Bo[ugh]t of Stroud[12] 4 Bath Stove grates at 11d pr Inch & ordered Davies to paper the two Chambers.[13]

[*p. 248*] April 14th. at ¼ past 12 o'Clock I deliverd my Sister Mary of a Daughter & her name was Rachell.[14] 23rd. John Jarvis was bound Apprentice to me for the sum of £50 for 5 Years.[15] 28th. Bo[ugh]t of Mr Wm Adnam the washing Copper, Locks, Bells &c. gave him £1 11s. 6d.

---

1. James Kingham (c.1769-1843) was the son of local farmer, Joseph Kingham (c.1736-1807) and his wife Esther, née Hester (c.1738-1806), who settled at Lower Farm, Farnborough in 1786, having migrated from Monks Risborough, Buckinghamshire, via Wick Farm, Radley. James Kingham would marry Sarah Hooper, née Reeves (1769-1861) in Huish, Wiltshire, in 1800. For the Hooper family, and for Sarah's brother, John Reeves, see [252 and *n*]. Savory's nephew, Silas Eagles (1795-1848), would marry James and Sarah Kingham's eldest child, Amy Kingham (1801-1842), at St Aldate's Church, Oxford, on 28 July 1821.
2. Buried at St Andrew's Church, Chaddleworth, on 23 February 1791.
3. William Adnam was the churchwarden at St James's Church, Leckhampstead.
4. John Blagrave is listed as an attorney in Newbury in the *UD*.
5. For more on this agreement, see [255], and for Savory's purchase of a washing copper from Adnam, see [248].
6. Charles Hamblin, carpenter and joiner; Thomas Whitewood, plumber and glazier; George Brown, bricklayer; and Daniel Brown, plumber and glazier: all listed in Newbury in the *UD*.
7. John Jarvis (1775-1867), son of John and Elizabeth Jarvis, was baptised at St Mary's Church, East Ilsley, on 31 October 1775. It is not clear whether he completed his apprenticeship with Savory (see Afterword), but he certainly became a surgeon. For many years he was in practice in Hart Street, Bloomsbury Square, London. He lived to the age of 92.
8. John Pratt, yeoman, buried at St John the Baptist's Church, South Moreton, on 19 April 1791.
9. i.e. Ecclesiastes 7:2, It is better to go to the house of mourning, than to go to the house of feasting: for that is the end of all men; and the living will lay it to his heart.
10. Thomas Whiting was buried at St Andrew's Church, Chaddleworth, on 16 April 1791. TNA PCC PROB 11/1206/129.
11. William Vincent and Co., linen and woollen drapers, Newbury, is listed in the *UD*. Savory probably means duffels/duffles, i.e. coarse woollen cloth.
12. Possibly Benjamin Stroud, listed as an auctioneer in Newbury in the *UD*.
13. Probably the same 'Davies' mentioned later (see [251]) but possibly William Davis, see [257 and *n*].
14. Rachel Norris was baptised at Brightwalton on 1 May but was buried on 13 October.
15. RBA D/EX2704/1, Apprenticeship Indenture of John Jarvis, son of John Jarvis of East Ilsley, bound to William Savory, Surgeon, of Newbury, for a period of five years (1791).

This Easter I agreed with Farmbro' & Leckhamstead parishes to attend the poor by the Year – Farmbro' for £2 12s. 6d. Small Pox Fractures & Midwifery excluded & Leckhamstead for £5 5s. 0d.

The following is a List of Farmbro'
poor I am to attend[:] Miss Partirdge, Jo. Dearlove, Liverd, John Hughes, Ab. Brown, Thos Williams, Wm Darling, Baydon, J. Painting, Eagleton, Hen[r]y Arter, Wm Moulden, Jo Sheppard, Jordan Fisher, Wm Willis, Mills & Wid Duck, Crosses, Taylor, Thos Hains, Jo. & Jas Selw[oo]d, Richardson, James Duck, John Hamblin, Jo. Fisher.

[*p. 249*]
In all 28 Families.

In Leckkamstead parish:[1]
<u>Hill Green</u> Bradfield, Carter, Heath, Yeatts, Fisher, Holmes, Sheppard, Hayes &c.
<u>Thickett</u> Chittar, Brooks, Froude, Wakefield, Marshall, Curtis's, Biggs, [?Bristor], Hamlin, Carter, Flower, Ball, Ducks.
<u>Leckhams[tea]d.</u> Old Lawrence, Js Head, Wm Hope, James Prince, Pearce Junr, Head &c. Kember, Webb, Is. Wakefield, Hatton, E. Lawrence, [E.] Church, Dolton, Hatt, Kings, Potter, J. Lawrence, Pearce Sen[io]r, Lewis, Fullers, Patience, Old Banger.
Egypt – Wakefield (Prices or Wakefields), Old Dolton.
In all 44 Families & 28 in Farmbro' so that I attend[e]d 72 Families dur[in]g the Year 1791.

[*p. 250*]
April 26th 1791.
We the Chapple Wardens, Overseer & chief inhabitants of the parish of Leckhamstead in the County of Berks, now assembled upon parish business, Do by these present jointly & severally grant unto Wm Savory Surgeon & Apothecary of Newbury in the same County, the sum of Five pounds Five Shillings, to be paid unto the said Wm Savory Yearly during the term of two Years for attending the poor of the parish of Leckhamstead aforesaid in all diseases respecting Surgery, Pharmacy & Midwifery, Fractures & Small Pox included.[2] In witness whereoff we have hereunto sett our hands the day & Year above Written.
Wm Adnum, Chapple Warden
Jesse Winkworth, Jos[ep]h Adnum, Overseers
Wm Bew, Jos[ep]h Chamberlain, Jos[ep]h Shuff, Tim[oth]y Bew.

[*p. 251*] May 1st. was baptized Rachel the daughter of Joseph and Mary Norris & the 28th <April> Was baptized Miriam the daughter of Thos & Ann Barratt of Shefford.[3] 11th. Bo[ugh]t of Mr Josh Adnum of Leckhamstead a 4

---

1. The remainder of the page is divided into three vertical columns listing the names.
2. The agreement with Farnborough, by contrast, apparently excluded such cases under its general terms.
3. The details of Rachel and Miriam's baptisms are confirmed in the parish registers of Brightwalton and Great Shefford respectively, though Miriam's surname is given as *Barrett*.

Year old Gelding for 27 pounds. 19th. Payd Davies for papering two Chambers £5 11s. 8d.

May 3rd. Went to Mrs Jones who keeps the Inn at Lilly[1] & who the preceeding Night fell in the fire, or by a Giddiness in her Head (some think by the Essence of Sr John Barley Corn[2] set herself on fire with the Candle[)]. however it was a very extensive burn. her right breast, Shoulder, posterior part of her Neck[,] one side of her face, her right Arm & both hands were scorchd & lookd as black as a Coal. I made an excellent Cure of it.

[*p. 252*] May 11th. Mr Wm Hooper of Puizey brother to Mr Hooper who lived at Farmbro' fell from his Horse & fractured his Scull near Dutsill[3] in the parish of Brightwaltham[,] as he was returning to puizey from farmbro' being intoxicated with strong Liquor[,] also a fracture of the Sternum[.] Mr Withers & Mr Stevens of Puizey likewise attended but could not get the grant of performing the operation, being of so stubborn & resolute disposition, & would go to puizey. however the Operation was performd at puizey & he died owing to his own misconduct & Mr Hooper of Farmbro' went to live at puizey and Reeves his brother in law came to Farmbro' to live.[4] 22nd. Went to London[.] my companion on the Coach was a painter & he told me the best thing to clean an old picture was the White of an Egg beat to a froth & well rub the pictures after [*p. 253*] being well scowered with New Urine, Warm Water or Warm Water and Soap, only mind the Soap should be wiped off. I ordered my stock of Drugs of Crawly & Adcock in Bishopsgate Street & Surgeons Instruments of Davenport in White Chapple, Oils &c. of Clarks in Red Lion Street, White Chapple.[5] I came from London on the Bristol Mail[.] sett off from Picadilly at 9 o'Clock at Night and was at Thatcham by 3 the next Morn[in]g. 24th. this Morning I attended Kembers Wife of Leckhamstead in Labour and delivered her of a boy about 2 o'Clock in the Afternoon.

June 2nd. Bo[ugh]t Glasses &c. of Goslings[.][6] being Newbury fair I had a great many guests at my new intended habitation[.] by this time I got almost all my things from Brightwaltham to Newbury.

[*p. 254*] 20th. Died Mrs Chittle[,] wife of Thos Chittle of Westbrook and sister to Mrs Jones, being maried 18 Years previous to her pregnancy & was

---

1. The Old Inn at Lilley was later known as the Fox and Cubs. It ceased trading in the 1980s.
2. 'Sir John Barleycorn' was a folk song, the protagonist of which personified barley and the alcoholic beverages derived from it (i.e. beer and whisky).
3. i.e. Dutshill.
4. William Hooper (c.1759-1791), of Pewsey, Wiltshire, died on 3 August 1791. His brother, Robert Hooper (c.1763-1795), whom he was visiting in Farnborough, had married Sarah Reeves (1769-1861) at Huish, Wiltshire, on 10 April 1785. The Hooper and Reeves families were Wiltshire farmers. The 'brother in law Reeves' whom Savory refers to was Sarah's brother, John Reeves (1756-1845), who settled at Upper Farm, Farnborough. In 1792 John Reeves married Ear(e)y Kingham (c.1770-1804), the daughter of neighbouring farmer Joseph Kingham, of Lower Farm, Farnborough, and his wife Esther, née Hester. In 1800 John Reeves's sister, Sarah, having been widowed when Robert Hooper died in 1795, would marry John Reeves's brother-in-law, James Kingham, whose accident Savory records above (see [246 and *n*]). A memorial tablet to the Hooper brothers (William, Robert and Richard) survives inside St John the Baptist Church, Pewsey.
5. John Clark, Oil and Colourman, Red Lion Street, Whitechapel, is listed in the *UD*.
6. Robert Gosling, tailor and shopkeeper, is listed in Newbury in the *UD*.

delivered of a Child about a week before she died.[1] 21st. My Nag died owing to a Wound on the hollow above its Eye which was done in the stable at Lilly. had of Mrs Trulock £25 the 14th. 29th. This Morning I attended Leah Prince of Leckhamstead in Labour[.] I was there about an hour.[2]

July 6th. Geo Whiting of Chaddleworth took to Trulocks Mortgage[.] my Uncle had £550 upon it[.] this Trulock lives at Charlton in the estate mortgaged. 8th. Payd George Brown 19 Guineas, Cha[rle]s Hamlin £31 & Fidler for bricks £6 6s.[3] 10th. Went to London[.] Bo[ugh]t the large Mortar w[i]d[th] 72# at 9d pr lb.

[*p. 255*] July 11th. John Jarvis, my Sister Jenny & Leah pointer came to Newbury to continue. I hired Leah Pointer at the Rate of 3½ Guineas pr Year but she was not fit for my service therefore staied but a few Weeks & her sister Martha came in her room. they are daughters of Thos Pointer of Leckhamstead Egypt[.][4] 20th. this Evening I slept at Newbury at my new Habitation & the 21st I opened Shop being Markett Day. 25th. Bo[ugh]t a Gray Horse of Mr Ward of Paughly[;] gave him 25 Guineas. 26th Bo[ugh]t of Ben Ford a New Saddle & Bridles.[5] 28th. Uncle, Adnam & myself met at Blagraves & settled about the House[;] gave adnam a bond for £200. 30th. this Morning I went to Reading. [*p. 256*] Bo[ugh]t of Mrs Collins Sp[iri]t Wine & Malaga Wine.[6] Went to the printing Office & gave Cowslade the following Address; Payd him for 3 times inserting in the paper 16/6:[7]

William Savory

Surgeon, Apothecary and Man Midwife

In Bartholomew Street Newbury

Begs leave to inform his friends & the public that he has attended the practice of St Thos & Guys Hospitals London & studied the several branches of Medicine, Surgery, Anatomy & Midwifery under the most able professors[,] an advantage which greatly facilitated his arival to that honor conferrd on him by the Corporation of Surgeons in London, in constituting him a Member of their body.

---

1. Mary Hughes was baptised at St Mary's Church, Boxford, on 23 April 1747 and married Thomas Chittle there, on 27 October 1773. Their child, Thomas Chittle, was baptised at St Mary's Church, Boxford, on 11 June 1791; he became a chemist and lived until 1867. Mary was buried at St Mary's Church, Boxford, on 20 June 1791, nine days after her son was baptised. She was aged 44.
2. William Prince, son of James and Leah Prince, was baptised at St James's Church, Leckhampstead, on 3 July 1791.
3. Savory records engaging their services on 23 March [247].
4. Leah Pointer was baptised at St Mary's Church, Chieveley, on 27 November 1774; and Martha, on 31 January 1768, the daughters of Thomas Pointer and his wife, Mary, née Deacon, who married at St James's Church, Leckhampstead, on 31 May 1764.
5. Benjamin Ford, a saddler, is listed in Newbury in the *UD*.
6. Jane Collins, distiller, is listed in Reading in the *UD*. Her premises were in Minster Street, Reading, but she gave up business in 1793.
7. This is Thomas Cowslade (1757-1806) who in 1785 commenced partnership with Anna Maria Smart (the widow of the ill-fated poet Christopher Smart who died in 1771, and daughter of William Carnan). Cowslade married Mrs Smart's daughter, Marianne. Mrs Smart was the businesswoman and Cowslade the printer of the *Reading Mercury*. When Mrs Smart died in 1809 the *Mercury* passed down the generations of the Cowslade family. They owned the paper until the start of the twentieth century. It ceased publication in 1987.

[*p. 257*] WmSavory [*sic*] returns his sincere thanks to his friends and the public for their past favours conferrd on him when residing at Brightwalton and assures them that no care nor attention shall be wanting on his part to render his endeavours satisfactory. [1]

Aug[us]t 24th. was the new bedstead & furniture put up in the best Room by Davies[.][2] Sept[embe]r 1st. was Young Cravens birth day[,] this present L[or]d Craven being 21 Years of Age[.] on this occasion was a great entertainment at the Mansion house.[3] 2nd. Webb furnished my dining Room.[4] 3rd. Bo[ugh]t a Licence of Danvers Greaves Curate at Chievely gave him £1.12s. 6d.[5] Bo[ugh]t a Ring of Thomson the Jeweller for 9/.[6] [*p. 258*] 5th. Bartholomew fair[.] at this time Bartholomew tradesmen & a few others keeps feast from one house to the other. 6th. was Greg's feast I could not go. the 8th I entered the altar of Hymen,[7] but as I entered into a new life I shall for such a memorandum enter into a new book,[8] and fill this Book with Genitures of the Prince of Wales, Jane the daughter of F & S Fordham, a figure sett at the time of the Kings Coronation &c.

*   *   *

---

1. The notice was duly published in the *Reading Mercury* (1, 8, 15 August 1791), see section xvi of the introduction.
2. Probably William Davis, upholsterer and cabinet-maker, listed in Newbury in the *UD*.
3. This is William Craven (1770-1825), the son of William Craven (see [154, 228]) and his wife, Elizabeth, née Berkeley (1750-1828). His parents separated in 1780. Young Craven would become the 7th Baron Craven (of Hampstead Marshall) on the death of his father on 26 September, less than a month after young Craven's 21st birthday. He was created 1st Earl of Craven in 1801. The mansion, built in 1774-1775 by the 6th Baron and designed by Henry Holland, was at Benham Park, Speen.
4. John Webb, upholsterer, cabinet-maker and auctioneer, is listed in Newbury in the *UD*.
5. Rev. Danvers *Graves* (1750-1805), curate of St Mary's Church, Chieveley.
6. For Thomson the jeweller, see also [145].
7. William Savory and Mary Tyrrell were married by licence at All Saints' Church, North Moreton, by curate William West Green, on 8 September 1791. The witnesses were Savory's brother-in-law Joseph Norris and Sarah Shepherd (probably the 'Miss Sheppard' referred to [50]). The *Reading Mercury* noted, 'Thursday last was married, Mr Savory, surgeon, of Newbury, to Miss Tyrrell, of North Moreton', *RM* (12 September 1791).
8. Peachey notes, 'Unfortunately the latter is not forthcoming': no further manuscript volumes by Savory have subsequently been traced: 'Savory's after history', Peachey concludes, 'has to be extracted from other sources', Peachey, *Life of William Savory*, 19: see the afterword.

[*p. 259*]

King Geo: 3rd
Crowned Sept 22nd
1761
3h 30' PM

{Moon} in {Cancer} in 7th signifies his Enemies in general to be victorious also in fear of his people {Saturn} {square} {Moon}.

    his parliament consisteth of very eloquent & learned Men as may be seen by {Mercury} in {Virgo}. {Jupiter} in {Pisces} in the 2nd declares him to be of an immense fortune &c.

[*p. 260*]

Geo: Prince of
Wales Born
Aug[u]st 12th 1762
7h 30' Morn

{Venus} Lady 2nd in Asc[endan]t weak. {Aries} in 2nd, {Saturn} L[or]d 5th & 6th in {opposition} to the 2nd declares our prince to be weak in substance, according to his dignity and by reason of things belonging to the 5'th 6th & 8th Houses as Gaming, Drinking, Women, Sickness, Servants & people under his Authority &c. {Jupiter} L[or]d 4 in {square} {Sun} &c. signifies he will not improve his partrimony & that he shall be little bettered [*p. 261*] thereby. the sign of the 7th a double bodied sign & {Jupiter} in {trine} to Asc[endant] denotes plurality of Wives providing he lives long enough. {Saturn} L[or]d 5th in 8th & 4th from the 5th in {Aries} denotes small Issue. {Mars} in {sextile} to {Venus}. {Venus} in Asc[endan]t & {Jupiter} & {Moon} casting a {trine} thereto declares him to be of a good disposition delighting in the Company of the female Sex. {Opposition} {Jupiter} & {Mars} denotes him ungratefull to his friends, a destroyer of his own substance & of a very mutable fortune &c.

*   *   *

[*p. 262*]

Jane the daught[e]r.
of F & S Fordham
Born: Mar 11. 1785,
5h 45' PM.

That the Child could not be of long Life is plainly seen by the above figures for we find {Sun} who has his exaltation in 8th is in {opposition} to Asc[endan]t & {Jupiter} L[or]d 4 in {opposition}[.] Likewise in {conjunction} with {Sun}. {Mercury} L[or]d Asc[endant] in the house of sickness. {Conjunction} {Saturn} & {Mars} are all testimonies of a short life.

*　　　*　　　*

[*p. 263*]
A few remarks on some of the Archbishops of Canterbury

The first Archbishop of Canterbury was St Augustine[.] he came into England in the year 596 & converted King Ethelbert & Queen Bertha & the King gave him the palace at Canterbury[.] he was succeeded by Laurentius, Melitus & Justus and from Justus we have no certain account till the year 673 when Theodore was Archbishop. this St Augustine bap[tize]d 10000 Saxons in one day. Theodore was succeeded by Berkwald, Tatwin, Nothelm, Cuthburt, Brethwin, [*p. 264*] Lambert, Athelard, Walfrid. this Walfrid was present at the Councill of Calchith in the year 824[.] from there I can find no account till the Year 900 when Phegmand was Archbishop of Canterbury. the reasan thereoff may be attributed to the Danes who put a stop to all Ecclesiastical Authority, destroying monastries &c with great fury as may be seen in the history of England. Phegmand was succeeded by Wulfhelm who died in the year 946 & was succeeded by Odo[.] this Odo was the 22nd Archbishop of Canterbury & was remarkable for his excommunicating Edwig K[in]g of England. [*p. 265*] Odo was succeeded by St Dunstan, that celebrated prelate. he reformed the English Clergy. he left the Court to embrace a monastic life. He expelld all the Clergy who would not condescend to embrace good manners. St Dunstan was succeeded by Ethelgar, Sigerick, Elferic & Alphage. this Alphage was a Monk and was murdered by the Danes in the year 1011 & was succeed[e]d by Levingus, Good Agelnoth, Eadsua, Rodbert, Stigand, Lanfrance & St Anselm who was a persecutor of the marriage Clergy, a great asserter of the popes rights[.] he wrote a number of Books & did many miracles[.] he was succeeded by Ralph, Corbeil, [*p. 266*] Theobald & Thos o Beckett who in 1161 was murdered by 4 Villains in his own Church[.] he was succeeded by Richard, Baldwin, Hubert, Stephen Langton, Richd le Grand, Edmand, Boniface, Rob[er]t Kilwarby, Rob[er]t de Winchelsey, Walter Reginold, Simon Nepham, John Stratford, Islip, Simon Sudbury, Wm Courtnay, Arundell, Henry Chicheley, Strafford, John Kemp, Thos Bourchier, Moreton, Henry Deane, Wm Wareham who was the last roman Catholic Archbishop of Canterbury who was succeeded by the 1st protestant in 1533 by Thos Crammer [*sic*], Cardinal Pole, Parfiar, Ed[war]d Grindall, John Whitgift, Abbot, Wm Laud, Juxon, Sheldon, Sancroft, Tillotson, Tanison, Wake, J[oh]n Potter, Thos Herring, Matt Hutton, Thos Secker & Thos Cornwalis the present Archbishop.[1]

---

1. Frederick Cornwallis (1713-1783) was Archbishop from 1768 until his death. Savory probably copied this account from an out-of-date source.

[*p. 267a*]

Contents

[*p. 268*]

---

1. The words '2 leaves cut out' have been pencilled in the margin in a different hand, possibly Peachey's or Rev. Howard's.

1. This page, and the one which follows it, was not numbered by Savory, see Editorial Note.
2. The page referred to is missing. It concludes [115].
3. The page referred to is missing.

Lottery Drawing _____ 199
Morris Dancing _____ 31
Mitchel Sam[ue]l died _____ 152
Nelston John _____ 56, 16
Norris Wm Savory born _____ 71
Observations on 1st person _____ 226

[*p. (271)*]
Potatoes 1st br[ough]t to brightwalton _____ 5
Pulv Sympathy _____ 232
Questions _____ 145
Ringers Brightwalton _____ 58
Savory　myself _____ 1
　　　　Grandfather to Father _____ 16
　　　　Uncle John　　30　　　Sisters　36 to　42
Songs _____ 12. 21. 32 44　38
Samson Dr _____ 48
Spirit to buy _____ 115
Scheme of Andrews Child _____ 130
Trulock Mrs_____ 108
Taylor a story _____ 148
Ung Mirabilis _____ 226
Verses _____ 8 _____ 129 _____ 141
Will made at Brightwalton _____ 49
Waters Dr _____ 118

*　　　*　　　*

Afterword

As William Savory makes note of his marriage, he draws his MS to a close with the promise that 'as I entered into a new life I shall for such a memorandum enter into a new book' [258]. No subsequent volumes have yet been traced so we must assume that they either did not get written or have been lost. 'Savory's after history', as George Peachey put it, 'has to be extracted from other sources'.[1] Although such sources are few and scattered, there is a significant body of material which helps us round off Savory's story.

We can only imagine how Savory and his wife Mary adjusted to married life in Newbury following their wedding on 8 September 1791. One thing we know Savory did was to embark on the creation of his commonplace book. On 13 October 1791, at a time when he was almost certainly writing it, he presumably attended the funeral of his niece, Rachel Norris, whom he had delivered six months earlier [248]. We know his household included a servant (Martha Pointer) [255] and a medical apprentice (John Jarvis) [248]. In the course of the next three years a son, William, and a daughter, Mary, were born to the Savorys. Their dates of birth are not known. If William Savory Jnr's age was correctly recorded at the time of his death, then he was born some time in the twelve months before 1 February 1793. Both children were baptised at a private ceremony in Newbury on 11 April 1795, and the process was repeated publicly at North Moreton at the end of the year, on 26 December.

The Bartholomew Street house, owned freehold, was described as a 'substantial, modern well built Dwelling House and Shop, with suitable and convenient offices, outbuildings, and garden walled in entire'.[2] It was elegantly furnished and comfortably stocked. It boasted

> bedsteads with mahogany and japann'd pillars, with dimity, Manchester and other furnitures, festoon window curtains to correspond; fine bordered and other feather beds, mattresses, and bedding; floor and bedside carpets; large painted floor cloth, pier and dressing glasses, mahogany dining and pembroke tables, and chairs, bureau, and bookcase with glass doors, an eight-day clock, general assortment of kitchen requisites, washing and brewing coppers, mash tub, coolers, wort pump, lead underback, upstand casks and barrels; bridle and saddle, hard wood, &c. a still fixed containing upwards of 20 gallons, &c. &c.[3]

In addition there was the 'Plate, Linen, China, [and] Books' that one might expect to find, plus an 'Electrifying Machine' and a 'capital Riding Horse'.

This suggests that Savory achieved a considerable measure of success and enjoyed the comfortable lifestyle of a young middle-class professional

---

1. G. C. Peachey, *The Life of William Savory, Surgeon, of Brightwalton (with Historical Notes)* (1903), 19.
2. *RM* (2 and 9 February 1795).
3. *RM* (22 February 1795).

surgeon-apothecary and man-midwife. On 9 April 1792 he concluded an agreement with the overseers of Newbury to superintend the medical care of the poor of the parish.[1] He also appears to have been paid by the overseers of Brightwalton to attend the poor there. The account books kept by the churchwardens record payments of £1 2s in 1792 and 4/6 in 1793.[2] Likewise, the overseers at Burghclere record in their ledger two payments made to Savory: one for £7 14s in March 1793, the other, an extraordinary disbursement, of £3 13s 6d in September 1794.[3] Such work was essential for a medical man. It conferred official recognition, guaranteed a regular income, and provided an opportunity to come into contact with potential private patients.

By 1794 Savory acquired a 'substantial new built Dwelling House, Offices and Premises, with about two acres of land adjoining, being copyhold of inheritance' just south of Newbury at Newtown Common, which he used as a smallpox inoculating-house.[4] Savory would have continued to practice variolation, a form of inoculation that involved injecting patients with a small amount of smallpox matter so that they would develop immunity after experiencing a mild form of the disease, safely isolated from the general population. Given that when he was a small child Savory had lost his own father to the disease, it is not difficult to appreciate his sense of mission in running his own inoculating house. In 1785 John Haygarth published his *Rules for Preventing the Smallpox* and they are worth quoting at length for the sense they give of the care and caution with which these early experiments in immunology were properly to be carried out.

1.   Suffer no person, who has not had the smallpox to come into the infection house. No visitor, who has any communication with persons liable to the distemper, should touch or sit down on anything infectious.

2.   No patient, after the pocks have appeared, must be suffered to go into the street, or other frequented place. Fresh air must be constantly admitted by doors and windows into the infected chamber.

3.   The utmost attention to cleanliness is absolutely necessary during and after the distemper, no person, clothes, food, furniture, dog, cat, money, medicine, or any other thing that is known or suspected to be bedaubed with matter, spittle, or other infectious discharges of the patient, should go or be carried out of the house till they be washed; and till they be sufficiently exposed to the fresh air. No foul linen, nor anything else that can retain the poison, should be folded up or put into drawers, boxes or be otherwise shut up from the air, but must be immediately thrown into water and kept there till washed. No attendant should touch what is to go into another family,

1. RBA D/P 89/J/2.
2. RBA D/P 24 5/1.
3. Hampshire Archives: 148M82/PO4: Burghclere parish overseers of the poor accounts, 1788-1801.
4. *RM* (2 and 9 February 1795).

till their hands are washed. When a patient dies of the smallpox, particular care should be taken that nothing infectious be taken out of the house so as to do mischief.

4.   The patient must not be allowed to approach any person liable to the disease, till every scab has dropt off; till all clothes, furniture, food and all other things touched by the patient during the distemper, till the floor of the sick chamber, and till the hair, face, and hands have been carefully washed. After everything has been made perfectly clean, the doors, windows, drawers, boxes, and all other places that can retain infectious air should be kept open, till it be cleared out of the house.[1]

We must hope that Savory was equally scrupulous in his approach.

On 28 April 1794 a boy from Newbury died 'at the inoculating-house', presumably Savory's. He was mistakenly buried at Burghclere instead of Newtown.[2] The burial register for Newtown itself shows that four out of seven deaths in the parish in 1794 were caused by smallpox: James Tyrrell (18 February), William Wilkins aged nine months (14 March), James Whale aged three (23 December), and Mary Whale aged eight months (28 December), and the first burial in the following year (but none thereafter) was likewise the result of smallpox: Thomas Whale aged seven (11 January 1795). Whilst there is no mention of an inoculating-house, it is certainly possible that these deaths were caused by variolation. If these events were connected with Savory and his inoculating-house – involving, as they did, the deaths of at least four children, three of them from the same family who tragically died in quick succession – it would have been unimaginably devastating for the parents who entrusted their children to Savory, especially John and Ruth Whale. This may in part explain how Savory's life came to be turned upside down by the start of 1795 when bankruptcy proceedings were set in motion against him. He must surely have been reminded of Mr Stanbrook, of whom he had noted on 27 January 1790, that he 'made his exit from Brightwaltham being very much in debt and the Auction was March the 1st of all his household Goods' [227].

The earliest notices of Savory's business failure, issued by Messrs Allen of Clifford's Inn, appeared on 2 January 1795. Savory was described merely as an apothecary, 'late of Newbury'.[3] The *Reading Mercury* directed him to appear before the Commission of Bankruptcy at the White Hart Inn, Newbury, on 14 January at 4pm, noon the following day, and at 10am on 14 February.[4] At the first of the three meetings Savory's creditors had to prove their debts; at the second Savory chose his assignees; at the third, he had to 'make a full discovery and disclosure of his estate and effects'. Anyone indebted to him was advised to contact Messrs Allen at Clifford's Inn, or Savory's attorney in Newbury, Mr G. W. Bulkley. Such appearances before

---

1. J. Haygarth, *Rules for Preventing the Smallpox* (1785), 118-120.
2. Letter to Stuart Eagles from Hampshire Record Office, dated 15 July 1997, ref. CAS/AS/GT.
3. E.g. *Chester Chronicle* (2 January 1795).
4. *RM* (5 January 1795).

the Commission must have been humiliating for the 26-year-old. Doubtless it put a considerable strain on his marriage. The financial uncertainty would have been enormously stressful. There was solace, though, in securing as assignees his uncle, John Savory, and George Whiting of Chaddleworth, probably a friend of his uncle's.[1] Savory refers to Whiting in his MS volume briefly on two occasions [157, 254].

Savory's properties and belongings were sold at three separate sessions at the White Hart Inn by the Newbury auctioneer, Benjamin Stroud.[2] The real estate was disposed of on Thursday, 19 February at 3pm, and his belongings at 10am on the following two days. Anyone who wished to view the premises had to apply to Mr Stroud, whilst particulars were available only from Mr Thompson of Wantage, solicitor to the assignees.[3] Catalogues giving details of the furniture and other personal possessions were made available from three different Bear Inns respectively at Reading, Wantage and Hungerford; the Swan Inn (one at East Ilsley and another at Kingsclere); Messrs Dickers at Woolhampton; the Marlborough Arms at Marlborough; and the auctioneers, at Newbury.

In April the *Reading Mercury* was still notifying anyone indebted to Savory to contact Samuel Slocock, Samuel Grigg, or Mr Bulkley at Newbury.[4] The final meeting of the Commission was advertised to take place at the White Hart at 11am on Monday, 21 September.[5] It was the last opportunity for any creditors to prove their debts and claim their dividend. Savory was described as an 'apothecary, dealer, and chapman'. It appears that the Certificate of Bankruptcy was issued on 28 September when Savory's creditors were invited to Mr Bulkley's office to collect a dividend of 6s 8d in the pound.[6] It is likely that Savory continued to work off his debts, however. Further dividends were paid out to proven creditors at the White Hart on Saturday, 24 September 1796 and Saturday, 13 May 1797.[7] There is evidence that a final Certificate of Bankruptcy was issued on 8 June 1799, suggesting that four-and-a-half years after the failure of his practice, his debts were finally cleared.[8]

It is likely that Savory had to let his apprentice go, or, more accurately, to let him down and, presumably, pass him into the hands of an alternative master. Happily, however, John Jarvis (1775-1867) did become a surgeon. He had moved to London by the second decade of the nineteenth century. He had at least three daughters and a son, Richard Taylor Jarvis, who became a solicitor. For many years John Jarvis was in practice in Hart Street, Bloomsbury Square. He lived to the age of 92.

---

1. *RM* (2 February 1795).
2. *RM* (2 February 1795).
3. This may be George Thompson, a witness to Savory's grandfather's will, proved at the PCC in 1786, TNA PCC PROB 11/1147/2.
4. *RM* (13 April 1795), notice dated 2 April.
5. *RM* (14 September 1795).
6. *RM* (28 September 1795).
7. *RM* (5 September 1796, 8 May 1797).
8. *Bath Chronicle and Weekly Gazette* (23 May 1799).

When Savory's paternal uncle, John, made his will on 7 August 1796, he gave no indication of feeling let down, though it must have been a strain to support his nephew through the bankruptcy. Savory was his principal heir and executor, but there were several legacies.[1] The main one was £10 per annum for life to his sister-in-law, Jane, Savory's mother, to be paid quarterly on 25 March, 24 June, 29 September and 25 December. In addition, there were one-off legacies of £10 each for his three nieces, Sarah Fordham, Jane Eagles and Mary Norris, and a further £10 apiece to each and every one of the children of his nieces and nephew, to be paid when they reached the age of 21. He bequeathed a further £10 to his niece, Jane Eagles, 'due to her on Ballance of a Bill' to be paid within three months of his decease. His sister-in-law would be given use of all plate, china, linen, bed and bedding, tables, chairs, and other household goods and furniture during her lifetime, and afterwards to be inherited by Savory. As we shall see, though, John Savory's sister-in-law, Savory's mother, predeceased him.

It is likely that Savory returned to Brightwalton after the forced sale of his Newbury and Newtown properties. Small payments to him are recorded in the churchwardens' accounts of the parish from 1800, presumably for medical attendance of the poor. By 1803 Brightwalton is given as his address in the registers of the re-named Royal College of Surgeons in London (later, of England), a body of which he automatically became a member by virtue of having been admitted into its less august predecessor, the Corporation or Company of Surgeons.

Savory's mother-in-law, Elizabeth Tyrrell, died at North Moreton, according to her gravestone, on 27 May 1799. She was buried 1 June. Savory's mother died at Brightwalton on 7 January 1802, at the age of 66, and was buried exactly one week later. Her gravestone does not appear to have survived, but the inscription is preserved in the file of miscellaneous records relating to the parish. It read, 'To the Memory of / Jane Savory / Who died 7th Jan 1802 / Aged 66 Years' and was followed by the verse:

Reposing here, beneath this verdant sod
I wait the summons of my Saviour God
Wait the dread hour when the holy trumpets blast
To [*illegible*] and dead proclaims "That time is past!"
Then shall my scattered dust again combine
The soul again its kindred body join,
Both shall appear before the Omniscient Eye,
The sentence here of bliss or misery
Then when the earth shall blaze from pole to pole
And Heaven's expanse "be gathered as a scroll"
May I, redeem'd from sin and from the grave
Hosanna shout to Him who died to save![2]

The quantity of lines here arguably outweighs the quality.

---

1. TNA PCC PROB 11/1460/1.
2. RBA D/EW/O8, 10-11.

William Tyrrell, Savory's father-in-law, died at North Moreton on 22 March 1803, and was buried five days later. He had made a will on 30 July 1801 appointing as his executors William Hazell of Sotwell, Gentleman, and William Toovey of Brightwell, whom he describes as his nephews.[1] He entrusted all his furniture and goods absolutely to them for the benefit of his daughter, Mary, Savory's wife. She should have full use and enjoyment of them until her son, William Savory Jnr, reached the age of 21, at which time such goods should be equally divided between mother and son and, on the mother's death, between Tyrrell's grandson and granddaughter, William and Mary Savory Jnr. Tyrrell bequeathed all his property in South and North Moreton, which included a malthouse, an orchard, garden and yard, severally occupied by Mary Bennett, Edward Inns and John Butcher, to his grandson, William Savory Jnr, who would also eventually inherit the Tyrrell family home in North Moreton, though his mother should live there during her lifetime 'if she think fit'. Tyrrell directed that within six months of his daughter's death, a legacy of £250 should be paid to his granddaughter, Mary Savory Jnr. But the most important clause in the will concerned his grandson, William Savory Jnr. Tyrrell desired that his estate should be used to fund his grandson's education. The will was duly proved in London by Hazell and Toovey on 9 August 1803.

John Savory, Savory's beloved bachelor uncle, died in Brightwalton on 7 December 1806, aged 79, and was buried on the 12th. His gravestone appears not to have survived, but the inscription has once again been recorded. 'To the Memory of / John Savory / Who died 7th Dec. 1806 / in the 80th year of his age' with the following verse:

> The present monument is all we can be
> sure of therefore let us
> study to improve it in preparing for
> death and judgment
> Awake thee, O my soul true wisdom learn
> Nor till to-morrow the great work adjourn.[2]

Savory apparently invested much of the money he inherited and earned from his professional activities to buy land and property. No doubt some of the land was used for the cultivation of plants, herbs, vegetables and fruit to supply ingredients for various medical distillations, compounds and mixtures. He rented three acres of land, called Long Ground, from Lord of the Manor, Bartholomew Wroughton, and he also seems to have owned land on Brightwalton's Holly Street. As a freeholder he had the right to vote, on 30 October 1816 he served on a jury, and a local census of Brightwalton conducted in 1821 states that he lived in a household of three women and three men, one of whom was a 'doctor's man', presumably an apprentice or assistant.[3]

---

1. TNA PCC PROB 11/1398/37.
2. RBA D/EW/O8, 11.
3. RBA D/EW/O8, 230.

Savory's sisters had relatively large families, and the lives of his nephews and nieces must in large part fall outside the scope of this afterword. Nevertheless, the Fordhams, the family of Savory's eldest sister, Sarah, merit particular attention, not least because of the lengthy period Savory spent living with them at the Flying Horse at Lambeth Street in Whitechapel when he was a student in the Borough in 1788-1789. Savory almost certainly made return visits to his sister and her family in Whitechapel in subsequent years. It would have been a convenient place to stay on trips to London for medical supplies, instruments and books. The Fordhams remained at the Flying Horse until at least February 1796 when Francis Fordham made an appearance at the Old Bailey at the second of two trials in which he gave evidence. Life in a public house in Whitechapel was rarely, if ever, dull. The first trial dates to 1 July 1795.[1] On the morning of Tuesday, 15 June 1795, during the period that Savory was dealing with the fall-out from his bankruptcy, Francis Fordham discovered that a cupboard had been broken open at the inn and that 960 copper halfpenny coins, wrapped up in papers and stored inside it, had been stolen. Fordham had been absent for most of the previous evening, but Sarah, who was on duty, pointed the finger of suspicion at John Martin, a 31-year-old journeyman sugar baker who had been drinking at the pub. He was suspected of concealing himself at the inn after closing-time in order to steal the money. Fordham tracked Martin down to the London Hospital. Martin had gone there for surgery on his leg. When he was confronted, the suspect denied the theft, but a law officer searched him and found a quantity of halfpenny coins in his pocket. A further 48 halfpenny coins wrapped in paper were found in his bedside cupboard. Seven additional papers of halfpennies were found with Mrs Ashton, the landlady of the London Hospital Public House, whom Martin had asked to look after them for him. The halfpenny coins had been wrapped up in five-shilling bundles by Fordham's brother, Thomas.[2] Thomas testified that he recognised the wrapping as his own. A device that might have been used to break open the cupboard at the inn was found in Martin's possession. Martin first claimed that the halfpenny coins found on him were the result of careful saving, that he had called in several debts from fellow sugar bakers, and that he had pawned some of his own belongings, including his watch, great coat, shirt 'and everything else' in order to pay for his medical care. However, one Francis Newham testified that Martin had in fact recently paid *him* a debt: five shillings in halfpenny coins wrapped in paper. Convicted of stealing 39 shillings'-worth of halfpenny coins, Martin was sentenced to transportation for seven years. The case is particularly relevant in the context of Savory's profession because it highlights the cost of medical care in this period and the lengths to which some people were prepared to go in order to pay for it, though it is clear that Martin took more than he strictly needed for that purpose.

In the course of giving his evidence, Francis Fordham made it clear that the Flying Horse was a busy place: 'we have different people that lodges in

---

1. See *Proceedings of the Old Bailey*, t17950701-26.
2. Another of Francis Fordham's brothers, Edward, became a victualler, and in the 1820s ran the Queen's Head, in Hoxton.

the house', he testified. When he stood witness in a second trial, on 17 February 1796, he was described as a 'headborough', a respected member of the community with some responsibility for policing. He would have been expected to report suspicious behaviour and criminal wrongdoing to a constable. That is precisely what he did in this case. He reported his suspicions to an officer at the nearest police-station which, like the Flying Horse, was on Lambeth Street.[1] The case involved Martha Dummert, the wife of John Daniel Dummert, the Anglicized name of a German immigrant who worked as a journeyman farrier. Mrs Dummert alleged that she was assaulted by James Riggs whom she also accused of stealing from her a box worth sixpence, with half a guinea and a shilling inside it which, by the law of the day, were the property of her husband. The theft was alleged to have occurred as she walked from her father's house in Little Prescot Street to her home in Gower's Walk. She claimed that Riggs had noticed her at a cheesemonger's shop on Red Lion Street. She refused his offer to carry her goods. He then assaulted her and robbed her at the end of the street on which she lived. The alleged victim and the accused were cross-examined fairly intensively. The defence attorney attempted to make much of a motto on the box which read, 'I love too well to kiss and tell'. Riggs was apprehended at the corner of Union Street and taken to the police-station where the case was put before Fordham who later found the box with the money still inside it. Riggs, who said he worked at the India Warehouse, and was also a warder, claimed that the woman deliberately brushed up against him and invited him 'to take liberties with her', a temptation he evidently did not resist, adding in implied mitigation that he 'kissed her afterwards'. He deliberately mentioned his wife and children in his testimony, underlining that he was a respectable married man and that this episode was an aberration. He maintained that Mrs Dummert had fitted him up after the assignation turned sour, and he accused Fordham and two members of the local Jewish community of joining in the alleged conspiracy against him. Riggs convinced the court of his good character and he was found not guilty. Whatever the merits of the case, it must have been a galling experience for Fordham and the two unnamed Jews for whom the benefit of any conspiracy is not obvious.

Perhaps this unhappy experience at the Old Bailey helps explain why the Fordhams had moved from the Flying Horse by the start of the new century.[2] Francis Fordham remained committed to innkeeping however. On 29 September 1797 he was admitted to the Freedom of the City of London as a member of the Company of Innholders.[3] The family's departure from the Flying Horse at least meant that they avoided an incident which occurred there during a storm in January 1802. When a hearse left the yard of the inn 'to receive the corpse of a Jew' in the neighbourhood, the winds became so strong that the horses and carriage were forced to the other side of the street. The pantiles were blown off part of the pub and stables, and the courtyard

---

1. See *Proceedings of the Old Bailey*, t17960217-23.
2. Land tax records suggest the Fordhams were in Aldgate High Street by 1800.
3. London Metropolitan Archives COL/CHD/FR/02, Freedom of the City Admission Papers.

gates were ripped apart.[1] One can only hope that when the hearse reached its destination the driver was not greeted by a householder telling him that the loved one had not, in fact, quite yet departed, something Fordham had experienced [127-128].

The Fordhams moved the short distance to the Turk's Head, a narrow four-storey public house at 71 Aldgate High Street. They were definitely there by June 1801 when Francis Fordham helped raise a subscription to those wounded, and the families of those killed, in the Battle of Copenhagen, under the command of Admiral Sir Hyde Parker (1739-1807) whose second-in-command was one Horatio Nelson.[2] In September 1802, the Fordhams were visited by Samuel Allsop, but he promptly 'dropped down dead, without a sigh'.[3] He had £60 on him which, it was reported, was duly 'delivered to his friends'. On 29 April 1805 'the family of Mr Fordham, of the Turk's head, Aldgate, were sitting at breakfast' when something highly irregular happened:

> they were alarmed by the descent of a young woman, belonging to an adjoining house, who broke through the sky-light into the breakfast-room. She received some injury by the glass cutting her, but we are happy to hear she is likely to do well.[4]

Perhaps Sarah Fordham had picked up some medical knowledge from her parents and brother and was able to offer first-aid?

Francis Fordham made a will on 21 June 1806, leaving his entire estate to his 'beloved Wife', Sarah. He was buried at St Mary's Church, Whitechapel, on 5 October 1806, just short of his 48th birthday. Probate of his will was granted to Sarah Fordham on 21 January 1807.[5] Sarah continued to run the pub after she was widowed. 'Mrs Fordham', of 'the Turk's Head, Aldgate High-street' provided a contact-point in the sale of the King's Arms, Fieldgate Street, Whitechapel in December 1807.[6] Mrs S. Fordham was also listed as the victualler at the Turk's in *Holden's Directory* for 1811. What happened to her after this is uncertain, but the burial at St Mary's Church, Whitechapel on 24 April 1837 of a Sarah Fordham, aged 80, recently resident in Clerkenwell, was probably her. The Turk's remained in business until at least the late 1880s.

To round off what might be said of the Fordhams it is worth taking a brief look at their son, John Savory Fordham (1788-1826), whom Savory records having inoculated with smallpox whilst training as a medical student in the first half of 1789 [203]. Savory Fordham had been baptised at St Mary's Church, Whitechapel, on 4 May 1788. He was therefore a baby when Savory

---

1. Quoted from the *European Magazine*: see
   <https://www.mernick.org.uk/thhol/miscellany04.html> (accessed 23 May 2023).
2. *Morning Post* (16 June 1801).
3. *OJ* (2 October 1802).
4. *Public Ledger and Daily Advertiser* (30 April 1805).
5. Consistory Court of London: Will of Francis Fordham, 'victualler of Aldgate High Street' (probate 21 January 1807).
6. *Morning Advertiser* (10 December 1807).

was living with the family. He was apprenticed to the vintner, Robert Joel Hilton, on 1 December 1802. Hilton died before the apprenticeship was completed so Savory Fordham was transferred to a new master, William Bellingham. On 6 December 1809 he was admitted a member of the Worshipful Company of Vintners. On 7 August 1813, Savory Fordham married Elizabeth Moore at St Olave's Church, Southwark (a church surely familiar to Savory from his days as a medical student). The couple had at least two children, Francis and Mary. Savory Fordham ran the tavern at Bull's Head Passage, in the parish of Allhallows, Lombard Street, where his sister-in-law, a spinster, and his widow appear to have continued as landladies after his death. The tavern had been a butcher's shop in the eighteenth century, and the passage had free-standing stalls much like nearby Leadenhall Market. In recent years, the entrance to the passage, beneath the famous Lloyd's Building, was used to represent The Leaky Cauldron in the 2001 film, *Harry Potter and the Philosopher's Stone*. Savory Fordham died aged 38 and was buried at St Mary's Church, Whitechapel, on 5 November 1826. He had made a will on 10 October, witnessed by his sister-in-law Mary Anne Moore and his cousin, William Savory Jnr, in which he bequeathed the tavern to his wife.[1] Intriguingly, he writes in his will, 'I should wish to be preserved my mothers portrait' which he bequeathed to his son Francis 'as a sincere token of my regard'. A portrait of Savory's sister, Sarah, might therefore have survived, but has not been traced. Mention is made of Savory Fordham's private method of transportation: his horse, chaise and harness. He desired that his children should be 'brought up and instructed in the Protestant Church' and become 'valuable members of society', and begged them, 'do not undertake to support any part of your family' except for his sister-in-law, Mary Ann Moore, 'who I hope you will provide for as long as you have the power'. He acknowledged a debt of £15 to his sister and £2 to his wife's brother, loans which, in light of his advice to his children, we might presume he regretted. Probate was granted on 21 May 1827.

On Monday, 16 August 1819 a crowd of around 60,000 people gathered in St Peter's Field, Manchester, to demand electoral reform, specifically the extension of the franchise to (non-propertied) working men. When the cavalry charged, hundreds of people were injured, and at least 18 were killed. It was a scandal that would be known as the Peterloo Massacre. As a freeholder, who already had the right to vote, Savory was not untypical of his class in standing behind King and Country and those people and groups that defended the rights of property. On 31 October a long list of Berkshire freeholders felt it their 'bounden duty to declare [their] sentiments [...] on the subject of the late occurrences'.[2] They declaimed their 'firm and unalterable attachment to the King and the Constitution of our country, as by law established, and all those invaluable rights and privileges which that Constitution has been formed to secure to us and our posterity'. Whilst they conceded that they 'most sincerely deplore[d] the unhappy events which [had] recently taken place at Manchester' they nevertheless insisted that it

---

1. TNA PCC PROB 11/1725/362.
2. *Windsor and Eton Express* (31 October 1819).

would be unjust to make any judgements about it before the 'legal investigation' was considered by a Jury, which they parenthetically but pointedly described as 'that great bulwark of English liberty', without acknowledging that it was composed of men conveniently just like themselves. The thrust of their opinion was made plain when they asserted that it was that jury which would decide whether 'those who are now so loudly accused by a portion of the community, of being the authors of these calamitous events, have or have not violated the laws of the country'. Those in Brightwalton who joined Savory in signing this letter were Joseph Jennaway, William Taylor, Joseph Mitchell, Thomas Landfear of Woolley, and in the neighbouring parish of Farnborough, farmers James Kingham and John Reeves. Whilst campaigning journalists and others were later jailed for their role in the terrible events in Manchester, a civil case against four members of the yeomanry ended in their acquittal.

Although Savory remained an Anglican, there is evidence that his religious beliefs shared much in common with his methodist brothers-in-law, John Eagles and Joseph Norris. When Stephen Britannicus Mathews (1790-1868), the curate of Stone in Buckinghamshire, published his *Sermons intended to explain and enforce some of the Leading Truths of the Gospels* in 1821, there were several subscribers from Brightwalton, including John Trumplet, William Whiter, John Eagles, Joseph Norris and Savory.

John Eagles forged a successful career as a carpenter and builder. His son, John Savory Eagles (1788-1866), who became a successful carpenter and builder himself, was probably apprenticed to him informally, but in 1800 Eagles also took on another local boy, William Church, aged 14 (the typical age at which to begin an apprenticeship).[1] John Eagles and his wife Jane (Savory's sister), whose first son William Savory Eagles had died of measles in infancy [141], went on to have three more children besides John Savory Eagles: Sarah, Silas, and Esther. Sarah Eagles (1791-1843) did not marry until 1841 when she was 49. She was wed at Brightwalton to a farmer from Speen, John Goddard, the son of another farmer, also John Goddard. Silas Eagles (1795-1848) followed his father and elder brother in undertaking carpentry work, but for most of his life he was a baker and shopkeeper. He married Amy Kingham (1801-1842), the eldest daughter of James and Sarah Kingham who ran Lower Farm, Farnborough.[2] We shall meet Esther Eagles later. John Eagles died, aged 63, on 11 April 1822, and was buried at All Saints' Church, Brightwalton, four days later. His gravestone has survived and reads 'Sacred / To the Memory of / JOHN EAGLES / who departed this Life / April the 11th 1822 / Aged 63 Years / Long didst thou drink of deep afflictions cup / But sweet divine were with the bitters had / It was blessed Religion bore my spirit up / And gave these comforts on a dying bed' and below it is one line, 'Blessed are the dead which die in the Lord'.[3]

Eagles's death in 1822 was just one in a series of bereavements to hit the Savory family around this time. Savory's nephew, William Savory Norris

---

1. RAI (30 November 1800).
2. For Savory's reference to James Kingham, see [246].
3. The verse is a variation on Psalm 73.

(1784-1821), died on 23 July 1821 aged 37 and was buried in Brightwalton three days later: in Savory's geniture horoscope, he notes that the 'general testimonies that declare the shortness of this Natives Life are many' [136]. Savory Norris had five siblings: the second-born, and the last, Miriam and Caleb, will feature later. The third-born, Rachel, whom Savory delivered into the world, died in infancy [248, 251]. The fourth child, Joseph Norris (1800-1866), became a smallholder and land surveyor and lived in Leckhampstead with his wife, Hannah (1792-1862). The fifth-born, Keturah (1805-1890), had two children with her husband, George Palmer (c.1801-1876), who worked variously as a farmer, grocer and baker. Of the other deaths around this time: Savory's sister, Mary Norris (1765-1822), died aged 57 on 16 November 1822 and was buried six days later. Mary's widowed husband, Joseph Norris, died on 19 March 1825 and was buried on the 27th. The *Berkshire Chronicle* described him as 'an old and respected inhabitant of Brightwalton'.[1] Their headstones, which bear simple inscriptions and are side-by-side, have survived.

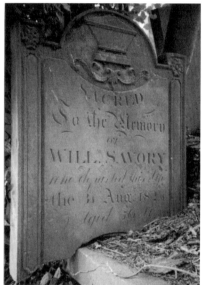

7. William Savory's headstone in the old churchyard of All Saints' Church, Brightwalton.
Photo: Stuart Eagles.

William Savory died on 31 August 1824. He was only 56 years old and left no will. Given this fact, and although we do not know his cause of death, it is fair to speculate that the end came suddenly. His widow, Mary, formally relinquished her right to file for letters of administration, in favour of the couple's son. William Savory Jnr called upon his cousin, John Savory Eagles, and his uncle, Joseph Norris, both Brightwalton free holders, to witness his application for letters of administration. The modest value of Savory's estate was estimated at under £600.[2] He was buried on 4 September in a grave alongside members of his wider family in a corner of Brightwalton's churchyard, and a simple headstone was dedicated 'SACRED / To the Memory / of / WILLM. SAVORY / who departed this Life / the 31st Aug. 1824 / Aged 56 Y[ears]'. No verse is visible. His widow lived a further 20 years. She died, aged 79, on 25 December 1844, and was buried on the 30th next to her husband, and a headstone in the same style was erected, still extant.

1. *BC* (9 April 1825).
2. RBA D/A1/237/149.

In his mother's lifetime, William Savory Jnr had married a distant relative. His father's maternal cousin, Miriam Barratt (1791-1869) had married Thomas Langford (1786-1857) in 1818, and Savory Jnr married Thomas's paternal cousin, Martha Langford (1799-1863). The wedding took place at All Saints' Church, Farnborough, on 1 June 1826. Martha was the daughter of the wealthy farmer of Great Shefford Manor, John Langford (1756-1821) and his wife, Mary, née Seymour (1762-1802), though both of them, like Savory Snr, were deceased by the time of Martha's marriage to Savory Jnr. Martha, in common with her other spinster sisters, had inherited £1,200 on her father's death in 1821 (those sisters who were already married were given the legacy minus the value of their marriage settlement).[1] William and Martha Savory would have only one child, a son, also christened William, the sixth generation of Williams born to the family. He was baptised at Brightwalton on 4 November 1828.

Savory Jnr followed in his father's footsteps and joined the medical profession. It is highly probable that he was informally apprenticed to his father whose notebooks and store of experience would in any case have benefitted him greatly. As he grew up he surely observed at least some of the medical cases attended by his father. He enrolled as a pupil of the eminent surgeon, Richard Clement Headington (1774-1831) at the London Hospital in Whitechapel. He was admitted on 22 October 1811 for a period of six months and was granted his certificate on 5 May 1812, two days short of exactly 23 years after his father was examined at Surgeons' Hall. Perhaps, during his studies, he stayed with his widowed aunt at the Turk's Head on Aldgate High Street.

Richard Headington and his brother, William, followed their father to train as surgeons. They were brought up in Spitalfields, and their father, William Clement Headington, was an active Governor of London Hospital. Richard Headington became a member of the Corporation of Surgeons in 1795. He was elected assistant surgeon at the London Hospital in 1797, and full surgeon in 1799. He was an active lecturer from at least 1804, and was an able surgeon. From 1805 he was Surgeon to the London Dispensary. In the 1820s he was criticised by colleagues on account of his view that coroners should not require professional qualifications. Thirty-eight of Headington's pupils, though disagreeing with his opinion, nevertheless praised 'the worthy surgeon' and expressed their 'pride in being under the tuition of such a master'.[2] When Headington died in 1831 he was President of the Royal College of Surgeons. The surgeon and medical author Samuel Cooper (1780-1848), speaking at the end of his Hunterian Oration in 1832, said of Headington, 'I regard him as one, whose merit as a lecturer, as an examiner, as a practical surgeon – and as a character adorned with the nicest sense of honour, will fully apologise for me having mentioned his name in this Address, composed in praise of the greatest man that ever adorned the medical profession'.[3]

---

1. WSA P1/1821/14.
2. *The Lancet, 1830-1* (2 vols, 1831) 95-96 (from the issue dated 9 October 1830).
3. Quoted in *London Hospital Gazette*, 17 (1992), 32-34, specifically 34.

Savory Jnr thus fully earned his professional membership of the Royal College of Surgeons according to the requirements of the day. In fact, he exceeded them, because before the passing of the Apothecaries' Act in 1815, these requirements were few and modest. In practice, he probably remained professionally in his father's shadow for as long as the senior practitioner was capable of working. Indeed, he seems to have led a quiet professional life, at least initially. Leaving aside his entries in the *Medical Register*, the first notable reference to Savory Jnr's career as a professional medical practitioner dates to 1835. The source is the meticulous record of medical provision organised under the Poor Law as amended the previous year. In *Early Medical Services: Berkshire and South Oxfordshire From 1740*, Margaret Railton noted that

> [d]uring the first few months [of Poor Law medical relief] problems arose with the organisation of medical attendance. In some instances Mr Robinson [of the Newbury Union] would visit a patient only to find another practitioner already there. He was advised that when this happened he should suspend his attendance except in 'peculiar circumstances'. When he was called to visit Elizabeth Stanbrooke at Leckhampstead in October 1835 and found Mr Savory [later of the Wantage Union] already there, the Guardians decided to notify the parishes that in cases of sudden and urgent necessity they might call the nearest practitioner. [...] No payment would be made for attendance in these circumstances for a period of longer than 24 hours.[1]

Devon-born Richard Rodd Robinson (1792-1883), who lived in Speen, had been a Member of the Royal College of Surgeons since 1810. He was appointed Medical Officer for all three districts of the Newbury Union on a salary of £385 *per annum*. Savory Jnr was not a poor law medical officer at the time of this incident in 1835. His tender for the second division of the Wantage Union was accepted on 6 March 1838. His terms were £36 plus 10/6 per case of midwifery. In 1840 his annual retainer was increased to £40. The division included Brightwalton, Peasemore, Chaddleworth, Fawley, Farnborough and Catmore.[2]

In March 1841, all five of the local medical officers – the others were William Barker, William Hewert, William Brathwayt and John Woodroffe Workman – petitioned the chairman and guardians of the Poor Law Union to abolish the annual tender and election, and thereby put their appointment on an equal footing with the clerk, relieving officer and other officials. They should, the medics contended, remain in office as long as they performed their duties to the guardians' satisfaction. Their submission was rejected

---

1. M. Railton, *Early Medical Services: Berkshire and South Oxfordshire from 1740* (Cranbrook, 1994), 59.
2. This information, and details subsequently given of Savory Jnr's contribution to medical relief under the Poor Law in Berkshire are derived from RBA G/WT/1/1-5 (Guardians' Records, Minutes, Wantage Union). For a history of the Wantage Poor Law Union, see H. Brown, *Gallon Loaves and Fustian Frocks: The Wantage Union and Workhouse, 1835-1900* (2008).

unanimously by the Board. A year later, however, on 8 March 1842, the plea was accepted on the recommendation of the Poor Law Commissioners. Savory Jnr was duly reappointed on this ongoing basis and on the same terms as before. He was also paid 1/6 for every successful case of vaccination he performed in his capacity as the division's Public Vaccinator. This was in line with the general Medical Order issued by the Poor Law Guardians.

The Public Vaccinator came into being as a result of the Vaccination Extension Act of 1840. The medical officers were responsible for encouraging their patients to be vaccinated for smallpox, but many patients resisted. In 1840, Savory was paid 17 guineas for his vaccination work, implying that 238 patients were persuaded to submit to the procedure. Voluntary vaccination of the poor represented a risk to public health where take-up was low, and such a highly communicable and deadly disease as smallpox could quickly threaten the whole community, including the better off. The controversial Vaccination Act of 1853 made compulsory the vaccination of babies under three months old, and authorised the sanctioning of parents with punitive fines for failure to comply. By the 1860s two-thirds of babies were vaccinated and the disease was becoming markedly less prevalent.

Compulsory vaccination, however, came too late in Savory Jnr's career. Although he officially continued to work as the divisional medical officer until his death in January 1854, he was unwell and unable to perform some of his duties during 1853. Nevertheless, his voluntary vaccination figures overall were respectable if rather erratic, but for the most part they remained above 100 patients a year. His annual retainer as medical officer was paid in quarterly sums of £10 from 1844, and he was paid additional fees for extraordinary cases. In March 1850, however, with expenses mounting, it was proposed that medical officers' pay should be cut. It was recommended that Savory Jnr's annual salary should be slashed by a quarter to £30. It was noted that he was responsible for a population of 1,756. Even after the reduction in pay, he would be the second best-paid *per capita*. On the other hand, in the area he covered, the households were somewhat more widely dispersed, yet the general health of his division was assessed to be above the average. In the event, the proposal was rejected, and the medical officers continued on the terms formerly agreed. The minutes of the Board of Guardians give details of medical cases which fell outside the parameters of the care for which the medical officer was contracted. Such cases, which necessarily merited additional payment, typically involved complicated fractures or prolonged and/or difficult labours which sometimes involved post-natal complications such as puerperal fever. Occasionally, as Railton noted, an extra payment was made because a patient had been attended who lived outside the boundaries of the division. In Savory Jnr's case, such incidents most often involved residents of Leckhampstead. Poor health evidently slowed Savory Jnr down considerably in the final months of 1853, and it was noted that he had not returned his vaccination books. On 7 February 1854, his death was recorded by the Board of Guardians and regret was expressed at his loss. Richard Rodd Robinson temporarily stepped in to take care of Savory Jnr's patients, before his successor, Bristolian surgeon, John Mills Probyn (1795-1867), was appointed later in the year.

Local newspapers provide some insight into the more extraordinary cases that faced Savory Jnr as a private medical practitioner on the Berkshire Downs in the 1840s and 50s. On Wednesday, 11 May 1842, for instance, an inquest was held at Leckhampstead Thicket on the body of six-year-old Charlotte Wakefield. Savory Jnr's 'prompt attendance and care' was commended, but the girl nevertheless died as a result of severe burns. The inquest heard that 'the mother left home on Monday morning to work in the fields, first putting out the fire; soon after the deceased's little brother rekindled the fire and the child's clothes igniting she was so dreadfully brunt that the poor creature expired after a few hours intense suffering'. A verdict of accidental death was passed.[1]

Another inquest, this time held in North Fawley on 20 January 1847, investigated the death of Ann Prince. Aged about 40, she was prone to epileptic fits. One day a neighbour, Charles Edlin, a middle-aged woodman and grocer, spotted 'smoke issuing from her doorway'. Edlin ran in and found the woman insensible on the floor with her clothing on fire. Although he 'immediately extinguished the flames', Prince's clothes were so badly burnt that they disintegrated and it was clear that the woman's body was extensively burnt. George Stone, the farmer of 1,200 acres in the parish, 'immediately sent his man for Mr Savory' while Stone's wife, Martha, 'with her usual kindness, employed two women to wait upon' the victim of the fire who sadly died shortly after the accident.[2]

Occasionally Savory Jnr was called in to give a medical opinion *post-mortem*. Thomas Crane, who worked as a bird-keeper on Whatcombe Farm at Fawley, was found by the farmer, Mr Turrell, in the early hours of a morning in August 1852 'lying on his back in a wheat field, with his gun by his side, and a large flat stone on his breast'. He was clearly dead. There was a wound near his eye and pieces of lead in his pocket. In Savory Jnr's opinion, the lad had died from 'a gun-shot wound commencing under the eye and terminating at the back of the ear. He had not been able to discover any substance in the wound'. The jury returned a verdict of 'Accidental Death'.[3]

A report that appeared under the title, 'A Melancholy Affair' in the *Berkshire Chronicle* in January 1853 concerned the fate of 31-year-old Louisa Langford, the eldest daughter of John Langford (1797-1876) of Great Shefford Manor, and his wife, Naomi. William Savory refers to John's uncle, Thomas Langford (1758-1851) and his second marriage, to Mary Mitchell (1761-1846), in a diary entry for 1782 [58]. In attending to Louisa Langford, Savory Jnr was in fact rushing to the aid of his wife's niece. Louisa was at the home of another of her uncles, William Froome (husband of Savory Jnr's sister-in-law, Hannah), in Little or South Fawley, where she spent an entertaining evening with friends. Although she joined in the dancing, it was not, the paper reported, 'to such an extent as to cause unusual fatigue or

1. *RM* (14 May 1842).
2. *RM* (23 January 1847).
3. *Oxford Chronicle and Reading Gazette* (28 August 1852).

excitement' and she appeared to be 'in her usual health and spirits'. However, at about two o'clock the following morning she suddenly became ill and complained of 'sickness and oppression of the chest'. Savory Jnr was 'immediately sent for', and whilst 'everything was done for her that medical skill could devise', by seven or eight o'clock that morning she was, in the newspaper's indelicate words, 'a corpse'. 'The awful and sudden affair has plunged the bereaved parents into deep grief', it was reported. It went on: 'their feelings may be more easily imagined than described'. Moreover, it had 'thrown a gloom over a wide circle of friends, by whom, from her urbanity and liveliness of disposition, she was deservedly be loved [*sic*] and respected'. The report concluded: 'There can be little doubt that so rapid a termination of life was the result of deep-seated disease of some standing'.[1] She is remembered today on a panel of her parents' box tomb in the churchyard at Great Shefford. The inscription concludes by quoting Mark 13:35-37, which underlines the suddenness of her death: 'Watch ye therefore: for ye know not when the master of the house cometh, at even, or at midnight, or at the cockcrowing, or in the morning: lest coming suddenly he find you sleeping.'

Savory Jnr was presumably responsible for introducing his aunt, Jane Eagles, to the Vegetable Universal Medicines of the British College of Health based on New Road in King's Cross. An advert in the *Berkshire Chronicle* shared 'a few of the many cases of cures obtained by the use of Morison's Pills'.[2] Among them was 'J. Eagles' of Brightwalton. The advertisement claimed that 'by taking two boxes at 2s. 9d. each, with a box of powders, according to the directions' she 'had her leg, which had several wounds in it, entirely healed in a fortnight, and her health much improved after suffering for three months'. Although she 'had the best advice' – not least from Savory Jnr himself – she obtained 'no relief until using the Universal Medicines'. Although she is only identified by an initial, she was the only female J. Eagles in Brightwalton at this time, and given that she was then aged 72, the problem with her leg is understandable. Perhaps the combination of her nephew's medical care, and her faith in these more or less harmless but pharmaceutically dubious medicines, helped her to live just over a fortnight past her 81st birthday.

The 1841 census shows her living on Brightwalton's Upper Street with the family of her youngest daughter, Esther (1803-1886) and her husband, Richard Green (1792-1881), a farm bailiff. She died on 25 October 1841. Her death was registered by her daughter-in-law, Mary Eagles, the wife of John Savory Eagles, and the cause of death was given as simple 'debility', i.e. old age. The *Reading Mercury* printed a notice of her death, in which she was described as the 'relict of Mr John Eagles, builder'; she was 'universally beloved and deeply lamented by her relations and friends'.[3] She had made her will on 19 March 1828 in which she bequeathed legacies of £100 to her

---

1. *BC* (29 January 1853).
2. *BC* (25 May 1833).
3. *RM* (13 November 1841).

children Sarah, Silas and Esther, to be paid within a month of her decease.[1] The executor, her eldest surviving son John Savory Eagles, inherited the remainder of her estate. The will was witnessed by Eliza Wicks and Jane's nephew, Caleb Norris. It was proved in London on 23 February 1842 by John Savory Eagles. Jane was buried in Brightwalton's churchyard on 30 October and her gravestone survives. It reads: 'Sacred / To the memory of / JANE, Wife of / JOHN EAGLES / who died Octr 25th 1841 / Aged 81 Years / Farewell conflicting hopes and fears / where lights and shades alternate dwell / How Bright and unchanging morn appears / Farewell inconstant world Farewell'.

Practically nothing can be said of William Savory's daughter, in stark contrast to the son. She did not marry until she reached middle age. Her father was long dead, but her mother was still alive. She married a younger man, William Henry Mitchell (1811-1879), who was in his late twenties and worked as a farmer. He was the son of Joseph Mitchell (d. 1845), a baker in Brightwalton, and his wife, Phoebe. The wedding took place at Brightwalton on 28 February 1838 and was witnessed by Thomas Whiter, Louisa Mitchell and Mary's cousin, Sarah Eagles. According to her brother's will, she was still alive in 1854 but it is unclear what happened to her. Her widowed husband died in Inkpen in 1879.

Savory Jnr invested his various inheritances and the money he made professionally in land and farming. In February 1841 he attended the AGM of the Daley General Association for the Protection of Property which met at the Swan in East Ilsley.[2] A report on the Newbury Agricultural Society and Fat Cattle Show in December 1843 noted that John Brown of Compton had reared 175 lambs from 410 ewes, with 112 twins (of which only one ewe died), a feat achieved on behalf of William Savory, of Brightwalton.[3] Savory Jnr's will, made on 30 January 1854, the day before he succumbed to bronchitis, enumerates some of the land and property he purchased.[4] This included a property in the possession of Mr Beeston, land in Upper Street in his own occupation, a cottage in the occupation of John Parrot, 14 acres of land called the Breaches, four acres of land called Yew Tree Field with its 'rickyard, barn, stable and appurtenances', all bequeathed to his wife, Martha, provided she pay £7 to his sister, Mary Mitchell, at Christmas and Midsummer. Six months after Martha's death, £175 should be paid to the couple's son, William. who would inherit all the land and property on his mother's death. William was bequeathed Folly Farm, and Row Down Bank situated between Brightwalton and Peasemore. William would also inherit a property on Pudding Lane in the occupation of shoemaker, John Lovell, plus an acre of land in Pudding Lane in his father's occupation. His executors were his wife, his cousin Joseph Norris, and his friend John Webb Ward, of Wyfield Farm, Boxford.

1. TNA PCC PROB 11/1957/335.
2. *BC* (6 February 1841).
3. *BC* (9 December 1843).
4. RBA D/A1/163/81. Some details have been added from particulars of an auction given in the *RM* (11 September 1863).

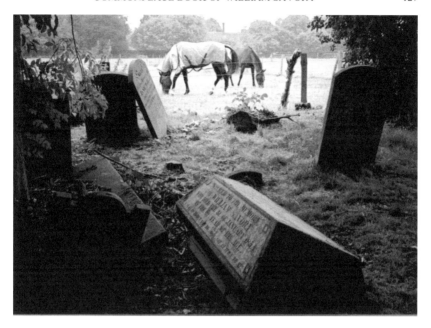

8. Graves of the interrelated Savory, Eagles and Norris families in the old churchyard of All Saints' Church, in Brightwalton. Savory Jnr's gravestone is the raised horizontal stone in the centre of the foreground. Photo: Stuart Eagles.

Savory Jnr died on 31 January 1854 and was buried near his parents, uncles and aunts, in the corner of Brightwalton's churchyard, on 6 February. A diagonally sloping coffin-style horizontal stone was erected, bearing a verse which reads: 'I shall go to him but he shall not return to me'. Martha made an agreement with her husband's successor as Brightwalton's medical officer, Henry A. Duncan, to lease to him the surgery and premises and sell him the stock of drugs and utensils, payments being made in instalments until 13 April 1857.[1] Described by George Peachey as 'a ship's doctor', Duncan had left the village by 1860.[2] The widowed Martha Savory and her son William farmed the 70 acres of Lime Tree Farm on Holt Lane until Martha's death on 25 May 1863 aged 64. She was buried with her husband, and a line inscribed for her on their shared gravestone reads simply, 'Blessed are the Dead who Die in the Lord'.

The early life of the last William Savory (1828-1870) in the family line can only be surmised. He was in his mid-20s when his father died, and his childhood and youth were doubtless in large part shaped by his father's work as a medical practitioner. Perhaps he became interested in his father's landholdings and farming interests early on. In 1864 he married his second

1. RBA D/EW/E25/2/34 (Wroughton, Norris and Tipping Papers, Estate Papers).
2. Peachey, *Life of William Savory*, 20.

cousin, Elizabeth Jane Goddard (1826-1891). Elizabeth was the daughter of Joseph and Mary Norris's second child, Miriam (1788-1848) who married farmer Stephen Goddard (1797-1882) at Brightwalton in 1821. The Goddards had four children, Elizabeth Jane, who married the last William Savory, being the second-born. Elizabeth inherited a moiety (a half-share) in the estate of her unmarried and wealthy uncle, Caleb Norris (1807-1855), a surveyor. From at least 1841 Norris lived in London at 10 Lancaster Place, off The Strand. His financial interests appear to have been many and varied. They included the Metropolitan Water Company and, from 1845, he held a managing directorship of the Exeter, Dorchester and Weymouth Railway Company and the Windsor, Slough and Staines Railway Company.[1] When he made his will on 13 October 1855, he bequeathed his entire estate equally to his niece, Elizabeth Jane Goddard, and his nephew James Norris during his lifetime (and thereafter to the remainder of Caleb's nephews and nieces, Elizabeth excluded).[2] Elizabeth Jane's life with Savory was unconventional. Although the couple married in 1864, Elizabeth had given birth to a baby daughter on 23 May 1856. Named Mary Ella Goddard (1856-1941), but known as Ella, the child was recorded on the 1861 census living with her mother and maternal grandparents at Brightwalton Holt Common.

The last William Savory did not follow his father and grandfather into the medical profession and instead managed the family's properties. Following his mother's death in 1863, he sold all the properties at auction. Messrs Alex. Davis & Thos. Palmer sold the freehold land and properties in nine lots at the Pelican Hotel at 3pm on 2 October.[3] Some land might have been acquired in the nine years since William Savory Jnr's death, but the lots mostly tally with what the son inherited on his mother's death. In summary, it included three dwellings, four lots of arable land, and building land with a barn, stable and other features. More specifically, there were parcels of arable land bounding the Woolley Park Estate: more than 13 acres to the north-west, just over four acres to the south-east and (in the same direction) 'building land, with front yard and orchard, excellent pond of water, with a brick, boarded, and thatched barn, stable for four horses, cow house, and a newly erected brick, boarded, and slate cart shed, containing together about one acre, more or less, near to the New Church'; also near the new Church, and near the road leading from Brightwalton to Farnborough, a 'modern built freehold brick and tile gentlemanly residence comprising dining and drawing room, five bed rooms, man servant's room, kitchen, pantry, brewhouse, knife house, larder, cellar, coachhouse, cart shed, stable for two horses, with brick and thatched gardener's cottage, court yard, fruit and back pleasure garden, excellent kitchen garden, orchard well stocked with fruit trees' (almost certainly the Lawns, the home and surgery his father is understood to have built) with more than two acres of arable land attached, then all in the occupation of Mr Ward; another acre or so of land in Pudding Lane, also in Ward's occupation, and bounded by the footpath from the Green; a 'very comfortable freehold

1. *Windsor and Eton Express* (26 September 1846).
2. TNA PCC PROB 11/2221/109.
3. *RM* (19 September 1863).

brick and thatched cottage, containing two bed rooms, attic, sitting rooms, pantry, brick and slate brewhouse, capital garden, well of water, in the occupation of Mrs Hatt'; and a 'brick, thatched, and slate dwelling house [...] containing four bed rooms, sitting room, kitchen, shoemaker's shop, and pantry' set in four acres of land and surrounded by hedges, and then in the occupation of John Lovell; and Row Down Bank, which straddled the parishes of Brightwalton and Peasemore, and was an area of more than an acre of rich arable land bounded on the west by the Newbury to Wantage road, and on the north by land in the ownership of the Marquis of Devonshire. It is worth pausing to note the mention of 'the new Church'. This was completed in 1863, designed in the style of the Gothic Revival by G. E. Street, then resident in Wantage. It was located in sight of the small Saxon church known to Savory, his son and his forebears, which had been located 200 yards to the north-east: it was demolished, but the site and its churchyard have been preserved to this day.

The last of the William Savorys served as an overseer of the poor in 1855-1856 and 1864-1865. He regularly attended the annual vestry meetings at Brightwalton from 26 March 1855, when records began, to 23 March 1866.[1] It was probably at this point, with his land and properties in Brightwalton all sold, and having recently married, that he moved to Shaw Crescent, Speen. It was at Shaw Crescent that he died on 19 November 1870. A notice in the *Reading Mercury* recorded that he had died 'after a long and painful illness, in the 43rd year of his age' and stated that 'Mr William Savory (son of the late Dr Savory, of Brightwaltham)' was 'much beloved and deeply lamented by his family and friends'.[2] He left an estate valued at £3,000. Elizabeth and Ella lived on in the house in Shaw Crescent, maintained by annuities Savory had provided for them.

Ella does not appear to have taken on Savory's name officially, except in the 1871 and 1881 censuses. He was almost certainly her father, however. By 1881 Ella and her widowed mother were living in Leckhampstead with Elizabeth's 84-year-old father and Ella's unmarried maternal aunt, Mary Goddard. Elizabeth Jane Savory died at Leckhampstead on 20 March 1891. In 1885, her daughter (Mary) Ella Goddard, had married Edwin Ford (1844-1925), a local smallholder from Frilsham. They lived in Leckhampstead for the rest of their lives. They had six children together, all sons. Their first-born was appropriately named William Savory Goddard Ford (1888-1973), partially preserving into the second half of the twentieth century a name with an unbroken lineage dating back to the middle of the seventeenth century.[3]

---

1. RBA D/P 24 8/1.
2. *RM* (3 December 1870).
3. For an anecdotal account of Ella and her descendants, see E. V. Satchell, *Leckhampstead Yesterday and Today: Leckhampstead, A Journey Through the Ages* (2010).

Appendix A:
Beating the Bounds of Brightwalton

[A transcript of RBA D/EW/O8, 47-51.]

*An edited transcript of this account was first published in G. C. Peachey,
'Beating the Bounds of Brightwalton', The Berks, Bucks & Oxon.
Archaeological Journal, x:iii (1904), 71-81 (and footnotes below taken from
Peachey are from this source). The transcript below has been made from the
MS, with the original pagination, spelling etc retained. Peachey attributes
this account of 'Processioning' to Savory's father, William Savory (1725-
1772). The original pages are unsigned, and Peachey does not explain his
rationale for the attribution. However, the handwriting appears to match that
used in the parish accounts up to 1772, and Savory, in the MS commonplace
book that forms the bulk of the present volume, explains: 'My father kept the
parish Accompts And took a Copy of the Register of Marriages, Christenings
& Burials in Brightwaltham parish which has been continued by my Uncle
John Savory to this time' [20-21], so the attribution appears to be sound.
Peachey should be consulted for the full historical context. For an account of
the beating of the bounds of Brightwalton in 1904, see RBA D/EX1805/1
(Papers of the Rev. Henry F. Howard) 49-55.*

[*p. 47*]

Processioning

Anciently among us there were, in each Parish, Customary Processions of
the Priest & the Patron of the Church, with the chief flag, or Holy Banner,
Attended by other Parishioners, each Ascension Week; to take a Circuit
round the limits of the Parish, and Pray for a Blessing on the fruits of the
Earth.

Of which Custom there still remains a Shadow in that Annual
perambulation, still called Processioning; though the order and Devotion of
the Ancient Procession be Almost Lost.

I Should be very Glad to see that Ancient Custom have a Renewal,
because I think it a very Necessary one, But at the same time, I am very Sorry
that so useful a thing, should be so much Neglected as it is[.]

The Last Perambulation round the Limits of this Parish (was according to
the best Account that I could get) was [*sic*] about the Year 1720;[1] which was
about two Years before the Decease of the Revd Mr House, Rector of this
Parish.[2] – Now I shall give you a short Description, but it's the best that I
could get, concerning the Custom of that Day's Perambulation.

[*p. 48*] The Farm carried Cake and Ale down to Lilly.

John Taylor, Sam[ue]l Taylor carried Cake and Ale down to the further
Holt Gate.

---

1. Peachey notes, 'The first Enclosure Agreement was 8 Geo. i, 1721'.
2. Rev. William House, Rector of Brightwalton, was buried at All Saints' Church, Brightwalton,
   on 27 November 1722.

Yew Tree carried Cake and Ale to the Upper end of the Lane next Thickett.

The Coombfarms[1] [*sic*] carried Cake and Ale down to the Cross at Stacorn.

The tythe of Rowdown Bank was Lost the Last Year as they went round, the Cross being made at the farther Holt Gate. Instead of going up to the Upper Corner of Taylors Ground.[2] there was Mr House and two Younger Daughters Ann and Sarah

Sarah 1689-1720 – 31

Ann 1686-1720 – 34

Henry Hatt & Joseph Sparrow carried Cake and Ale to the Knole by Holley street Lane.

Mr Giles Blagrave carried Cake and Ale to the Cross at the Boarded House.

John Tame, Thos Blackney, R[ichar]d Fulbrook carried cake and Ale to Knights Cross.

Rob[er]t Brown & Henry Bonner Carried Cake and Ale to the Cross in the Green where the stocks stands.

[*p. 49*] Then begun at Dunmore all round by Stacorn, by the Boarded House to Lilly to the Holt and round by Thicket Lots to Dunmore then to Knights Cross the Green and the Knole by Hatts. [3]

[*p. 50*]

Rowdonw Bank

peasmor hath the Tithe above the rising ground and Brightwalton below.

White Lands pays 1/4 pr Ann[um] Quit Rent to the Dean & Chapter of Westminster all the tythe of White Lands belongs to peasmore.[4]

R[ichar]d Birds, Hughes, Herberts, Esqr Tippings and Taylers Half the Tithe to peasmore and the other Half to Brightwalton.

Lilly Hill the Tithe of the lower part to Brightwalton the Upper part of peasmore, it was lost by peasmore Carrying a Corpse from Brightwalton up to the Certain place on Lilly Hill – before this time all the Tithe of Lilly Hill belonged to Brightwalton.[5]

---

1. Peachey notes: 'There were two farms at Combe, in the parish of Brightwalton, from early days until the first part of the nineteenth century.'
2. Peachey notes: 'The Tithe of Rowdown Bank may have been forfeited for the year in question by some custom imposing such a penalty; if so, it was discovered later. For "cross" one should probably read "crossing".'
3. The rest of the page is blank.
4. Peachey notes: 'The Priory of Poughley owned a small manor in Peasemore, of which Whitelands probably composed a part. After its dissolution by Cardinal Wolsey, and his subsequent fall, its possessions were given to the Abbot and Canons of Westminster, and to the present day the rectory of Chaddleworth (and until recently [Peachey was writing in 1904] Poughley Farm), is the property of the Dean and Chapter of Westminster, but Whitelands was long past out of possession.'
5. Peachey notes: 'The only corroboration of this is furnished by Roque's map (1759) which places the boundary on the top of Lilly Hill, but its accuracy is doubtful.' The rest of this page is blank.

Appendix B:
Residents of Brightwalton, 1768

[RBA D/EW/O8, pp. 188-190:
probably written by William Savory (1725-1772).]

[*p. 188*] The Number of Souls in Brighttwalton May 1768

Edwd Bartholomew his Wife, 3 Sons & 2 Daughters & 1 Niece	8
Thos Dearlove his Wife 5 Sons, 3 men servants & 1 Maid	11
Wm Hawkins: one Son and two Daughters	4
Franci Horton, his Wife and two Daughters	4
Widow Sansom one Son and two Daughters	4
Richard Aldridge	1
John Harris his Wife and two Daughters	4
John Norris his Wife and four Daughters	6
Major Sellwood, 3 Maid Servants & 12 Men Servants	16
Revd Dr Eyre & his Lady, 2 men & 2 Maud Servants	6
Henry Chandler his Wife 5 Sons & 1 Daughter	8
Thos Tomlin his Wife 2 Sons & 1 Daughter	5
Roger Guyer his Wife and one Daughter	3
Humphry Rivers his Wife 3 Sons & 2 Daughters	7
John Elkins his Wife and 2 Daughters	4
John Holmes his Wife one Son & 4 Daughters 1 Man	8
Widow Deacon, one Son & 2 Daughters	4
Joseph Gray his Wife, 4 Sons & 2 Daughters	8
Arthur Whiter his Wife & Mother & 2 Men	5
Grace Blackney	1
Jno. Oakley his Wife & 2 Sons	4
Widow froud, Widow Roach and Francis Purton	3
Joseph Mouldy his Wife 1 Son & 1 Daughter	4
Wm Fisher his Wife 2 Sons & 3 Daughters	7
[*p. 189*]	
Rob[er]t Bradley his Wife & one Daughter	3
Widow Cox and one Daughter	2
Sam[ue]l Ballard his Wife, 2 Men & one Maid Servant	5
Henry Hatt his Wife & one Maid	3
Wm Savory Junr his Wife 3 Daughters, 4 Men & one Maid	10
John Cullom and his Wife	2
Wm Savory Senr Mary weakfield & Daugher & a Boy Nurse-Child	4
Joseph Mitchell his wife 2 Sons, 2 Daughters & 1 Man	7
Jno. Tillen his wife 2 Sons & 4 Daughters	8
Widow White and one Daughter	2
Thos Taylor his Wife 6 Sons & 3 Daughters	11
Widow Bonner & 3 Grand Daughters	4
John Venn & his Wife	2

Andrew Cowley his Wife, 2 Sons & 1 Daughter	5
Hugh Turner 2 Sons 2 Daughters & a Woman housekeeper	6
R[ichar]d Bonner his Wife 2 Sons & one Daughter	5
Thos Adams his Wife 1 Son & 2 Daughters	5
Wm Fuller his Wife 1 Son & 2 Daughters	5
Widow Horner one Son, one Sister, one Man	4
Richd Fulbrook his Wife 1 Daughter & 1 Man	4
Willm Winkworth his Wife 2 Sons and a Mother	5
Widow Knight & her Brother	2
John Trumplet his Wife, 1 Son, 1 Daughter, 1 Man	5
Laurence Fulbrook	1
R[ichar]d Barnot and his Wife	2
[*p. 190*]	
Wm Fulbrook his Wife 4 Sons & one Daughter	7
Thos Brown his Wife and one Son	3
John Blackney, 2 Sons & 3 Daughter & one Man	7
Moses Bond his Wife 2 Sons & 2 Daughters	6
Richd Bird	1
Henry Horton his Wife, Niece, 2 Grand Daughters, & 2 Men	7
John Bird, 3 Sons & one Daughter	5
R[ichar]d Spokes his Wife one Son & 5 Daughters	8
Wm Sirmond his Wife one Son & 4 Daughters	7
Mary Deacon & one Man	2
Wm Flower & John Lovage	2
Thos Iremonger & his Wife	2
Wm Hicks his Wide 1 Son & 3 Daughters	6
Charles Collins his Wife & 2 Sons	4
Joseph Winter his Wife & Kinswoman	3
Thos Taylor his Wife, 5 Sons & 4 Daughters	11
Stephen Taylor & his Wife	2
Robt Bradley his Wife 2 Sons & 2 Daughters	6
Lot Lanfear his Wife 1 Son & 4 Daughters	7
Jane Marshall 2 Sons & one Daughter	4
John Huzzy, his Wife	2
Male In all	178
Female In all	171
Total	349

Appendix C:
Residents of Brightwalton, 1790

[RBA D/EW/O8, pp. 182-185:
probably written by William Savory (1768-1824).]

[*p.* 182] **The List of Souls in Brightwaltham Oct[obe]r 1790**

Timothy Bartholomew his Wife 3 Sons 4 Daug[hte]rs 2 Men and 2 Maid Ser[van]ts	13
Thomas Dearlove his Wife 2 Sons 4 Daugh[te]r 1 Man Ser[van]t 1 Maid	7
Widow Hicks 1 Daughter & 1 Son	3
Charles Collins his Wife 4 Sons	6
Joseph Stagg his Wife 2 Sons 1 Daugh[te]r 2 base born daughters	7
Widow Harris 1 Daughter 1 Son and 1 Grand Daughter	4
Henry Mitchel – Wm Frowde his Wife 4 Sons 2 Daughters	9
John Norris his Wife and 1 Daughter	3
Widow Brown Widow Spokes and Daughter	3
Mr Harbert his Wife 2 Sons 4 Daugh[te]rs 2 Maid Ser[van]ts 8 Men Ser[van]ts	18
Revd Mr Boucher his Lady 2 Maid Ser[van]ts 2 Men Ser[van]ts	6
Wm Whiter	1
Thos Tillon his Wife	2
Richd Rowe his Wife 2 Sons 1 Daughter	5
William Cooper his wife = Wm Butter his Wife and 1 Son	5
Thomas Pickett ~~his Wife~~ 3 Daughters 1 Son	5
Thos Stanbrook his Wife & Niece	3
[*p. 183*]	
John Holmes his Wife 2 Sons & 2 Daughters	6
Widow Deacon – Jas Brooker his Wife 3 Daugh[te]rs 1 Son	7
Joseph Gray & Richd Mills his Wife 1 Son 2 Daughters	6
Widow Whiter	1
Grace Taylor	1
Widow Sansom	1
John Oakley his Wife 1 Son 2 Daughters	5
Joseph Slade his Wife 1 Son 1 Daughter	4
John Crips his Wife 1 Son 5 Daughters	8
James Jackson his Wife 2 Sons 1 Daughter	5
Moses Bond his Wife & Brother	3
John Mouldy his Wife 2 Sons 5 Daughters	9
Widow Fisher and 2 Daughters	3
Fruin Wicks his Wife Mother 3 Daugh[te]rs 1 Son 1 Man Ser[van]t 1 Maid	9
John Savory=Wm Savory 1 Nephew 1 Maid Ser[van]t	5
Joseph Norris his Wife and 1 Daughter	3
Widow Tomlin and Daughter	2

John Tomlin his Wife & 2 Sons	4
John Brooks his Wife 2 Sons 1 Daughter	5
John Hazel his Wife 3 Sons 2 Daughters	7
Laurence Puizy his Wife & 1 Daughter	3
Lot Lanfear his Wife 1 Son 1 Daugh[te]r & Hopes Daughter	5
Widow Church 1 Son 1 Daughter	3
Willm Church his Wife 1 Maid Ser[van]t 4 Men Ser[van]ts	7
[p. 184]	
Richard Gibbons his Wife 2 Sons and 3 Daughters	7
Edward Wooldridge his Wife 1 Son	3
Moores Wife 1 Son 1 Daughter - Mary Blackford and Daughter	5
Henry Chandler 3 Sons 2 Daughters 1 Grand Son 1 Grand Daughter	8
Thos Church his Wife	2
John Cooper his Wife 1 Daughter	3
John Eacot his Wife 3 Sons 3 Daughters	8
Widow Bonner & 1 Son 1 Daughter & Wm Hawkins	4
Widow Adams – Wm Stevens 2 Daughters 1 Son	6
Richard Painter his Wife 4 Sons 2 Daughters & 1 Man	9
Thos Horne his Wife Mother & 1 Man Ser[van]t	4
John Fulbrook his Wife & 1 Son	3
Luke Finch his Wife & 3 Daughters	5
Taylor's Wife 3 Daughters & 2 Sons	6
John Trumplet 1 Son 1 Maid Servant	3
Hugh Turner his Wife & 1 Daughter	3
Thos Taylor his Wife 1 Son 3 Daughters 1 Grand Daughter	7
John Parrot his Wife 1 Son 1 Daugh[te]r Sarah Ellet Son & Daughter	7
Thos Brown his Wife and Son	3
Thos Palmer his Wife and 2 Daughters	4
Stephen Taylor & his Wife	2
John Tillon his Wife 1 Son and Widow Fuller	4
Wm May his Wife 3 Sons and 2 daughters	7
[p. 185]	
John Eagles his Wife and 1 Son	3
Francis Holder his Wife and 2 Daughters	4
Mary Deacon and Son = Widow Bird 2 Daugh[te]rs 1 Son	
– Sar[a]h Wilts & <Son>	8
Widow Sirman & 2 Daughters	3
William Dance his Wife and 2 Sons	4
Joseph Mitchel his Wife 1 Son 2 Daugh[te]rs & 1 Man Ser[van]t	6
Richd Frowde his Wife 5 Sons 3 D[aughte]rs	10
John Deacon his Wife & 1 Son	3
John Eades his Wife & 2 Sons	4
Arthur Whiter his Wife 2 Sons & 3 Daughters	7
William Janaway his Wife 1 Son & 1 Apprentice	4
Edward Avery his Wife 4 Sons & 1 Daughter	7
Thos Tayler his Wife & 3 D[aughte]rs	5
John Bennet 2 Sons 1 Daughter 1 Maid Ser[van]t	5
Francis Day his Wife & 1 Daughter	3

Males in all	191
Females in all	210
Total	401
Number of Souls encreased since the Year 1768 is	52

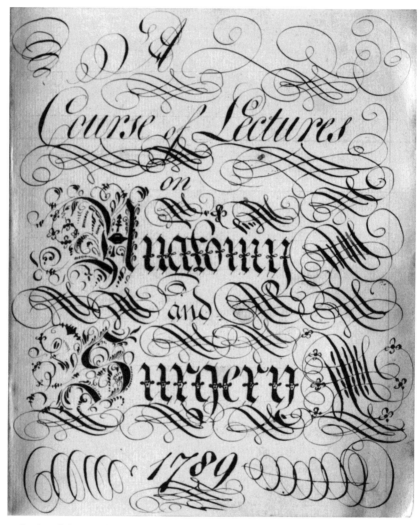

6. The elaborate title-page of Savory's student notes on Henry Cline's 'A Course of Lectures on Anatomy and Surgery', delivered at St Thomas's Hospital, London, in 1789. King's College London Archives, St Thomas's Hospital Medical School, TH/PP/54/1 (reproduced with thanks).

Appendix D:
Other Manuscripts by William Savory

[This appendix includes material from William Savory's student notes on lectures delivered by Henry Cline at St Thomas's Hospital and William Saunders at Guy's Hospital: King's College London Archives, St Thomas's Hospital Medical School, TH/PP/54/1 and 2 (with thanks to KCLA for permission to publish quoted material).]

In addition to his commonplace book, transcribed above, Savory wrote out at least eight volumes of medical lectures and notes. Of these, six appear not to have survived, and we only know about them because Savory refers in the commonplace book to 'the pharmacopeae of St Thomas['s] Hospital', 'Clinical Cases at Guys Hospital', and 'Dr Louders Lectures' on midwifery [195] (see also [195*n*]); 'the Lectures on Chymistry by Dr Saunders and Wm Babington' [196]; and his own 'Book of Clinical Cases' [234] kept as a junior medical practitioner. Of the remaining three volumes, comprising Savory's notes on lectures he attended as a medical student, two have survived: the first volume of his notes on Henry Cline's 'Lectures on Anatomy and Surgery', but not the second volume, containing the remainder of the anatomy lectures and all of the lectures on surgery. The other volume to have survived is Savory's notes on William Saunders's 'Lectures on the Theory and Practice of Physic'. These extant volumes seem to have been passed between successive medical practitioners based in Brightwalton – Savory's son, William Savory Junior (c.1792-1854), Henry A. Duncan, William James Wood (c.1834-1890), and George Peachey – the last of whom recognised their value to posterity and, in April 1903, entrusted them to the care of the St Thomas's Hospital Medical School. They remained there until the volumes were transferred with the rest of the Medical School's archive to the Archives of King's College, London, in 2002 (King's College London Archives, St Thomas's Hospital Medical School, TH/PP/54/1 and 2). As student notes, these volumes represent painstaking effort. Savory presumably compiled them ostensibly as medical reference works for his own use: a resource to be consulted in the course of his professional career.

The notes on Cline's lectures are in a bound quarto volume, with green boards, 266 pages in extent, and includes both a contents list and a sketch index. The cover-page, written in Savory's version of classic Gothic blackletter calligraphy (see illustration on previous page), bears the title, 'A | Course of Lectures | on | Anatomy | and | Surgery | 1789'. Each letter of the word 'Anatomy' incorporates a simple figure resembling a small tied bow, whilst each letter in the word 'Surgery' incorporates at least one simple figure of a human skull. The motif used in the word 'Anatomy' thus appears better to represent surgery, and that in the word 'Surgery' better to represent anatomy. Whether this was consciously ironical is impossible to say. The title-page bears the words, 'The | Anatomy | of the | Human Body | By | Henry Cline | Vol: 1st. | The Spring Course 1789 | WS'. These final initials form a monogram that Savory does not use in the commonplace book.

Fortunately, the contents of the missing second volume are listed at the beginning of the first (with page numbers).

The extant volume, which is remarkably well-preserved, begins with 'Notes taken from the Clinical Lectures of John Rutherford M.D., Edinburgh' and a note promises their continuation in the missing second volume. Savory does not mention Rutherford in the commonplace book. John Rutherford (1695-1779), an eminent Professor of Medicine, and a member of the Royal Society of Physicians in Edinburgh, died nearly a decade before Savory arrived in London to study medicine, so these notes were presumably based on a printed source.

The contents of Savory's notes on Henry Cline's lectures (with page numbers) are as follows: 'The General Introduction, 1; On the Blood, 4; On the Structure of the Arteries, 9; On the diseases of the Arteries, 13; Of the structure of the Veins, 14; Of the diseases of the Veins, 16; Of the Absorbent Vessells, 17; Of the Cellular Membrane, 24; Of the Nerves, 28; Of the Muscles, 34; Of the Glands, 40; Of the structure of the Bones, 46; Of the Appendages of the Bones, 51; Ossteology, 66; Of the diseases of the Vertebra, 71; Bones of the Pelvis, 75; Bones of the Thorax, 80; Bones of the Sup[erio]r Extremity, 89; Bones of the Inf[erio]r extremity, 101; Bones of the Head, 112; Of the Descriptions of the Muscles, 131; Of the Ligaments, 180; Male Organs of Generation, 191; Of the structure of the testicle, 196; Of the urinary organs, 200; The Penis, 204; Of the Urinary Bladder, 210; Of the Diseases of the Urinary Bladder, 215; Of the Viscera, 218; Of the Female Organs of Generation, 233; Of the structure of the liver, 241; Of the Gall Bladder, 241; Of the pancrease [sic], 245; Of the Female Breast, 248; Of the structure of the lungs, 250; Of the Structure of the Heart, 255; Of the Alimentary Canal, 258'.

The contents of the missing second volume are given as follows: 'Book 2nd. Of the Teeth and their growth, 3; Of the Common Integuments, 8; Of the distribution of the Arteries, 12; Of the distribution of the Veins, 31; Of the Absorbing System, 37; Of the Circulation of the Blood, 43; Of the distribution of the nerves, 48; Of the Brain & its Membranes, 57; Of the Eye and its Appendages, 65; Of the Organ of Vission, 75; Of the Organs of Taste, 83; Of the Lips, Cheeks, Gums, Glands &c, 86; Of Anatomical Preparations, 90; Of the Organs of Smelling, 96; Of the Organs of Hearing, 100; Of the Diseases of the Heart, 111; Of the Hystory of Anatomy, 118; Surgerical [sic] Lectures Commenced, 125; Of the Diseases of the Bones, 125; Of Sutures, 137; Of the Cessarian [sic] Operation, 143; Of the Gastroraphy, 146; Of the Hare lip, 148; Of the Bronctrometry, 151; Of the Wry Neck, 153; Of the Fistula Lacrymalis, 154; Of Ext[raction of] the Cataracts, 82; of Couching; 157; Of Cutting the Iris, 158; Of Removing the Eye, 158; Of Castration, 159; Of the Empyema, 163; Of Calculi, 164 Searching, 169 & performance of operations, 173; Of Amputations, 174, its Apparatus, 177, & tying Vessells, 182; Of Removing the Tonsil Glands, 185; Of Removing the Pelvis, 188; Of the polipus uteri, 189 & taking off pr of the uvula, 190; Of the polips in the nose, 191; Of the Scirrh[o]us Breast, 192; Of the fistula in Ano, 195; Of the paracentesis & Ascites, 199, Aneurism, 201; Of the phymosis, 203, Paraphymosis, 204; Of Amputating the Penis, 205, Suppression of Urine,

207; Of the Stone in Woman, 209; Of the Hydrocele, 210; Of the Trephine, 215; Of Hernias, 222; Of Trepanning the Sternum, 234; Of Carbuncles. Eusephelus &c, 234; Of Diseases of the Bones Contr., 236; Of Bandages, 247.'

Savory's notes on Saunders's lectures comprise one bound quarto volume with brown boards. There is no cover-page but the title-page reads 'Lectures | on the | Theory and Practice | of | Physic | by | William Saunders MD | 1788'. It consists of 362 pages, plus four pages at the end listing the volume's contents. Pages 305-362 consist of additional notes, headed 'Appendix to the Antecedent Lectures or Notes on the Spring Course of Lectures on Physic, By WSaunders MD, Physician to Guys Hospital, 1789'. On page 362 Savory notes, 'For the remainding [*sic*] part of the Course of Lectures see Saunders Elements of Physic.' This may refer to a ninth volume of Savory's notes, or to a printed source, as yet not identified. On the rear endpaper Savory notes, 'Two Lectures on Electricity given by Dr Saunders is Written in The Desideratum of Electricity', almost certainly a reference to a printed volume.

The Introductory Lecture with which the volume begins is worth quoting at some length for what it tells us about the view of medicine propounded at the time of Savory's studies.

By the Practice of Medicine, I understand the Art of preserving Health, prolonging Life and curing Diseases. Medicine is considered as one of the most liberal Arts. A knowledge of Mathematics, natural phylosophy, Chymistry, Optics, Hydrautics [*sic*], Botany, Anatomy &c is necessary. The necessity of understanding Anatomy is too obvious at first sight to everyone, It leads us to a knowledge of Physiology. various changes are daily produced in consequence of Chymistry: In the first place we are aided by Chymistry in discovering the means of counteracting many poisons, likewise we are indebted to Chymistry for the most active remedies we possess, as Mercury, Antimony &c. likewise we are enabled to point out the efficacy of medicines and to analyse any compound, and are indebted to it for a knowledge of the empirical medicines; Chymistry is not only applicable to Pharmacy & Medicine, but is also applicable to Surgery & Anatomy. An Animal Machine differs from an Inanimate one so far as sometimes to Cure a Disease without Aid, hence nature is to be called in, in the case of Diseases.' (1-2)

A look at the list of contents reveals the range of subjects Saunders covered in the course of his lectures and in which Savory was thus versed. The page number comes first, and the subject second, a reversal of Savory's approach in the volumes relating to Cline's lectures: '4, Physiology; 9, On the Circulation; 16, On the Pulse; 21, On the nature & properties of the Blood; 24. On the diseased state of the Blood; 28, On the Chymical properties of those fluids separated from the Blood; 30, Of the Secretions; 31, Urine; 32, Milk; 34, The Mucus of the Body; The Saliva; 35, Bile; 37, Phlogiston; 41, Direct Debility; 52, On the Elements of the Practice of Physic, Introduction; 53, Pathology; 63, Remote Causes are ... ; 54, Predisposing Causes; 67, Proximate Causes; 68, Of the Symptoms of Diseases; 69, Of the Crisis of Diseases; 72, Of the Diagnosis; 73, Of the Prognosis; 75, On the General Doctrine of Fevers; 84, Of the Remote Causes;

88, Of the Prognosis in Fevers; 92, Of the General Cure of Fevers; 107, Of the General Division of Fevers; 109, Of the Inflammatory Fever; 112, Cure; 113, The low Nervous Fever; 115, The Cure; 121, Of the Putrid, Malignant or Pectoral Fevers; 124, Prognosis; 125, Cure; 128, Of Intermittent Fevers; 131, Of Inflammation in general; 146, Phrenitis; 147, Ophthalmia; 150, Of the Inflammatory Angina; 153, Of the Malignant Angina; 155, Of the Angina Trachealis; 157, Inflammation in the Cavity of the Thorax; 164, Of the Peripneumonia Notha; 165, Of the Phthisis Pulmonalis; 171, Inflammation of the Cavity of the Abdomen; 176, Inflammation of the Liver; 177, Inflammation of the Kidney; 179, Of the Strangury "painfull discharge of urine"; 182, Of the Rheumatism; 190, Of the Gout; 201, Of the Erysipelas; 213, Of the Measels; 215, Of the Dysentary; 220, Of the Cholera Morbus; 222, Of Haemorrhagy [*sic*]; 224, Of the Scurvy; 227, Of the Dropsy; 235, Of the Asthma; 237, Of Indigestion; 240, Of the Haemorrhoides or Piles; 242, Of the Jaundice; 246, Of the Diabetes; 245, Of Calculus Concretions; 249, Of the Cholic; 252, Of the Apoplexy; 255, Of the Palsy; 258, Of the Epilepsy; 261, Of the Chorea Sancti Vite [*i.e. convulsive disease*]; 262, Of the Tetanus, Opisthotonus & [?Empiro-othismos]; 264, Of the Catalepsy; 265, Of Hysterical & Hypochondriacal Disorders; 271, Of the Lues Venerea; 279, On the Diseases of Woman; 283, Of the Chlorosis; 287, The Fluor Albbus [*i.e. Leukorrhea*]; 289, Disease Peculiar to Children; 290, Defect of Evacuations; The Jaundise; 291, Aphthae or Thrush; 292, Fitts; 293. Acidity. Eructations &c; 294, Teething; Worms; 296, Of the Rickets; 298, Hydrocephalus; 301, Of the Hooping Cough; 302, Scrophula.'

Given that Savory's commonplace book was completed no later than 1792, it seems probable that further volumes of case-notes were kept in the course of a career which seems to have ended only with his death in 1824. We can but hope that some of the missing volumes will yet come to light.

Index to Persons

Index to Places

Berkshire Record Society: volumes in print

Berkshire Glebe Terriers, 1634, ed. Ian Mortimer (1995)

Berkshire Probate Accounts, 1583-1712, ed. Ian Mortimer (1997)

Enclosure in Berkshire, 1485-1885, ed. Ross Wordie (1998)

Reading Gild Accounts, 1357-1516, ed. Cecil Slade (2 vols, 1999-2000)

Accounts of the Kendrick Charity Workhouse, Newbury, 1627-1641, ed. Christine Jackson (2001)

Berkshire Nonconformist Meeting House Registrations, 1689-1852, ed. Lisa Spurrier (2 vols, 2002-3)

Thames Navigation Commission Minutes, 1771-1790, ed. Jeremy Sims (2 vols, 2004-5)

The Diocese Books of Samuel Wilberforce, 1845 and 1854, ed. Ronald and Margaret Pugh (2006)

Berkshire Religious Census, 1851, ed. Kate Tiller (2007)

Berkshire Archdeaconry Probate Records, 1480-1652: Index, ed. Pat Naylor (3 vols, 2008-9)

Diaries and Correspondence of Robert Lee of Binfield, 1736-1744, ed. Harry Leonard (2010)

Reading St Laurence Churchwardens' Accounts, 1498-1570, ed. Joan Dils (2 vols, 2011-12)

The Church Inspection Notebook of Archdeacon James Randall, 1855-1873, and other records, ed. Sabina Sutherland (2013)

Newbury to Chilton Pond Turnpike Records, 1766-1791, ed. Jeremy Sims (2014)

Berkshire Feet of Fines, 1307-1509, ed. Margaret Yates (2 vols, 2015-16)

Reading Abbey Records: a New Miscellany, ed. Brian Kemp (2018)

Berkshire Schools in the Eighteenth Century, ed. Sue Clifford (2019)

Hungerford Overseers' Accounts, 1655-1834, ed. Peter Durrant (2021)

Tudor Windsor, ed. David Lewis (2022)

Stanford in the Vale Churchwardens' Accounts 1522-1705, ed. Joan Dils (2023)

To order volumes, and to join the Society, please use the links on the website www.berkshirerecordsociety.org.uk. Postal enquiries to the Berkshire Record Society, c/o Royal Berkshire Archives, 9 Coley Avenue, Reading, Berkshire RG1 6AF.